An Atlas of Mitral Valve Imaging

Milind Desai · Christine Jellis
Teerapat Yingchoncharoen
Editors

An Atlas of Mitral Valve Imaging

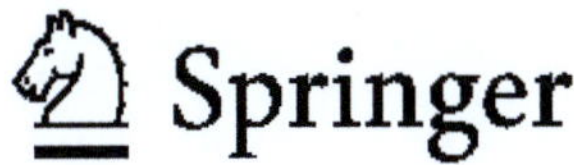 Springer

Editors
Milind Desai
Department of Cardiovascular Medicine
Cleveland Clinic
Cleveland, OH
USA

Teerapat Yingchoncharoen
Cleveland Clinic
Cleveland, OH
USA

Christine Jellis
Cleveland Clinic
Cleveland, OH
USA

Additional material to this book can be downloaded from http://extras.springer.com

ISBN 978-1-4471-7046-4   ISBN 978-1-4471-6672-6   (eBook)
DOI 10.1007/978-1-4471-6672-6

Springer London Heidelberg New York Dordrecht

Printed on acid-free paper

Springer-Verlag London Ltd. is part of Springer Science+Business Media (www.springer.com)

I would like to acknowledge my wife, Rajul, and my kids, Ria and Rohan, for their tremendous support in life.

MD

To my husband and son, Dan and Hamish Waters, for their unwavering love and support. Their ongoing encouragement, understanding, and sacrifice allow me to pursue my academic dreams.

CJ

To the memory of my respected father, Adisak Yingchoncharoen; my beloved mother, Sumalee Phiphitwattanaphan, for her unconditional love, encouragement, and unfailing optimism; to Professor Suradej Hongeng who always believes in me and has been more than an inspiration and tireless supporter through these many years; to all my teachers and lastly all my patients who have taught me a lot about cardiology and echocardiography.

TY

Imaging and assessment of the mitral valve provides ongoing challenges due to its complicated structure and physiology. For decades, echocardiologists have been seeking new methods to evaluate the mitral valve and quantitate valve dysfunction. From the era of M-mode through development of two-dimensional Doppler and now three-dimensional techniques, echocardiography has remained the imaging modality of choice. The fact that there are still so many measures employed to assess the mitral valve illustrates that it remains a complicated process, which is not well performed with any single parameter.

The purpose of this Atlas is to provide readers with a case-based overview of mitral valve structure and echocardiographic evaluation. The clinical scenarios illustrate how the various echocardiographic parameters provide incremental value in the accurate assessment of mitral valve dysfunction. Detailed, noninvasive assessment of the mitral valve remains integral for planning and performance of mitral valve surgery. Increasingly, echocardiographic assessment and real-time guidance are also required to facilitate percutaneous treatment options. We highlight important imaging aspects of these cases, along with salient teaching points and further recommended reading.

We have aimed to make this contemporary style of Atlas interactive and useful for individual learning as well as group teaching purposes, with the inclusion of numerous video files. Real-world examples of both common and rarer conditions are included to illustrate the breadth of mitral valve pathology and the challenges faced in acquiring optimal images. We hope that readers will enjoy exploring the mitral valve with us in this format.

Cleveland, OH, USA

Milind Desai
Christine Jellis
Teerapat Yingchoncharoen

Acknowledgments

We would like to acknowledge the sonographers, cardiologists, and imaging fellows who comprise the team behind the Cleveland Clinic Cardiovascular Imaging Center. Their tireless efforts, experience, enthusiasm, and expertise on a daily basis are proudly represented by the images comprised within this Atlas. We also acknowledge the advice and assistance provided by Lee Klein and the editorial team at Springer Publishers.

Contents

List of Videos

Mitral Valve Nomenclature

Christine Jellis

The mitral valve was the first valve to be evaluated echocardiographically and has remained a priority of evolving echocardiographic techniques. Besides the multiple primary diseases of the mitral valve, it can also be impacted secondarily by other remote cardiac diseases. The mitral valve is the left-sided atrioventricular valve and separates the left atrium from the left ventricle. Embryologically, it forms from the endocardial cushions between the 5 and 8 weeks of development and is bicuspid, consisting of anterior and posterior leaflets (Fig. 1.1). These valve leaflets are attached to the ventricular walls by thin, fibrous chords, the chordae tendineae, which insert into small papillary muscles that are sculpted from the ventricular wall.

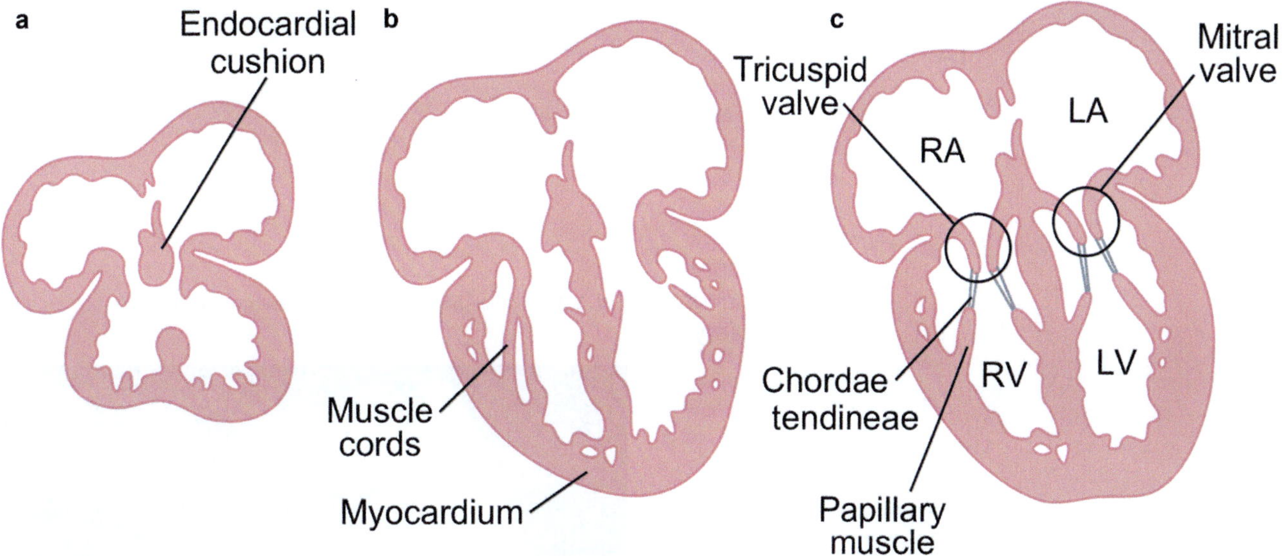

Fig. 1.1 Endocardial cushion embryological development of the atrioventricular valves occurs between gestational weeks 5 and 8 [Figures a–c]

C. Jellis
Department of Cardiovascular Medicine, Cleveland Clinic,
9500 Euclid Avenue, Cleveland, OH 44195, USA
e-mail: jellisc@ccf.org

M. Desai et al. (eds.), *An Atlas of Mitral Valve Imaging*,
DOI 10.1007/978-1-4471-6672-6_1, © Springer-Verlag London 2015

The mitral valve apparatus is a complicated structure consisting of the leaflets, the annulus, the chordae tendineae, and the papillary muscles. Pathology of any of these aspects can result in mitral valve dysfunction. Chordae attach along the entire leaflet coaptation line and insert into the papillary muscle heads (Fig. 1.2). The primary or "marginal" chordae insert on the free margin of the valve leaflets. Rupture of these chordae always causes valve insufficiency, which is often severe. The secondary chordae ("strut chordae") insert on the rugged ventricular surface of the leaflets. The secondary chordae may promote contraction of the ventricular longitudinal fibers, supporting the ventricular contraction. The tertiary chordae originate directly from the ventricular wall and insert only in the basal part of the posterior leaflet. The function of these chordae is unknown; they seem to reduce leaflet mobility by anchoring the leaflet to the ventricular wall.

The papillary muscles, which are the muscular part of the mitral apparatus, originate from the distal one third of the ventricular wall. There are two dominant papillary muscles, anterolateral and posteromedial. These provide chordae to a portion of each leaflet. The posteromedial papillary muscle is perfused only from the right coronary artery, so it is more susceptible to ischemic insult than the anterolateral papillary muscle, which has a dual blood supply.

The mitral annulus is part of the fibrous skeleton of the heart. It is a complex, saddle-shaped, nonplanar geometric structure with greater commissure-commissural diameter (long axis) and smaller septolateral diameter (short axis) (Fig. 1.3). The leaflets do not normally protrude above the annular plane. Three-dimensional (3D) echocardiography has revolutionized visualization and appreciation of the mitral valve annulus (Fig. 1.4).

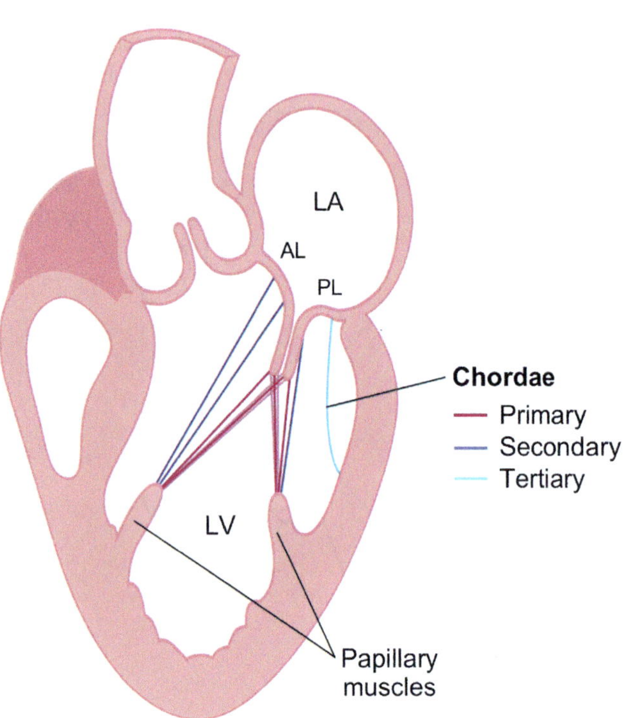

Fig. 1.2 Mitral subvalvular apparatus including chordal attachments

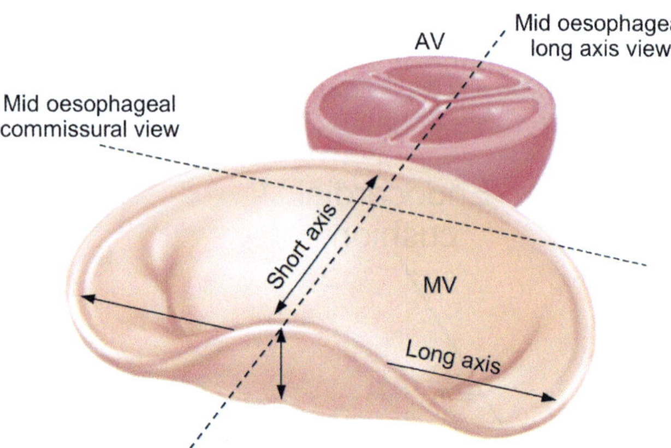

Fig. 1.3 Saddle-shaped structure of the mitral valve

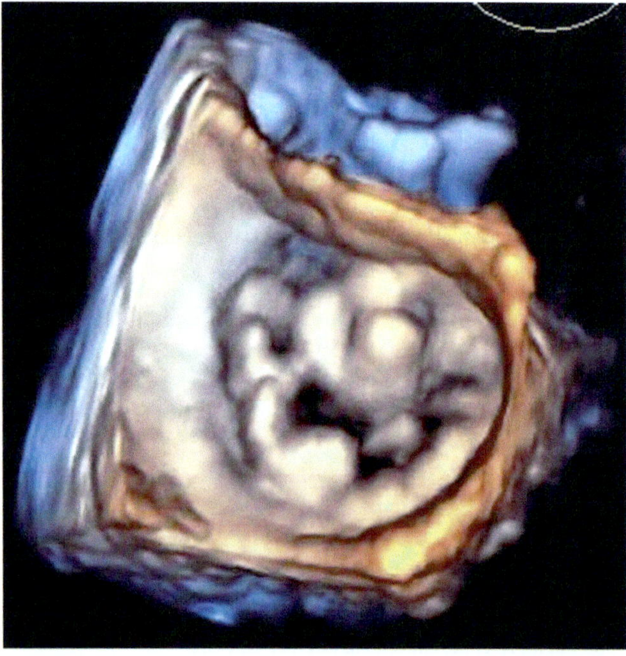

Fig. 1.4 Three-dimensional (3D) transesophageal echo (TEE) image of the mitral valve

Mitral valve leaflet structure is also complex. Each leaflet comprises a multiscallop structure (Fig. 1.5). For descriptive purposes, the leaflets are typically divided into six discrete scallops: A1–3 for anterior, P1–3 for posterior. Scallops A1 and P1 are lateral, A2 and P2 are central, and A3 and P3 are medial.

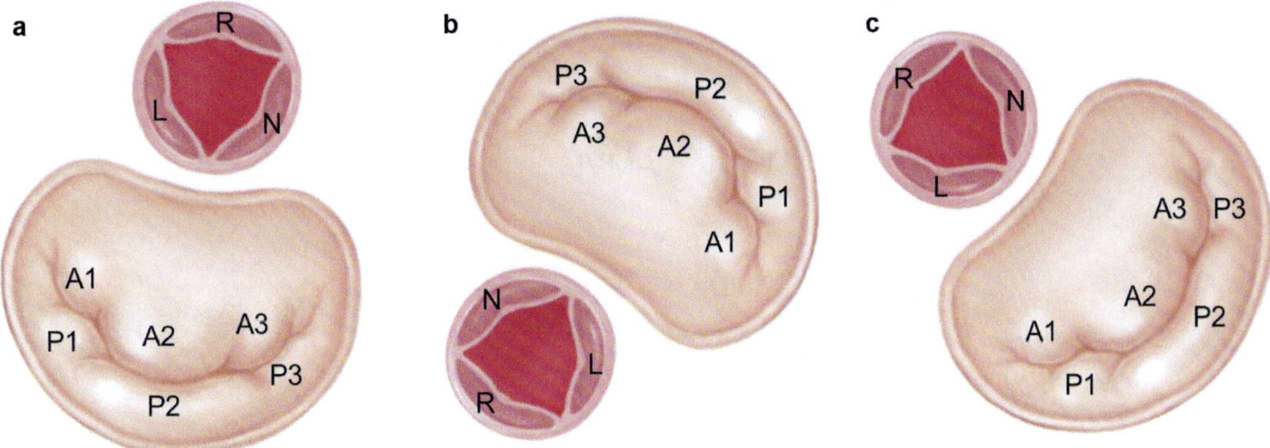

Fig. 1.5 Scallops of the mitral valve when viewed using different methods. (**a**) Surgical. (**b**) Transesophageal. (**c**) Transthoracic

Alternative descriptive nomenclature of the mitral valve scallops includes the anatomic and Duran classifications (Fig. 1.6).

The C-shaped coaptation line results in variable portions of each valve being visible on different cross-sectional imaging planes (Fig. 1.7).

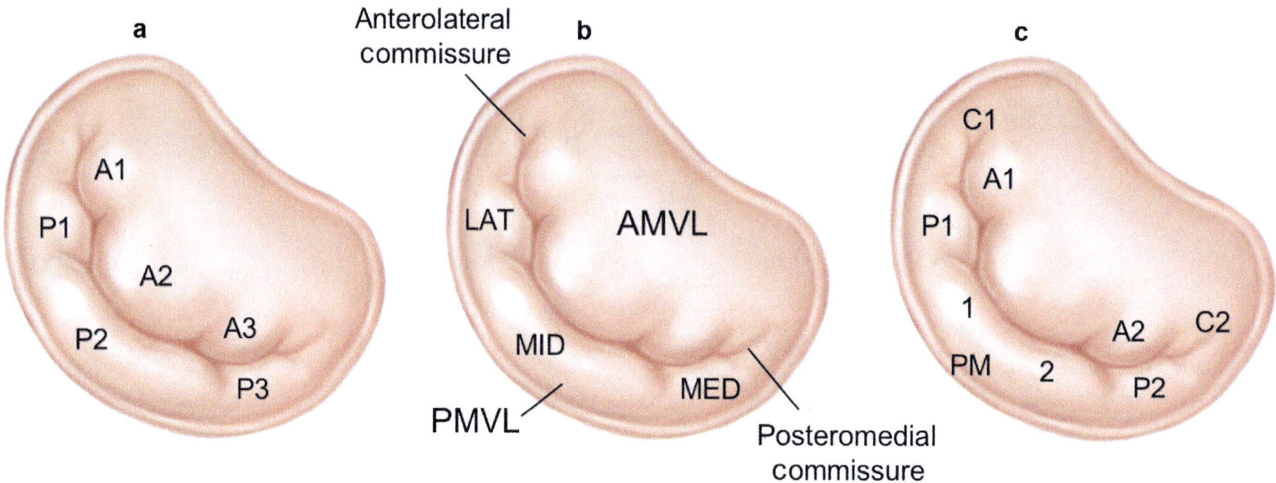

Fig. 1.6 Labeling systems for the mitral valve scallops. (**a**) SCA-ASE (Society of Cardiovascular Anesthesiologists – American Society of Echocardiography) or Carpentier classification. (**b**) Anatomic classification (**c**) DURAN classification

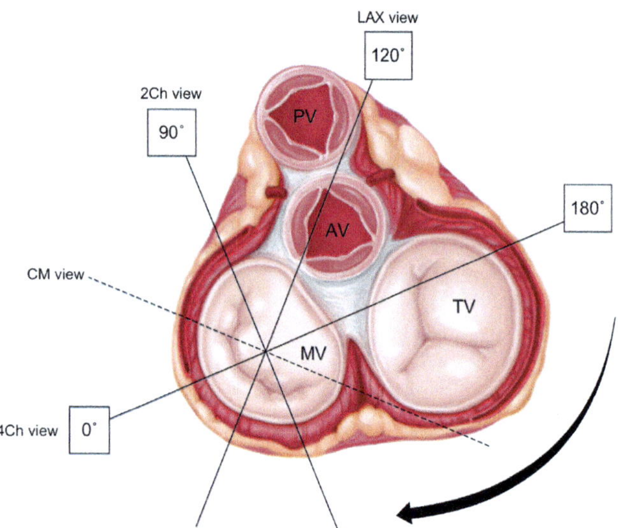

Fig. 1.7 TEE imaging planes

1.1 Representative Views: Transesophageal Echocardiography (TEE)

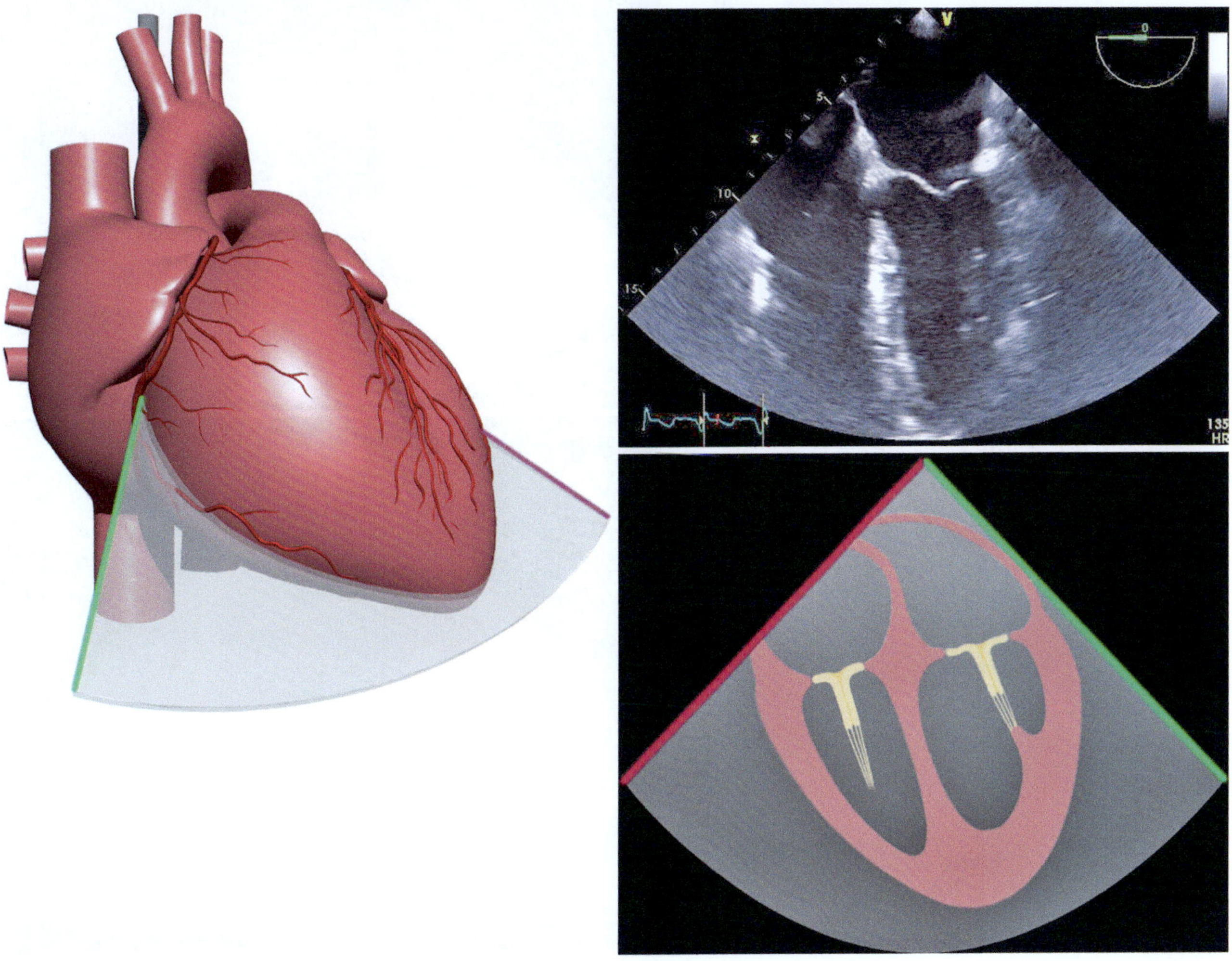

Fig. 1.8 Four-chamber view (0°, midesophageal)

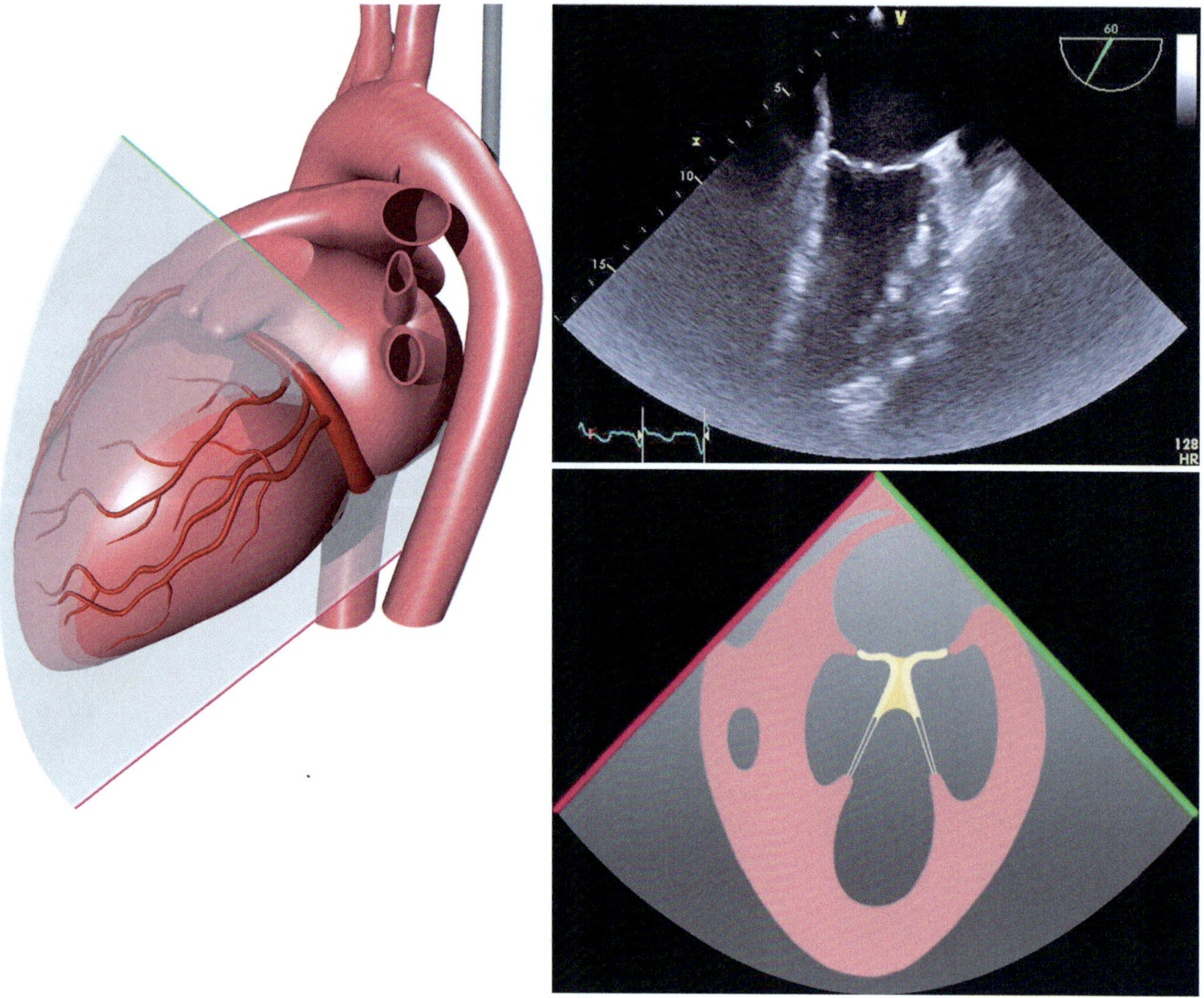

Fig. 1.9 Mitral commissural view (60°, midesophageal)

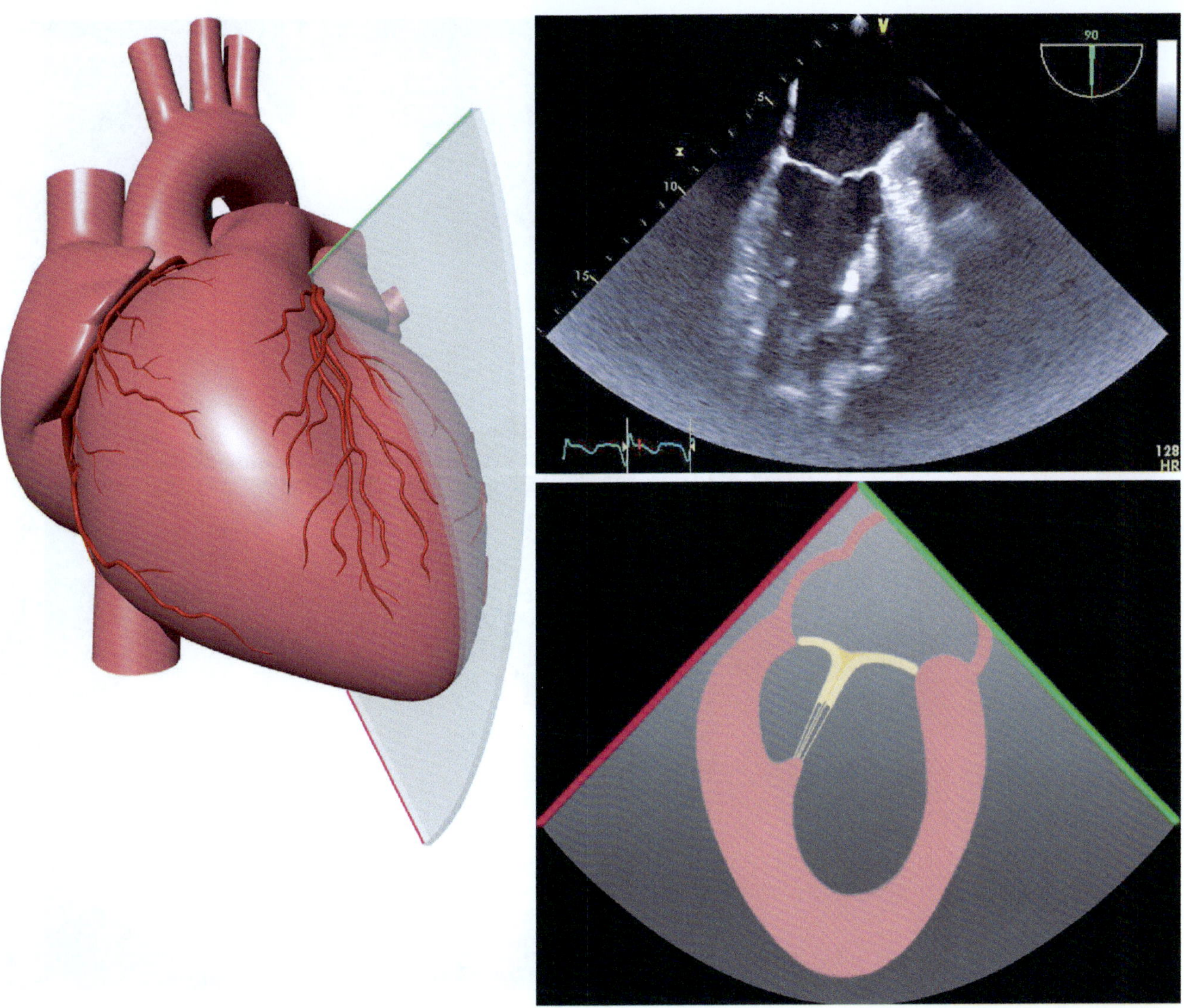

Fig. 1.10 Two-chamber view (90°, midesophageal)

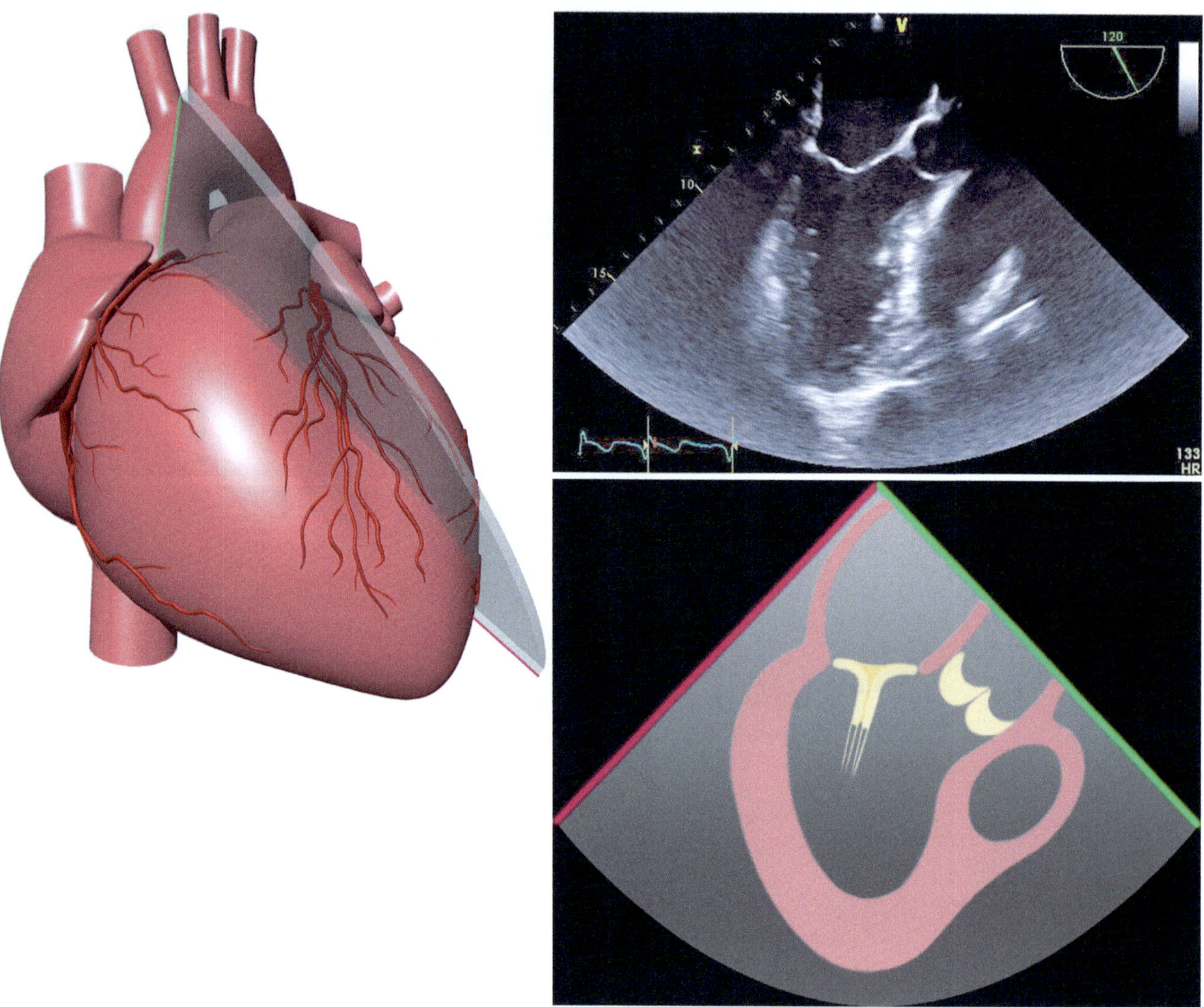

Fig. 1.11 Three-chamber, long-axis view (120°, midesophageal)

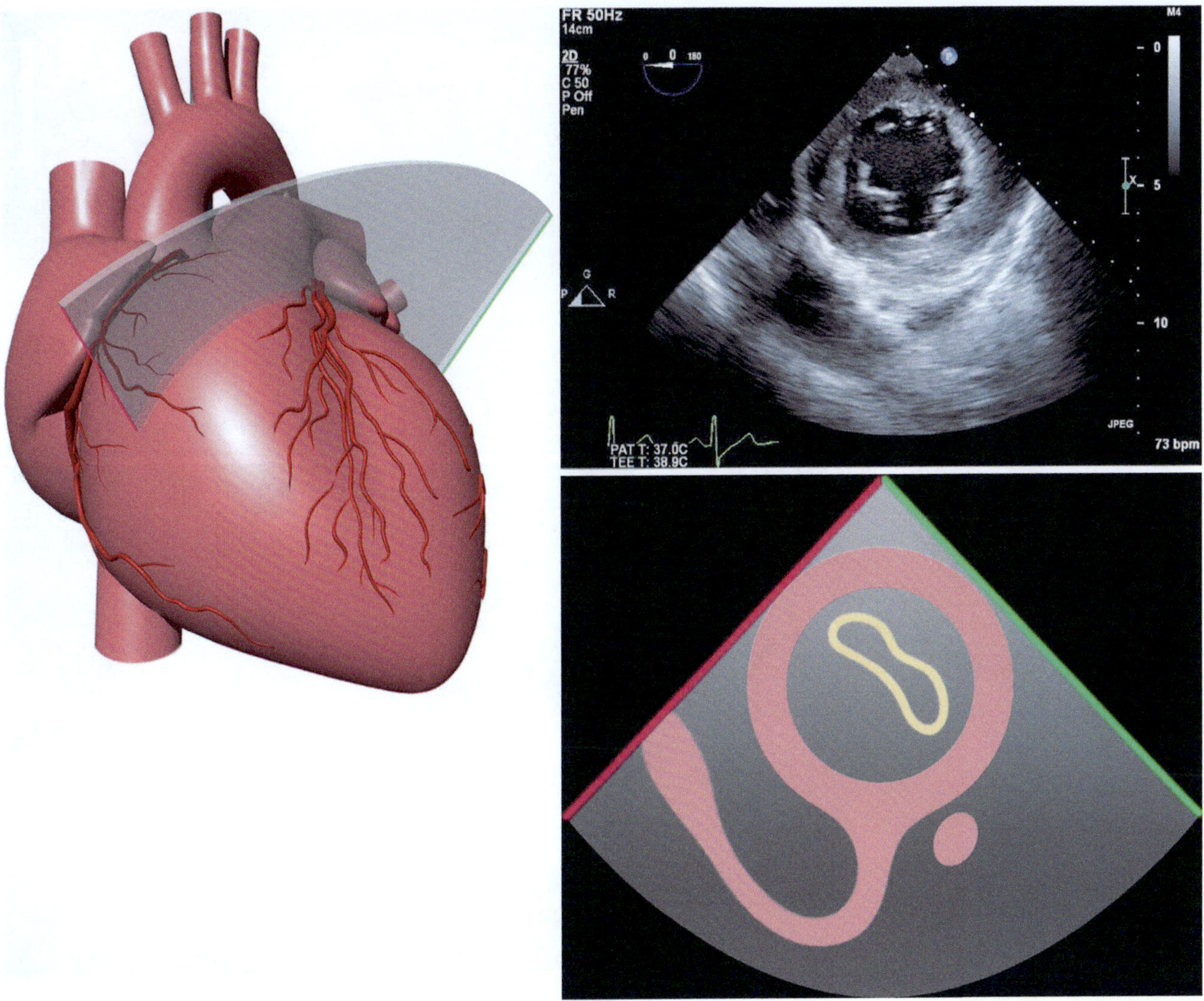

Fig. 1.12 Basal short-axis view (0° with anteflexion, transgastric)

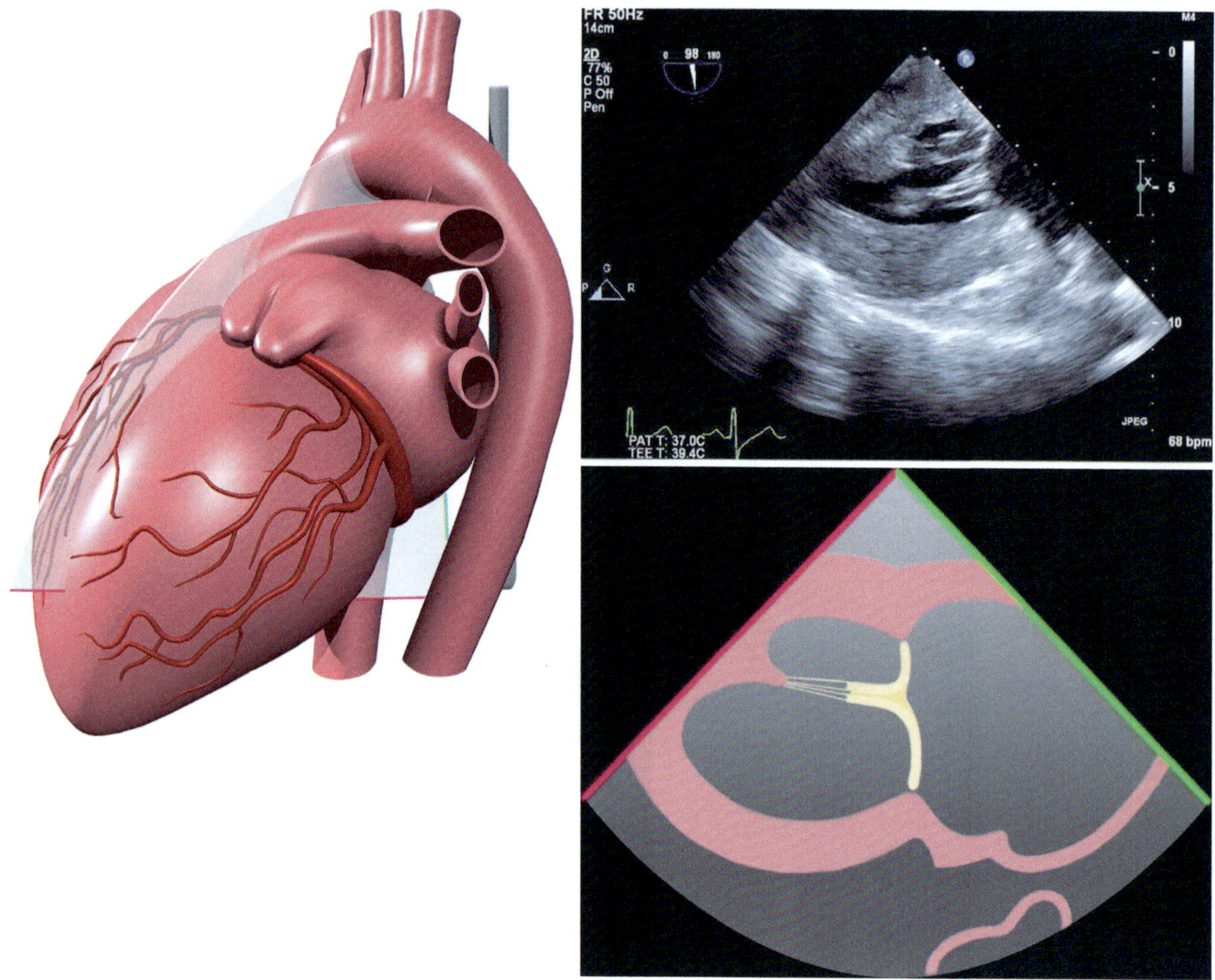

Fig. 1.13 Two-chamber view (90° with anteflexion, transgastric)

1.2   Representative Views: Transthoracic Echocardiography (TTE)

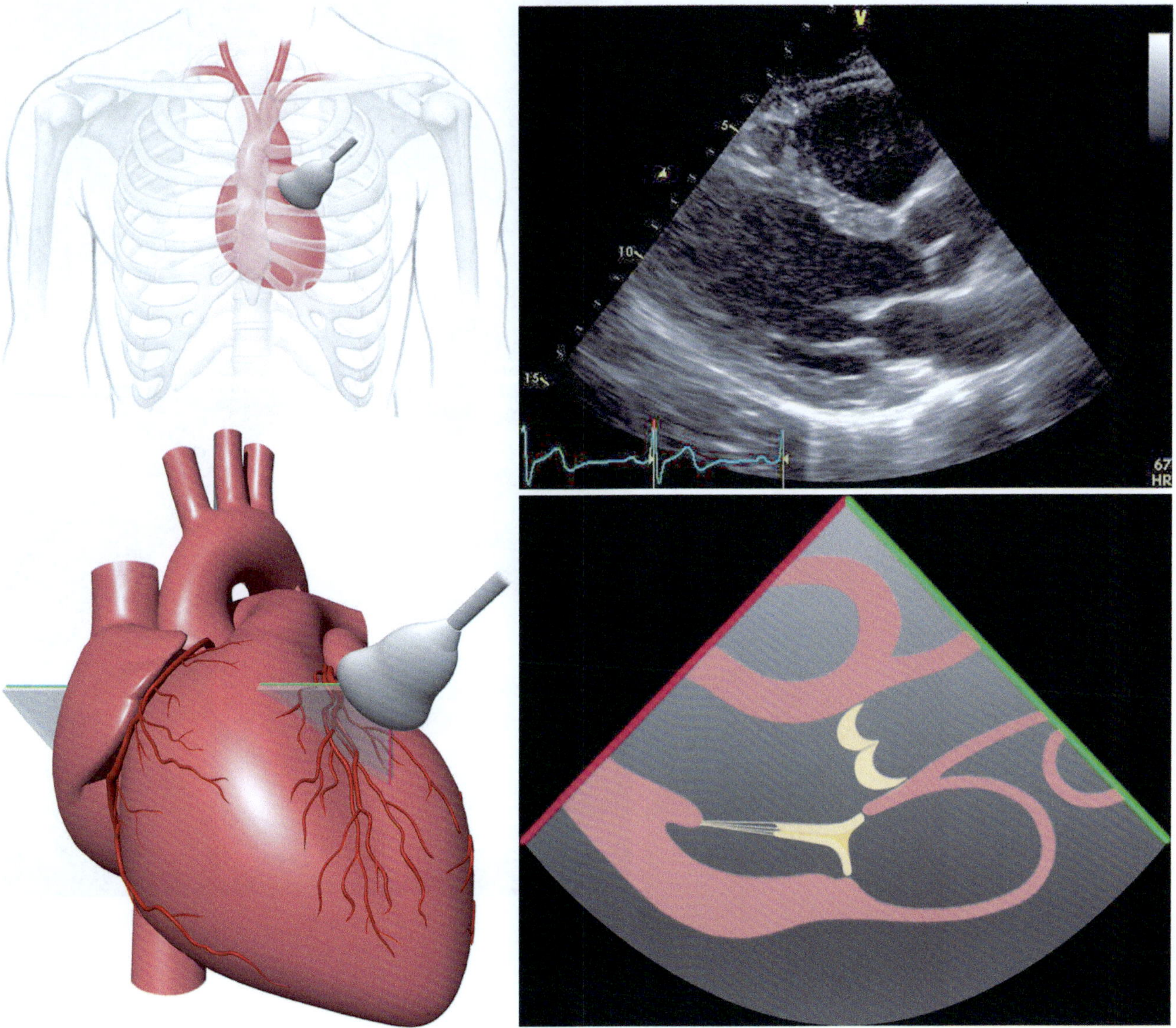

Fig. 1.14 Parasternal long-axis view

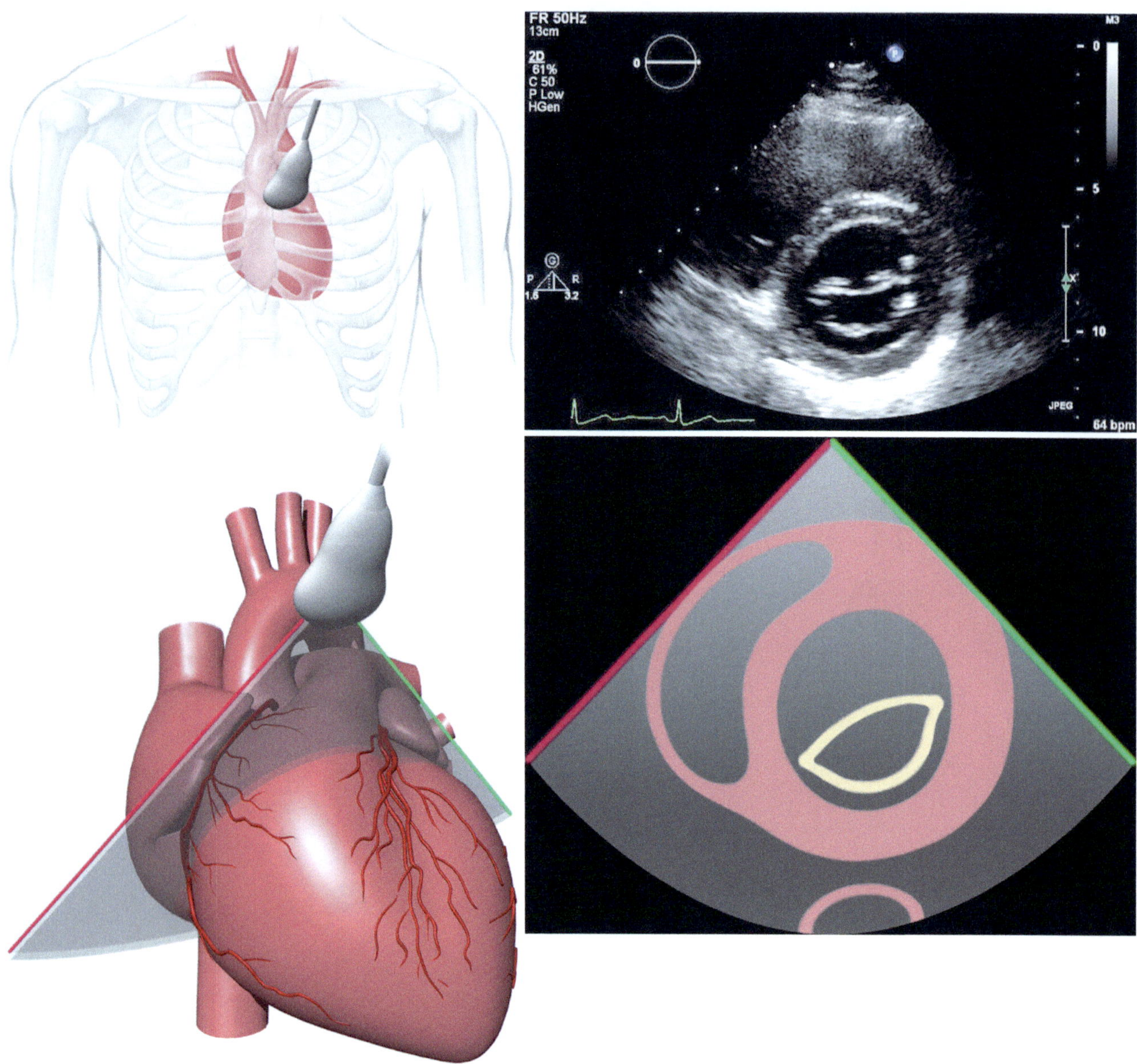

Fig. 1.15 Parasternal basal short-axis view

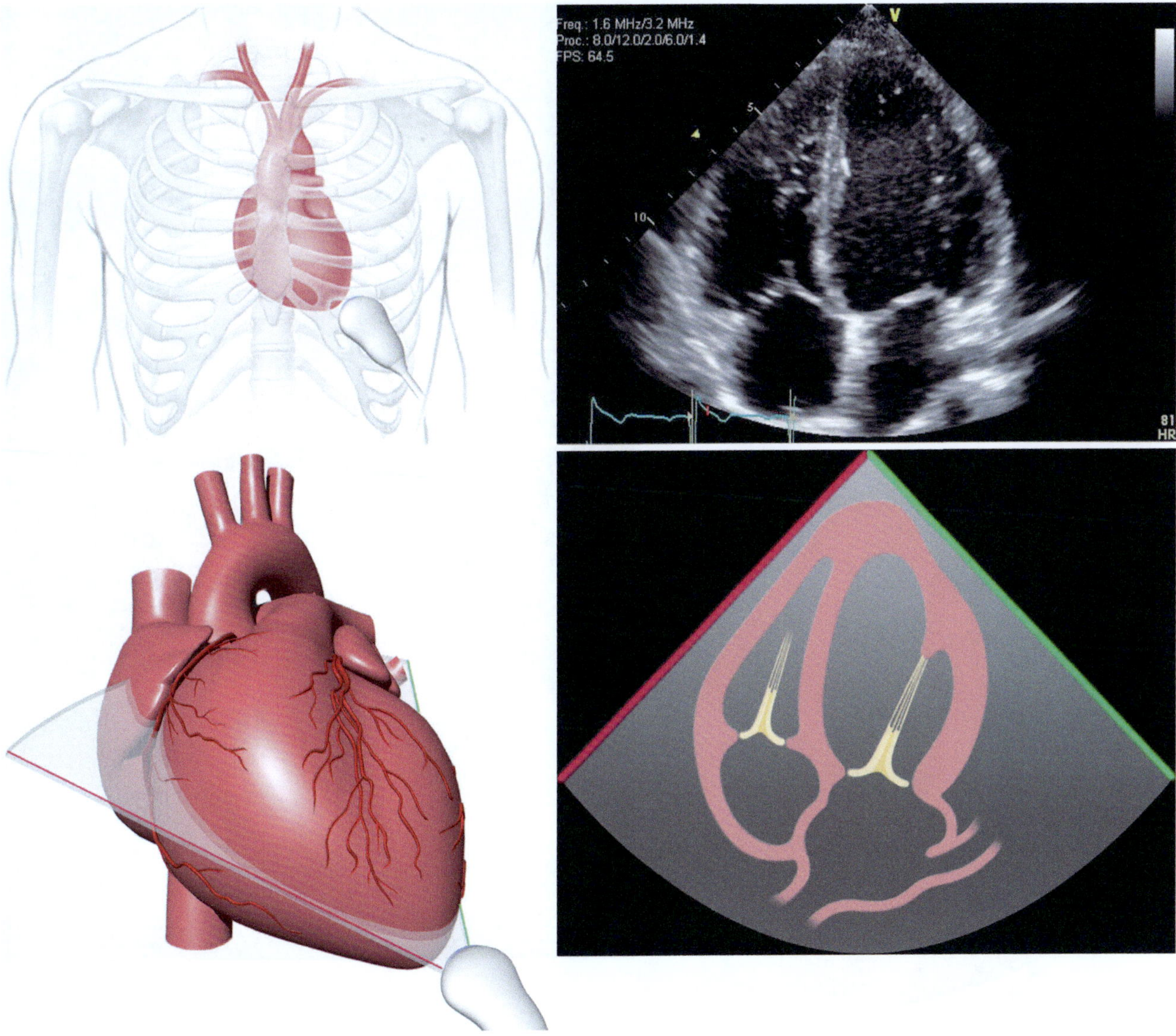

Fig. 1.16 Apical four-chamber view

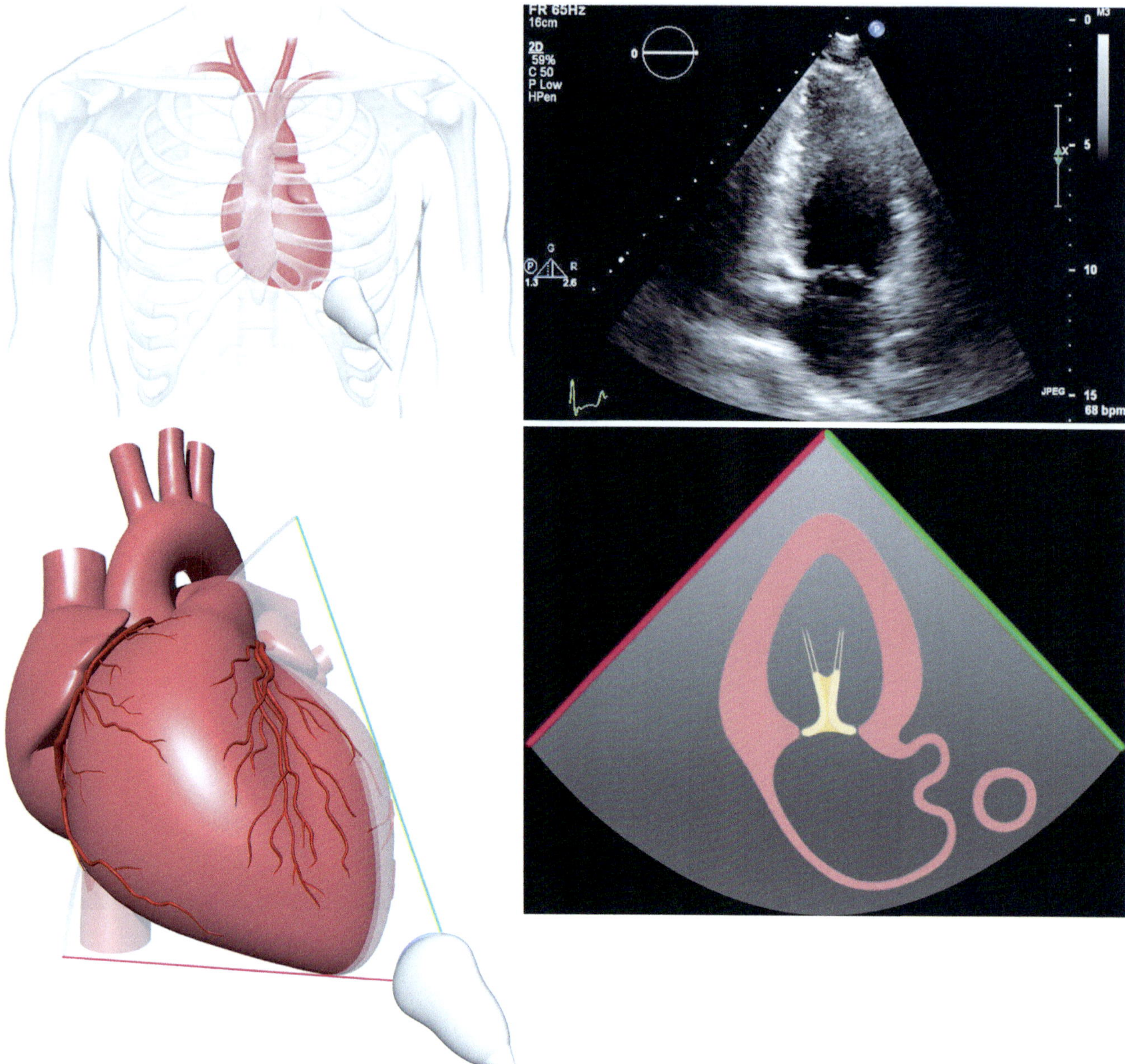

Fig. 1.17 Apical two-chamber view

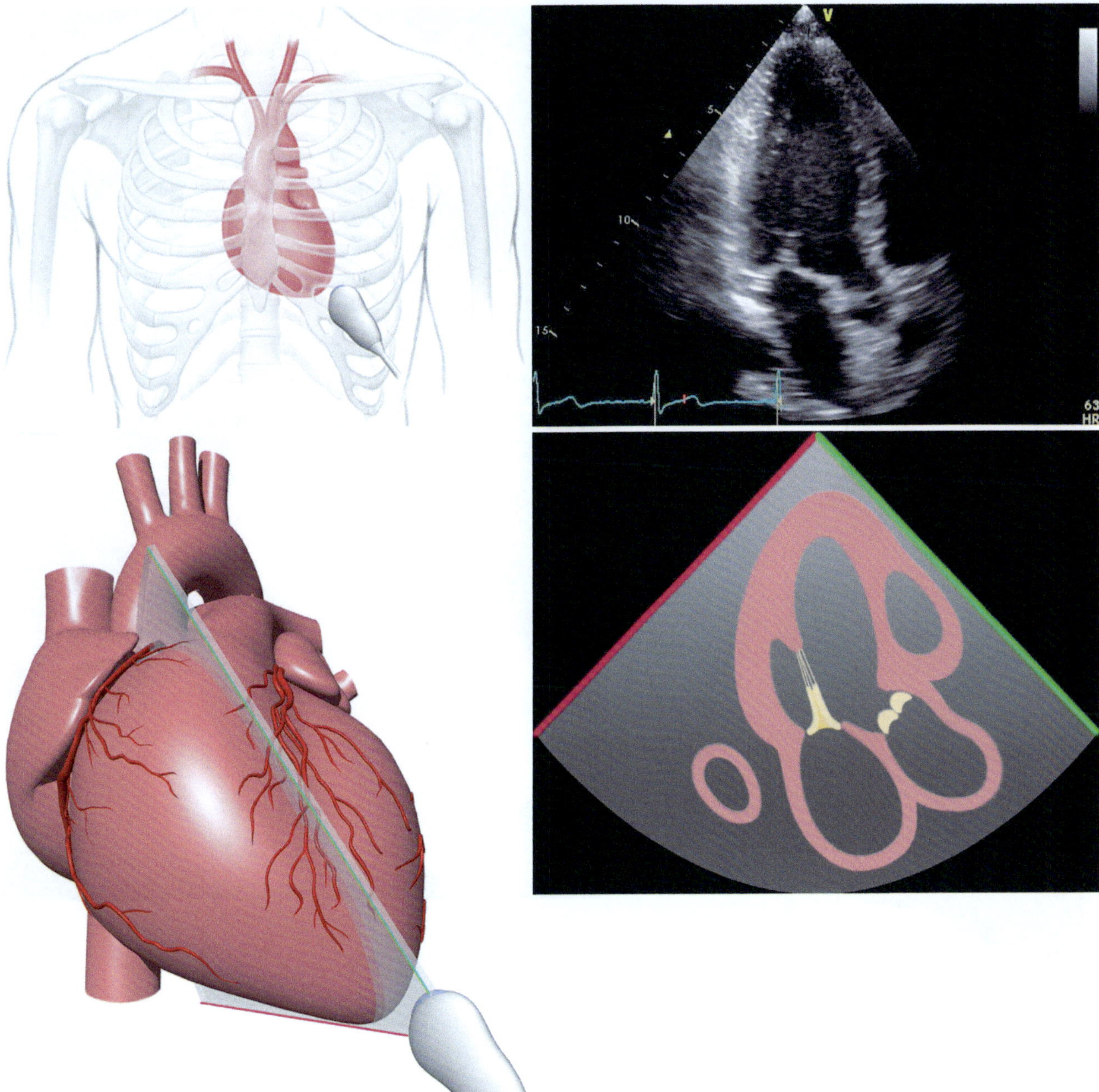

Fig. 1.18 Apical three-chamber view

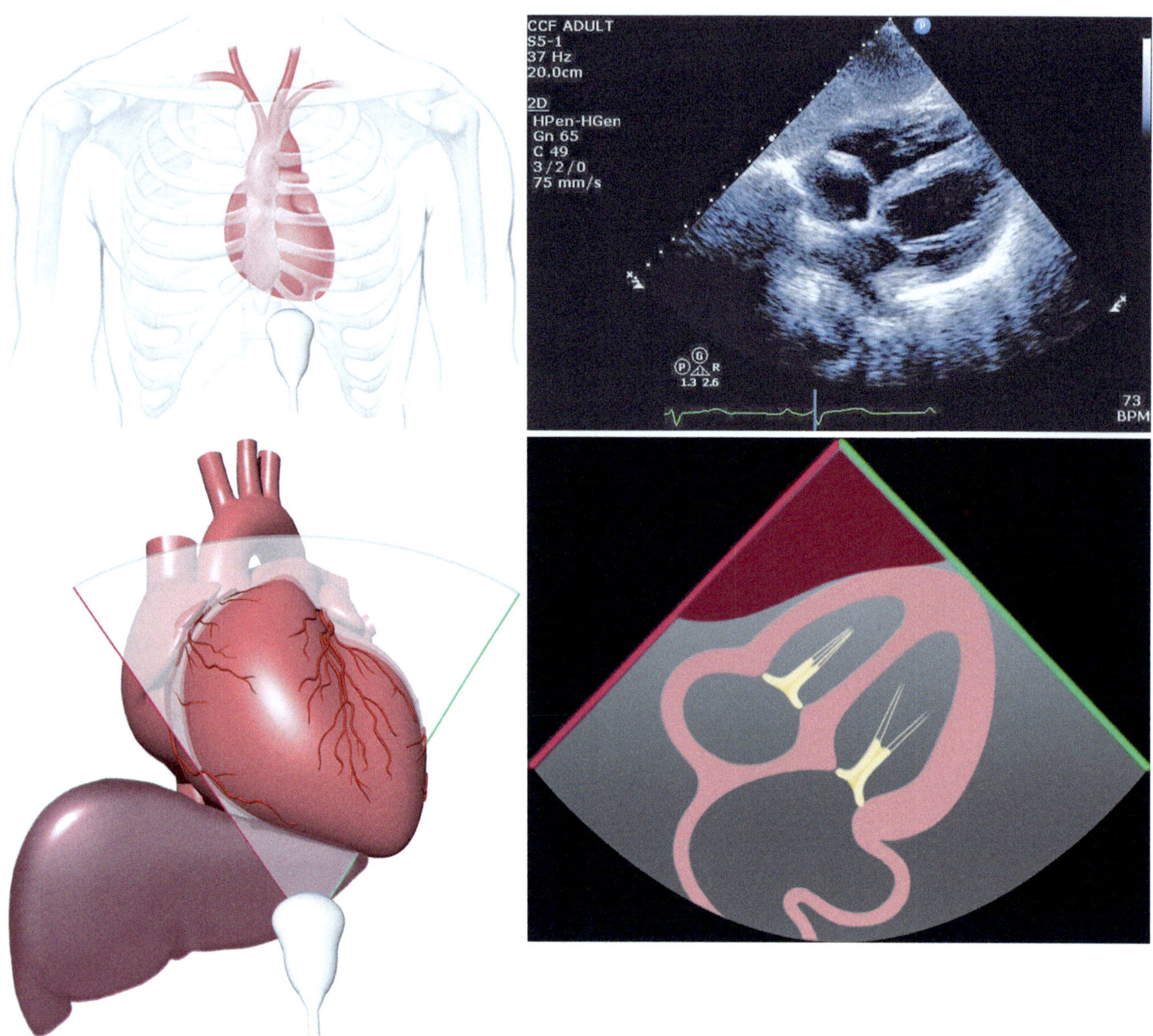

Fig. 1.19 Subcostal four-chamber view

Assessment of Mitral Valve Function

Christine Jellis and Teerapat Yingchoncharoen

Complete echocardiographic assessment of the mitral valve is achieved using a combination of techniques:

- Two-dimensional (2D) imaging
- M-mode imaging
- Doppler imaging—spectral and color

2.1 Two-Dimensional Imaging

Mitral annular dimensions can be best measured from the apical four-chamber and two-chamber views. Area planimetry can be performed on a short-axis view, although this method depends on image quality and correct measurement of the orifice at the level of the leaflet tips.

2.2 M-Mode Imaging

M-mode imaging of the mitral valve at the level of the leaflet tips delineates mitral valve motion (Fig. 2.1). The E-F slope reflects the partial closure of the anterior mitral valve leaflet during early diastole. The slope is dependent on the rate of left atrial emptying and is therefore prolonged in the setting of mitral stenosis. The E-F slope can be affected by other factors including cycle length, valvular calcification, and reduced left ventricular compliance. Because of the one-dimensional nature of M-mode imaging, a falsely normal E-F slope may be recorded if beam alignment is not maintained at the leaflet tips. M-mode imaging is also valuable for detection of systolic anterior motion (SAM) of the anterior mitral valve leaflet typically seen in hypertrophic obstructive cardiomyopathy (HOCM). In HOCM, a Venturi effect is created within the left ventricular outflow tract (LVOT), and the mitral valve apparatus is sucked into the LVOT during systole. This abnormal anterior motion contributes to both LVOT obstruction and mitral regurgitation.

M-mode imaging can be performed across the mitral valve from the apical approach with the addition of color Doppler (Fig. 2.2). The resultant trace enables the propagation velocity of blood to be calculated as it moves towards the apex. The M-mode cursor is placed in the center of the mitral valve, parallel to the transvalvular flow. Employment of a fast sweep speed (100–200 mm/s) and an aliasing velocity of 0.5–0.7 m/s will result in a vertical diastolic color pattern in the absence of mitral regurgitation. A line drawn along the initial early-diastolic slope of this color M-mode signal determines the propagation velocity. This measure of flow is reduced in the setting of elevated left ventricular pressure and is increased with constrictive physiology. In the setting of mitral regurgitation, a color M-mode signal will also be observed during systole. The density of this color jet is proportional to the degree of valvular incompetence.

C. Jellis (✉)
Department of Cardiovascular Medicine, Cleveland Clinic,
9500 Euclid Avenue, Cleveland, OH 44195, USA
e-mail: jellisc@ccf.org

T. Yingchoncharoen
Division of Cardiology, Department of Internal Medicine,
Faculty of Medicine, Ramathibodi Hospital, Mahidol University,
Bangkok, Thailand
e-mail: teerapatmdcu@gmail.com

M. Desai et al. (eds.), *An Atlas of Mitral Valve Imaging*,
DOI 10.1007/978-1-4471-6672-6_2, © Springer-Verlag London 2015

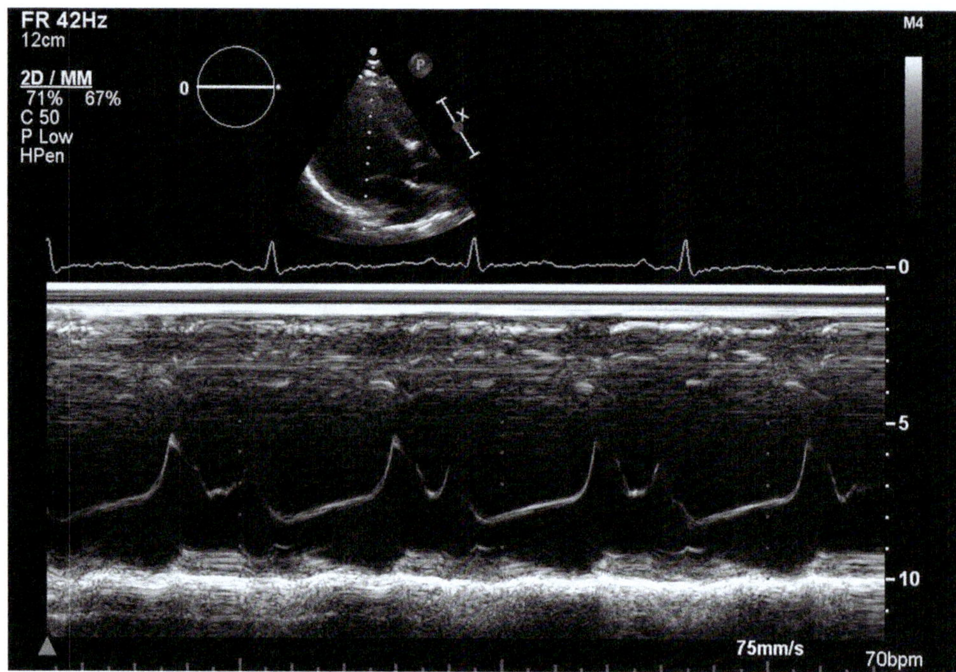

Fig. 2.1 M-mode imaging at the mitral valve tips

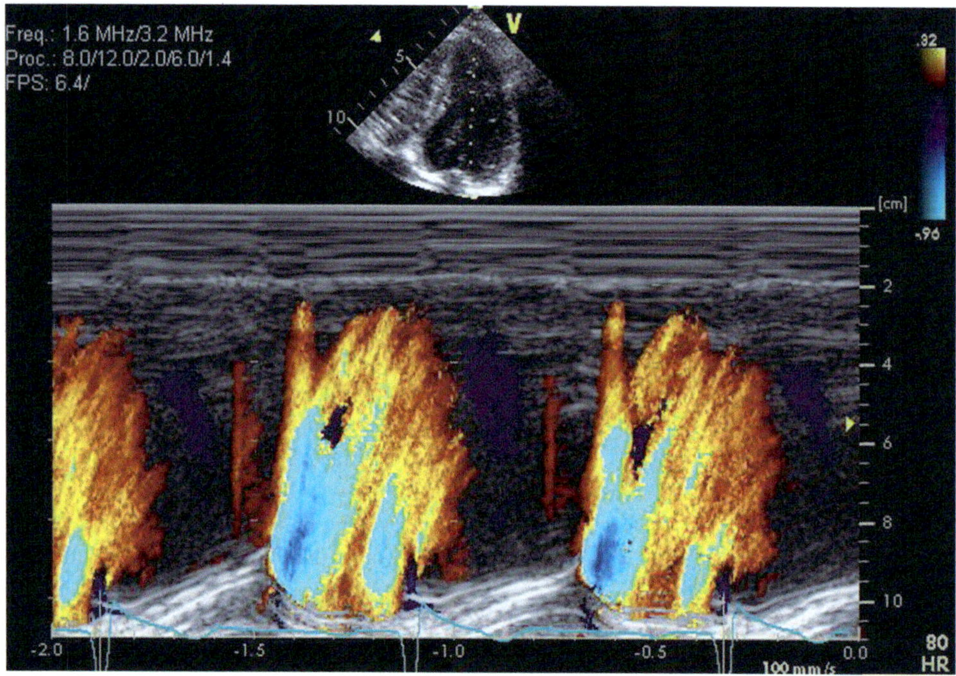

Fig. 2.2 Normal color M-mode through the mitral valve with transvalvular flow during diastole only

2.3   Spectral Doppler Imaging

Spectral Doppler imaging consists of both pulsed wave (PW) and continuous wave (CW) Doppler. Doppler interrogation of the mitral valve is optimized when flow is parallel to the ultrasound beam. Typically, this is best achieved on the apical four-chamber view. The PW sample volume is placed within the left ventricle at the level of the open mitral valve leaflet tips. Normally, antegrade blood flow through the mitral valve should occur during diastole (above the baseline), with no flow during systole (below the baseline) (Fig. 2.3). The E wave measures the velocity of rapid, passive transmitral flow during early diastole, whilst the A wave reflects active transmitral flow secondary to late diastolic atrial contraction. The mitral inflow profile therefore reflects left ventricular diastolic pressures and function. Increased antegrade velocity, seen by an elevation of the peak E wave, is also suggestive of increased transvalvular flow in the setting of mitral regurgitation. In mitral regurgitation, retrograde flow will also be noted (below the baseline) on CW imaging. The timing, wave profile, wave slope (dP/dt), peak velocity, and signal intensity of this spectral envelope can be used to help stratify the severity of the mitral regurgitation (Fig. 2.4).

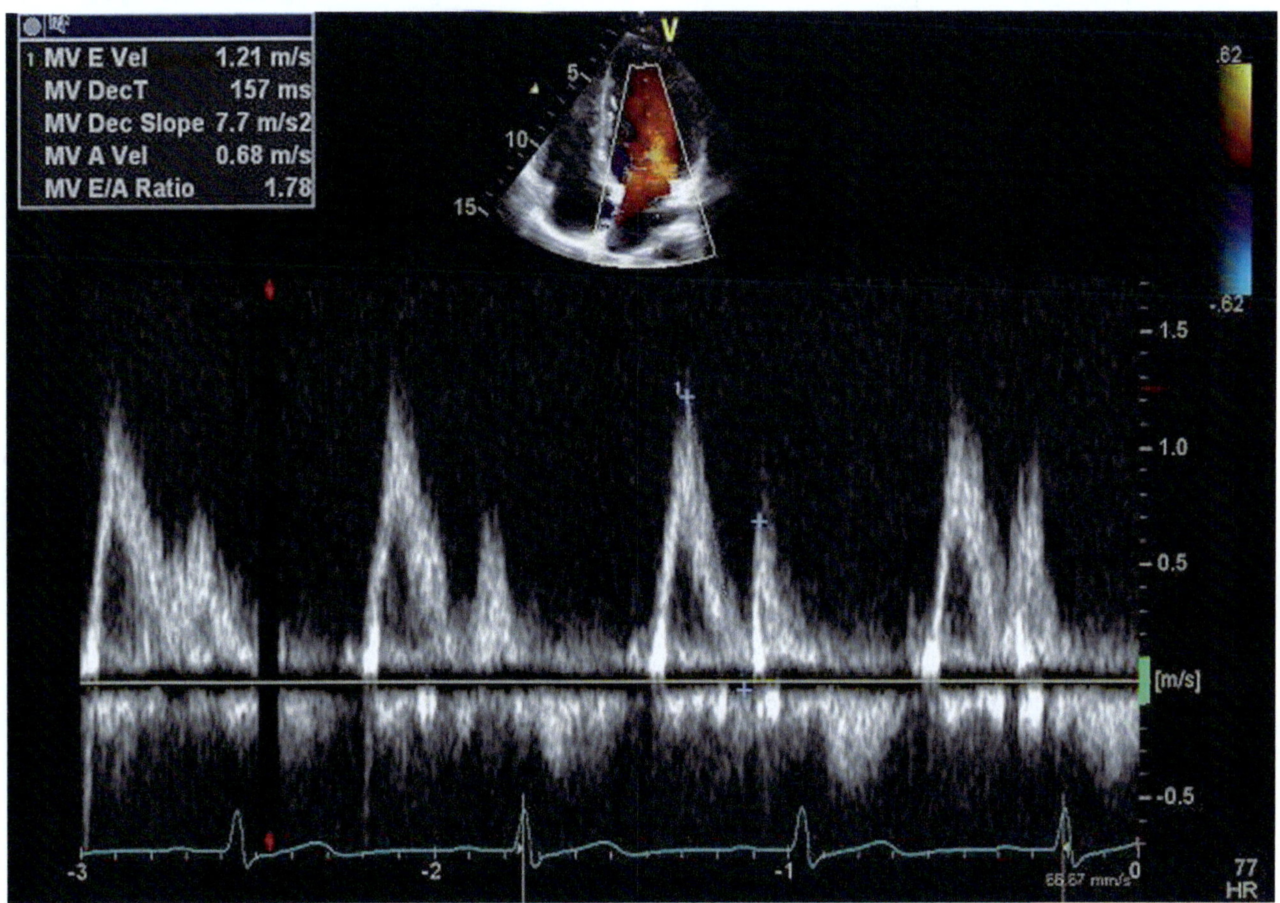

Fig. 2.3 Spectral Doppler image demonstrating inflow through the mitral valve during diastole

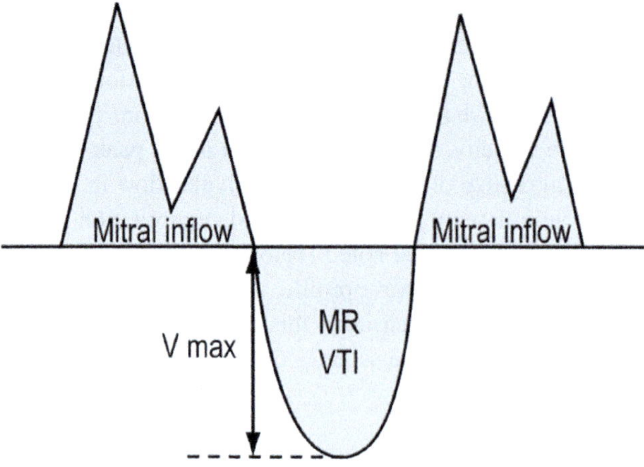

Fig. 2.4 The relationship and direction of diastolic mitral inflow and systolic mitral regurgitation

2.4 Color Doppler Imaging

This Doppler technique, which enables a color pattern of blood flow volume and direction within the heart to be superimposed on a 2D image, is particularly useful in the assessment of mitral regurgitation. The color Doppler jet pattern can be visually characterized with respect to the origin, direction, timing, and extent of reverse flow or turbulence of flow in different imaging planes. Quantitative assessment of the color Doppler jet can be employed for more formal classification of mitral regurgitation severity. Quantitative measures include jet width at the vena contracta, proximal isovelocity surface area (PISA), regurgitant volume (RVol), and regurgitant orifice area (ROA).

The PISA method uses the principle of conservation of mass by analyzing flow convergence of the regurgitant jet just proximal to the valve orifice on the left ventricular side of the mitral valve (Fig. 2.5). This radius can be used to calculate the severity of mitral regurgitation because acceleration of blood occurs further from the orifice in severe regurgitation than in mild regurgitation. A larger PISA corresponds to more severe mitral regurgitation. This method relies on a central circular valvular orifice for hemispheric measurements and is hence less accurate for eccentric or multiple jets. Adjustment of the aliasing velocity can be performed to optimize a hemispheric convergence zone. The PISA radius can then be used to estimate the regurgitant flow via the regurgitant flow (RF). In combination, the PISA radius and the peak velocity (V_{max}) or velocity time integral (VTI) of the regurgitant jet on CW Doppler can be used to estimate the regurgitant volume (RVol) or the effective

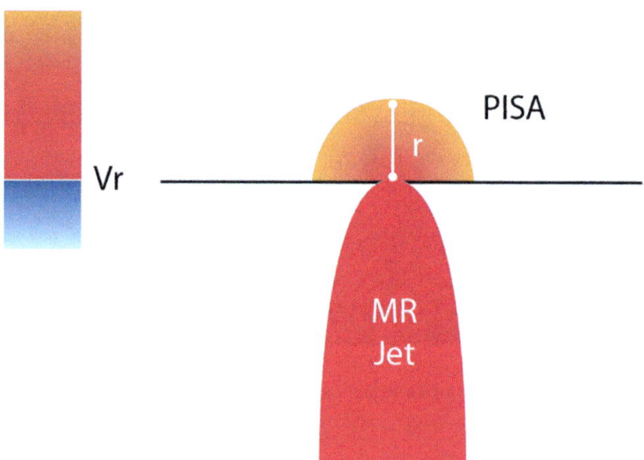

Fig. 2.5 Illustration of the PISA method

regurgitant orifice area (EROA) of the regurgitant jet, as shown in the following equations:

$$RF = 2\pi \times r^2 \times V_a$$

where r = PISA, RF = instantaneous regurgitant flow, and V_a = aliasing velocity.

$$EROA = \left(2\pi r^2 \times V_a\right) / V_{max}$$

where V_{max} = peak velocity of the regurgitant jet assessed by CW Doppler.

$$RVol = EROA \times VTI$$

where VTI = time-velocity integral of the regurgitant jet obtained by CW Doppler.

Table 2.1 shows the values for the PISA classification of mitral regurgitation.

Table 2.1 PISA classification of mitral regurgitation severity

Severity	ERO (mm²)	RVol (mL/beat)
Mild	<20	<30
Mild–moderate	20–29	30–44
Moderate–severe	30–39	45–59
Severe	≥40	≥60

ERO effective regurgitant orifice, *PISA* proximal isovelocity surface area, *RVol* regurgitant volume

2.5 Classification of Mitral Regurgitation

Mitral regurgitation is typically stratified as mild, moderate, or severe using the spectral and color Doppler methods illustrated above. Further classification includes assessment for reversal of pulmonary venous flow (via PW Doppler at the ostium of a pulmonary vein as it enters the left atrium) and assessment of LV size, ejection fraction, and contractile reserve.

Once severity is determined, classification of the cause of valve dysfunction is then typically performed visually from 2D images according to a standardized format. The most commonly employed classification system was described by Carpentier, as shown in Table 2.2.

The types of mitral regurgitation in the Carpentier classification are illustrated in Figs. 2.6, 2.7, 2.8, and 2.9.

For a referenced, complete, and up-to-date overview of mitral regurgitation assessment, readers should refer to the most current Guidelines and Standards by the American Society of Echocardiography available at http://www.asecho.org/clinical-information/guidelines-standards. The most current Guidelines and Standards at the time of publishing were recommendations for evaluation of the severity of native valvular regurgitation with 2D and Doppler echocardiography, found in the *Journal of the American Society of Echocardiography*, 2003;16:777–802.

Table 2.2 Carpentier classification of mitral regurgitation

Dysfunction	Lesions	Etiology
Type I:	Annular dilatation	Ischemic cardiomyopathy
Normal leaflet motion	Annular deformation	Dilated cardiomyopathy
	Leaflet perforation	Endocarditis
Type II:	Chordal elongation	Degenerative mitral disease
Increased leaflet motion (leaflet prolapse)	Chordal rupture	Fibroelastic deficiency
	Papillary muscle elongation	Barlow's disease
	Papillary muscle rupture	Marfan's disease
		Endocarditis
		Rheumatic disease
		Trauma
		Ischemic cardiomyopathy
Type IIIA:	Leaflet thickening	Rheumatic disease
Restricted leaflet motion (restricted opening)	Leaflet retraction	Carcinoid disease
	Chordal thickening	
	Chordal retraction	
	Chordal fusion	
	Calcification	
	Commissural fusion	
	Ventricular fibrous plaque	
Type IIIB:	Leaflet tethering	Ischemic cardiomyopathy
Restricted leaflet motion (restricted closure)	Papillary muscle displacement	Dilated cardiomyopathy
	Ventricular dilatation	
	Ventricular aneurysm	
	Ventricular fibrous plaque	

Fig. 2.6 Type I mitral regurgitation

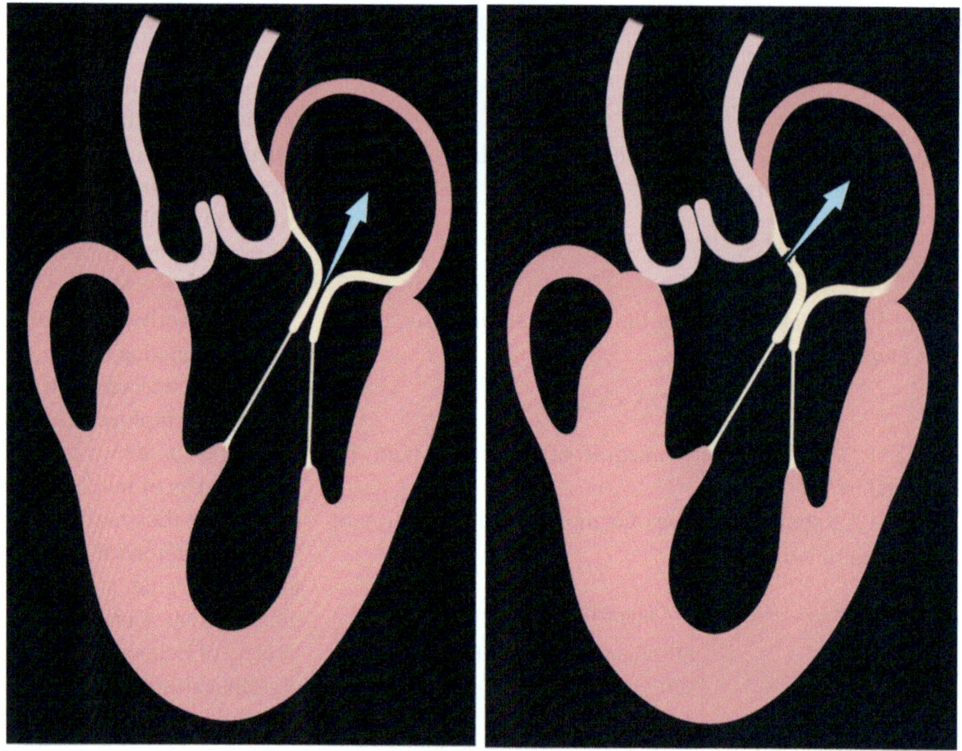

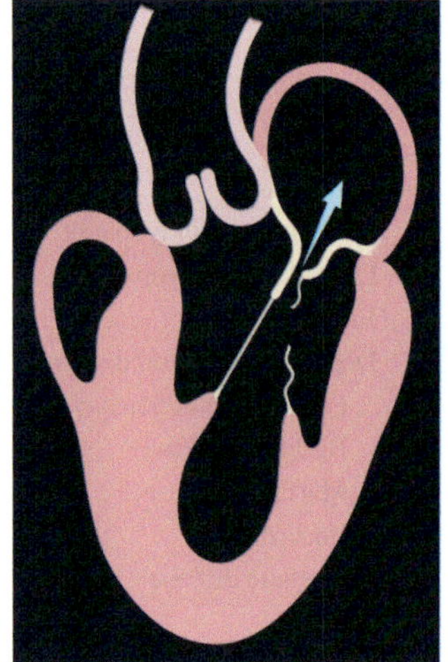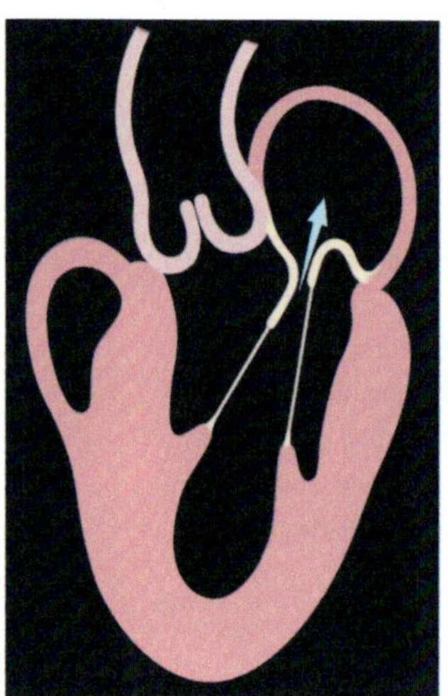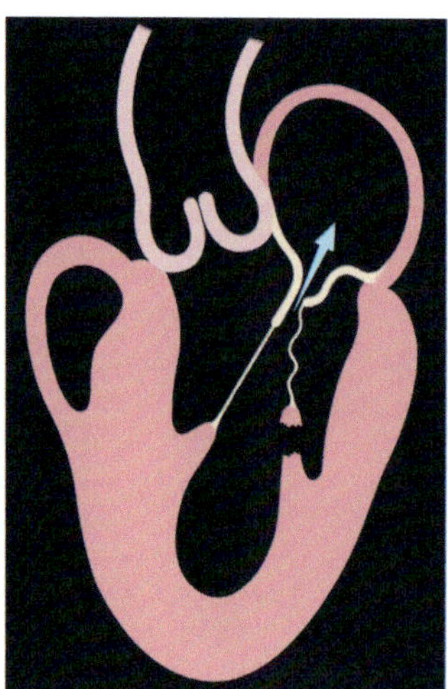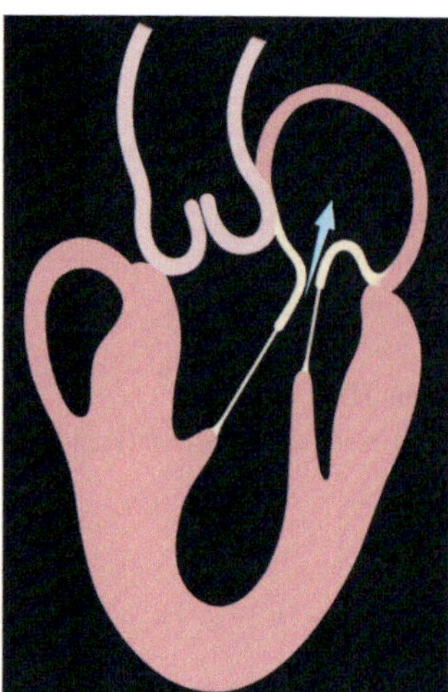

Fig. 2.7 Type II mitral regurgitation

Fig. 2.8 Type IIIA mitral regurgitation

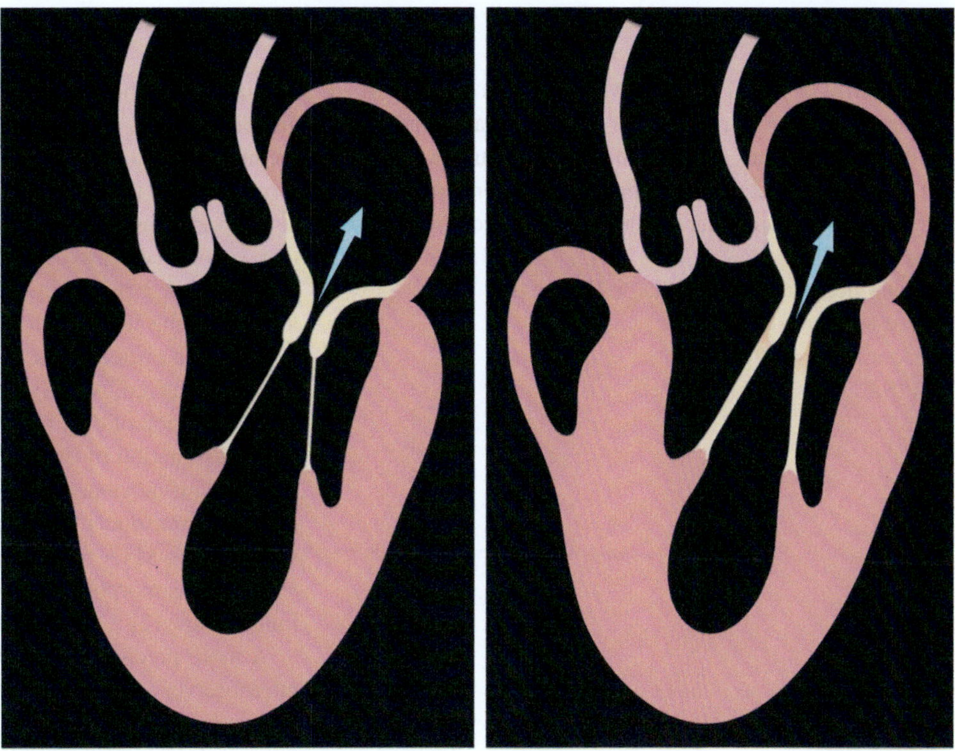

Fig. 2.9 Type IIIB mitral regurgitation

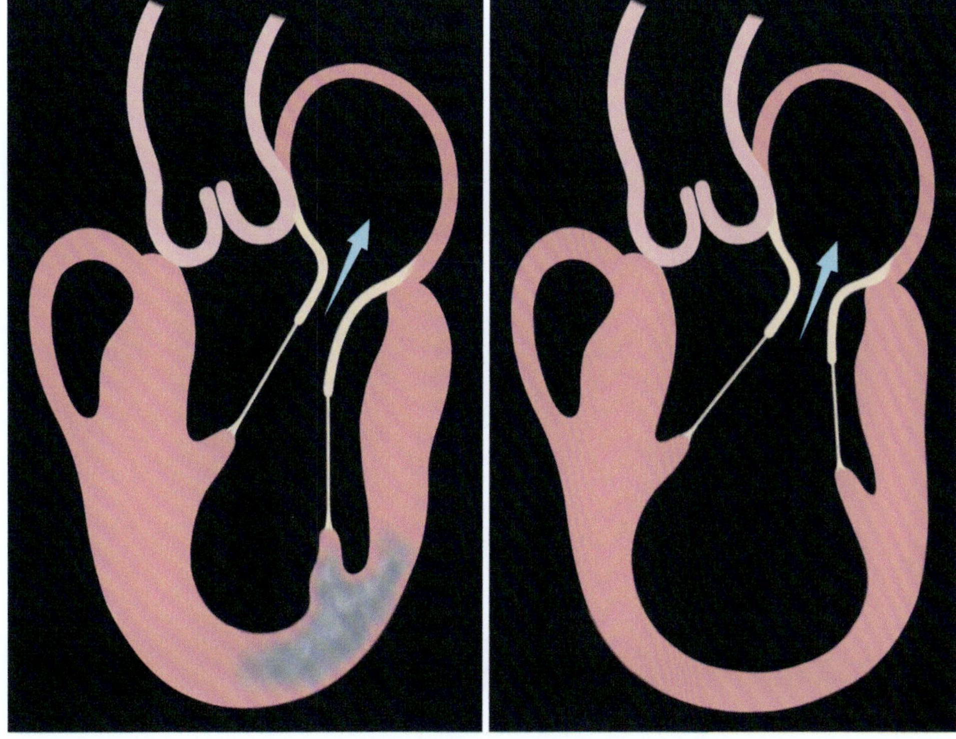

2.6 Mitral Stenosis

The severity of mitral stenosis (MS) should not be identified by single parameters, but rather should be assessed using multiple approaches that can determine mitral valve area (MVA), transmitral mean and pressure gradient, and pulmonary artery pressure. Four methods are most commonly used to assess MVA:

- Planimetry using either 2D or 3D imaging
- Pressure half-time (PHT)
- Continuity equation
- PISA

2.6.1 Planimetry

Planimetry has been shown to have the best correlation with anatomic MVA, as assessed by explanted valve [1]. This method requires no geometrical assumption or mathematical formulae. The technique is largely independent of hemodynamic variables, left ventricular compliance, and concomitant valvular disease. The 2D planimetry of the MVA is performed in a parasternal short-axis view at the tip of the leaflets during the maximal opening. The inner edge of the mitral valve orifice is traced in mid-diastole with the entire orifice visualized. A study in 48 consecutive patients showed that a deviation of only 6° from the optimal plane may result in overestimation of the MVA by 63 %, which increases to over 88 % if movement of the angle also leads to repositioning of the transducer by 2 mm. The influence of image plane variations on MVA measurements is more pronounced if the mitral valve morphology is prominent doming rather than funnel shape [2].

A more precise and reproducible method, with excellent interobserver and intraobserver agreement, uses 3D echocardiography (Figs. 2.10 and 2.11), which provides better alignment of the image plane at the mitral tips [3–5].

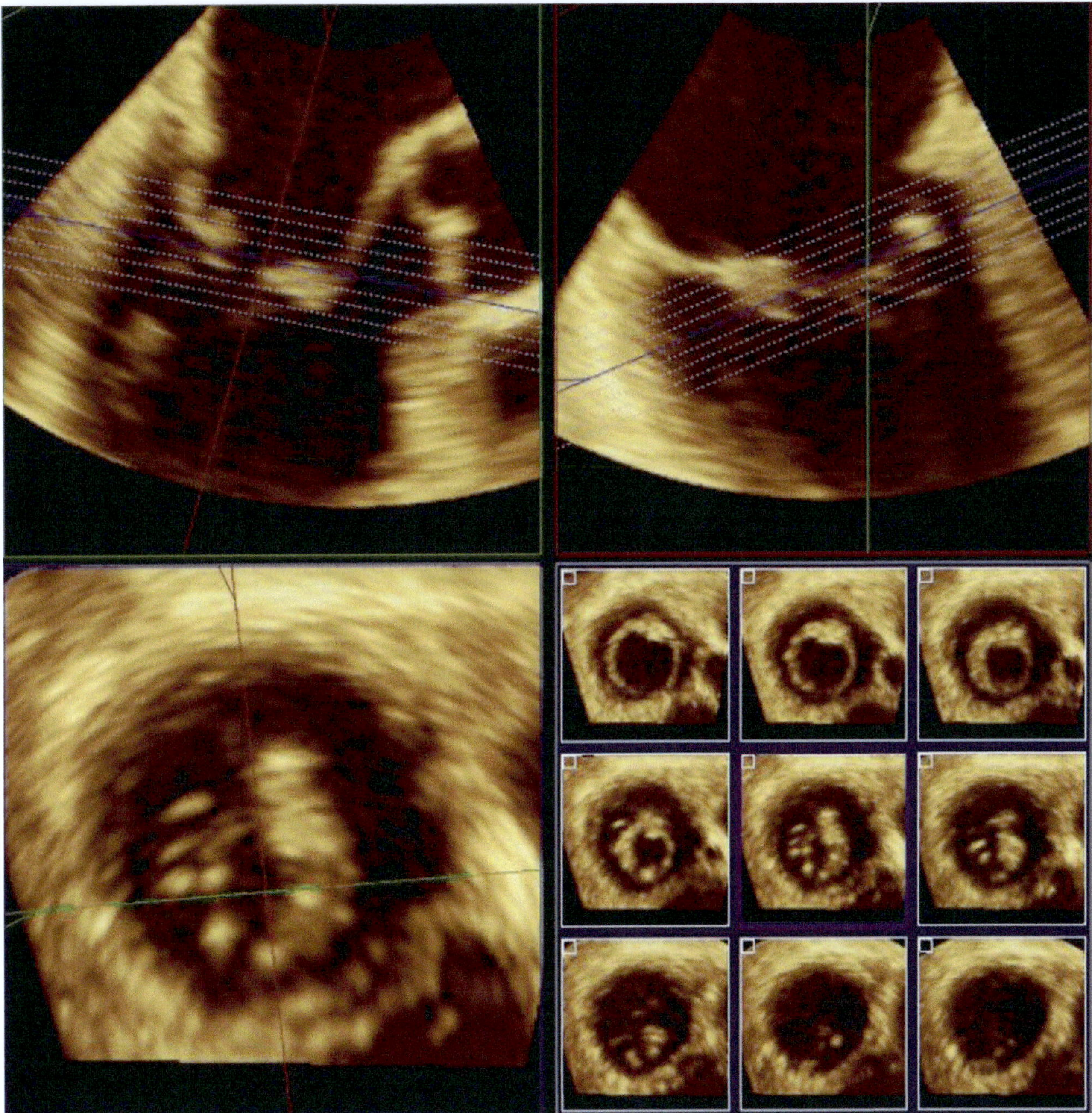

Fig. 2.10   3D transesophageal echo image of a stenotic mitral valve

Fig. 2.11 3D reconstruction of a stenotic mitral valve using QLAB quantification software (Philips, Amsterdam)

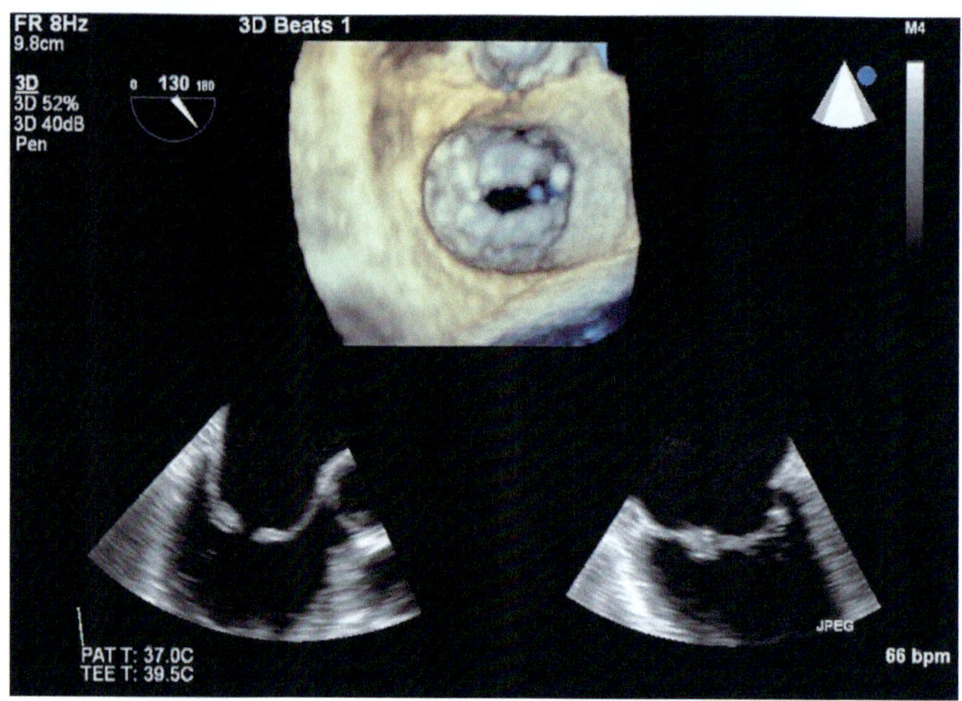

2.6.2   Pressure Half-Time

The PHT method relies on the fact that the rate of pressure decline in the left atrium during diastole is inversely proportional to the severity of mitral stenosis. PHT is obtained by tracing the deceleration slope of the E-wave on a Doppler spectral display of transmitral inflow (Fig. 2.12). The MVA can be calculated using an empirical formula: 220/PHT or 759/Deceleration time (DT). If the E-wave Doppler profile is bimodal, it is preferable to trace the deceleration slope in mid-diastole rather than using an early deceleration slope (Method 3 in Figure), as this slope was shown to have the best correlation with MVA by the Gorlin equation [6]. In patients with atrial fibrillation, the tracing should be done in long diastoles and use the average from multiple tracings. In patients with concave shape on the Doppler tracing, this technique cannot be reliably used. PHT is also affected by the net left atrial (LA) and left ventricular (LV) compliance and the square root of the peak transmitral gradient [7]. Therefore the reliability of PHT for the assessment of MVA is limited in settings of altered LA/LV compliance, including (but not limited to) aortic insufficiency, atrial septal defect, and following mitral valvuloplasty, especially in the first 24–48 h [8–12].

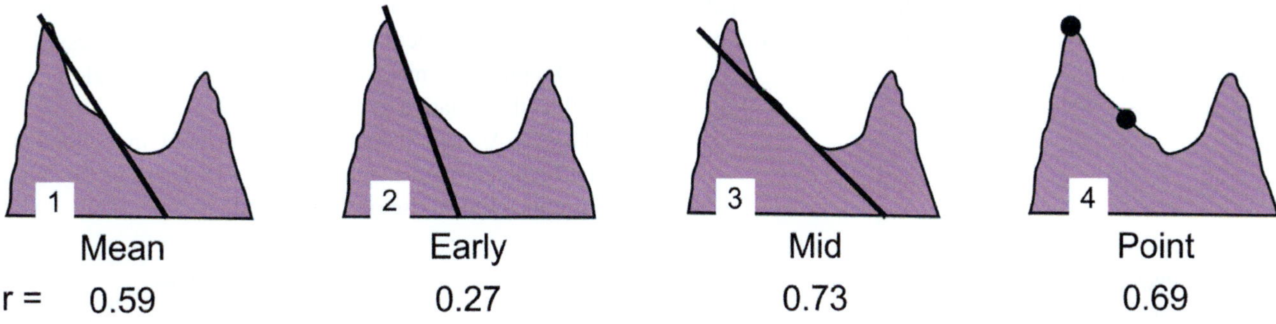

Fig. 2.12 Pressure half-time estimation of mitral valve area in mitral stenosis

2.6.3 Continuity Equation

The continuity equation relies on the conservation of mass theory, based on the assumption that the filling volume of diastolic mitral flow is equal to aortic stroke volume. The formula for calculation of MVA is

$$MVA = \pi \left(D^2 / 4\right)\left(VTI_{aorta} / VTI_{mitral}\right)$$

where D is the LVOT diameter and VTI is the velocity time integral in centimeters.

The main disadvantage of this method is the probability of errors in measurement, especially measurement of the LVOT diameter. The technique cannot be used in patients with atrial fibrillation or associated significant mitral or aortic regurgitation.

2.6.4 PISA Method

As described for the assessment of mitral regurgitation, it is possible to calculate the blood flow across a stenotic or regurgitant orifice based on the hemispheric shape of the convergence zone of mitral flow formed during diastole on the LA side. In mitral stenosis, the PISA formula must be adjusted for the angle formed by the leaflets ($\pi/180°$), yielding this formula:

$$MVA = \pi\left(r^2\right)\left(V_{alias}\right) / PeakV_{mitral} \times \alpha / 180$$

where r is the radius of the hemispheric convergence zone in centimeters, V_{alias} is the aliasing velocity (in cm/s), $PeakV_{mitral}$ is the peak velocity of mitral inflow assessed by CW Doppler (in cm/s), and α is the opening angle of the mitral leaflets relative to flow direction.

The PISA method requires a number of measurements and is technically demanding (Fig. 2.13). These factors limit the routine clinical use of this method.

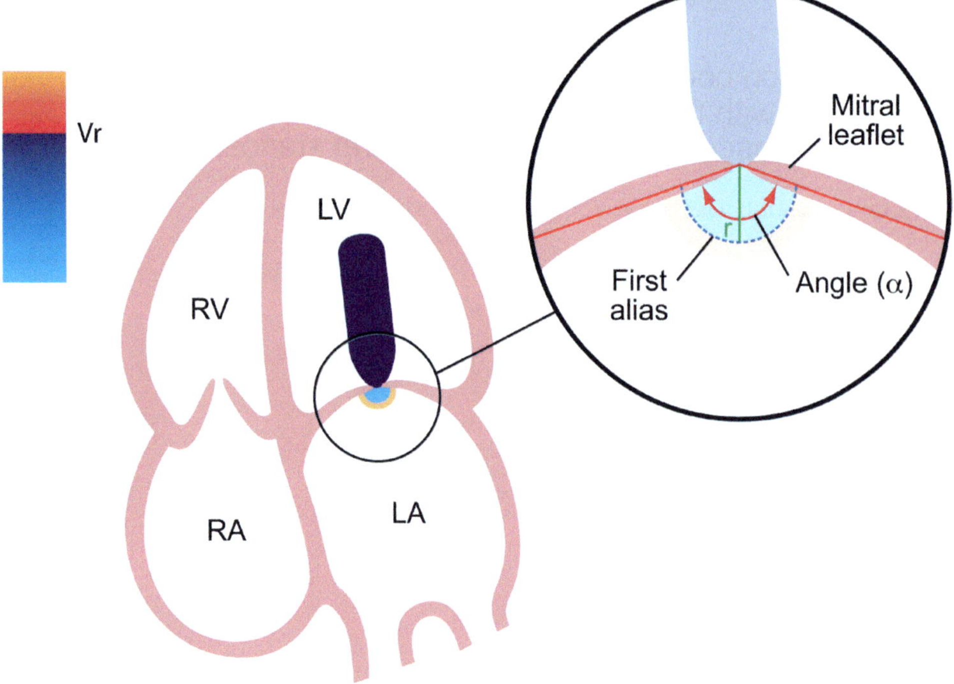

Fig. 2.13 PISA estimation of mitral stenosis

2.6.5   Mean Pressure Gradient

The transmitral pressure gradient can be obtained by tracing the transmitral CW Doppler. The mean gradient is the main hemodynamic determinant of MS severity. Because the transmitral gradient is a function of the square of the transvalvular flow rate, these measurements are highly dependent on heart rate and flow [13]. Patients in atrial flutter may have a nonlinear CW Doppler profile (Fig. 2.14), and patients in atrial fibrillation represent a challenge in measurement of the transmitral gradient because of beat-to-beat variability. In these patients, several beats should be averaged.

2.6.6   Pulmonary Artery Pressure

The degree of pulmonary hypertension is an indicator of the overall hemodynamic consequences of MS, and severe pulmonary hypertension is associated with worse clinical outcomes [14]. Right ventricular systolic pressure (RVSP) is obtained by adding the right atrial pressure (RAP) to the transtricuspid peak pressure gradient, which can be derived from the peak velocity of tricuspid regurgitation (TR_{Vmax}) using the simplified Bernoulli equation:

$$RVSP = 4\left(TR_{Vmax}\right)^2 + RAP$$

In the absence of right ventricular outflow tract obstruction, RVSP corresponds well to pulmonary artery systolic pressure [15].

For a referenced, complete, and up-to-date overview of mitral stenosis assessment, please refer to the most current Guidelines and Standards by the American Society of Echocardiography, available at http://www.asecho.org/clinical-information/guidelines-standards. The most current guidelines and standards at the time of publishing appeared in 2009 [16].

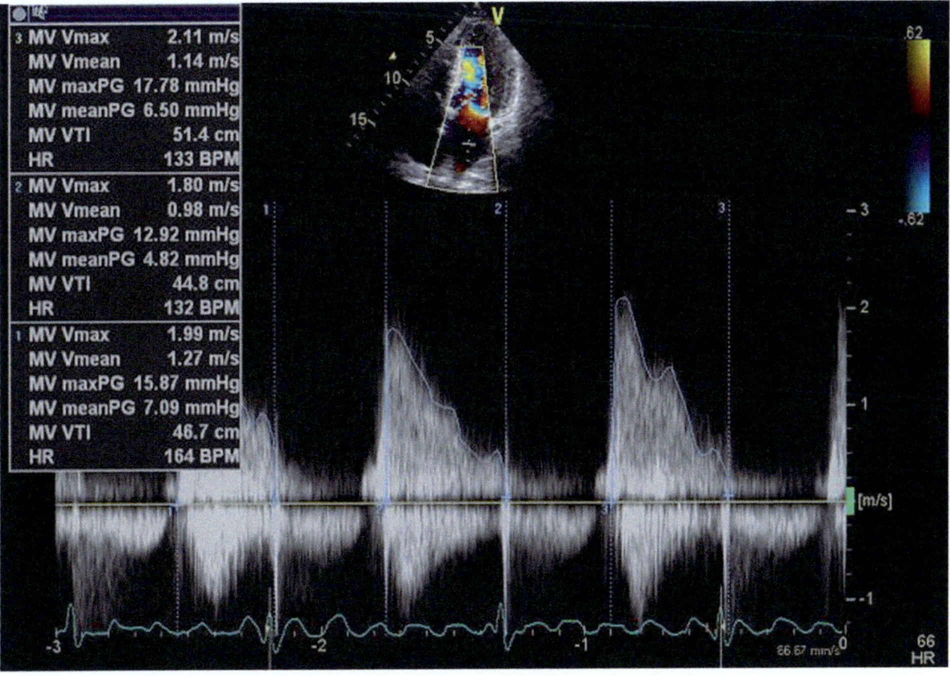

Fig. 2.14 Transmitral pressure gradient via transmitral continuous wave (CW) Doppler

References

1. Faletra F, Pezzano Jr A, Fusco R, Mantero A, Como R, Crivellaro W, et al. Measurement of mitral valve area in mitral stenosis: four echocardiographic methods compared with direct measurement of anatomic orifices. J Am Coll Cardiol. 1996;28:1190–7.
2. Binder TM, Rosenhek R, Porenta G, Maurer G, Baumgartner H. Improved assessment of mitral valve stenosis by volumetric real-time three-dimensional echocardiography. J Am Coll Cardiol. 2000;36:1355–61.
3. Min SY, Song JM, Kim YJ, Park HK, Seo MO, Lee MS, et al. Discrepancy between mitral valve areas measured by two-dimensional planimetry and three-dimensional transoesophageal echocardiography in patients with mitral stenosis. Heart. 2013;99:253–8.
4. Schlosshan D, Aggarwal G, Mathur G, Allan R, Cranney G. Real-time 3D transesophageal echocardiography for the evaluation of rheumatic mitral stenosis. JACC Cardiovasc Imaging. 2011;4:580–8.
5. Sugeng L, Weinert L, Lammertin G, Thomas P, Spencer KT, Decara JM, et al. Accuracy of mitral valve area measurements using transthoracic rapid freehand 3-dimensional scanning: comparison with noninvasive and invasive methods. J Am Soc Echocardiogr. 2003;16:1292–300.
6. Lang RM. American society of echocardiography. Dynamic echocardiography. 1st ed. Saunders/Elsevier: St. Louis; 2011.
7. Thomas JD, Weyman AE. Doppler mitral pressure half-time: a clinical tool in search of theoretical justification. J Am Coll Cardiol. 1987;10:923–9.
8. Hatle L, Angelsen B, Tromsdal A. Noninvasive assessment of atrioventricular pressure half-time by Doppler ultrasound. Circulation. 1979;60:1096–104.
9. Nakatani S, Masuyama T, Kodama K, Kitabatake A, Fujii K, Kamada T. Value and limitations of Doppler echocardiography in the quantification of stenotic mitral valve area: comparison of the pressure half-time and the continuity equation methods. Circulation. 1988;77:78–85.
10. Thomas JD, Wilkins GT, Choong CY, Abascal VM, Palacios IF, Block PC, et al. Inaccuracy of mitral pressure half-time immediately after percutaneous mitral valvotomy. Dependence on transmitral gradient and left atrial and ventricular compliance. Circulation. 1988;78:980–93.
11. Flachskampf FA, Weyman AE, Guerrero JL, Thomas JD. Influence of orifice geometry and flow rate on effective valve area: an in vitro study. J Am Coll Cardiol. 1990;15:1173–80.
12. Karp K, Teien D, Bjerle P, Eriksson P. Reassessment of valve area determinations in mitral stenosis by the pressure half-time method: impact of left ventricular stiffness and peak diastolic pressure difference. J Am Coll Cardiol. 1989;13:594–9.
13. Gorlin R, Gorlin SG. Hydraulic formula for calculation of the area of the stenotic mitral valve, other cardiac valves, and central circulatory shunts. Am Heart J. 1951;41:1–29.
14. Ward C, Hancock BW. Extreme pulmonary hypertension caused by mitral valve disease. Natural history and results of surgery. Br Heart J. 1975;37:74–8.
15. Chan KL, Currie PJ, Seward JB, Hagler DJ, Mair DD, Tajik AJ. Comparison of three Doppler ultrasound methods in the prediction of pulmonary artery pressure. J Am Coll Cardiol. 1987;9:549–54.
16. Baumgartner H, Hung J, Bermejo J, Chambers JB, Evangelista A, Griffin BP, et al. Echocardiographic assessment of valve stenosis: EAE/ASE recommendations for clinical practice. J Am Soc Echocardiogr. 2009;22:1–23.

Calcific Degenerative Mitral Disease

3

Teerapat Yingchoncharoen

3.1 Case 1. Caseous Calcification of the Mitral Annulus Masquerading as a Cardiac Mass

A 70-year-old woman presented to her primary physician with progressive shortness of breath. She was found to have atrial fibrillation and 2/6 pansystolic murmur at the left lower parasternal border on physical examination. Transthoracic echocardiography (TTE) showed mild mitral regurgitation and a cardiac mass at the atrioventricular (AV) groove area. She was referred to our institute for cardiac mass removal (Figs. 3.1, 3.2, 3.3, 3.4, 3.5, 3.6, and 3.7).

Video 3.1 Transthoracic echocardiography (TTE), parasternal long-axis view showing a mass with round, smooth borders and a heterogeneous echo density located at the posterior mitral annulus (AVI 5136 kb)

Video 3.2 TTE, apical four-chamber view showing a posterior mitral annulus mass (AVI 6292 kb)

Video 3.3 TTE, apical two-chamber view showing a posterior mitral annulus mass (AVI 5368 kb)

Video 3.4 Three-dimensional (3D) TTE, parasternal long-axis view again showing a mass with round, smooth borders and a heterogenous echo density located at the posterior mitral annulus (AVI 1511 kb)

3.1.1 Learning Points

Caseous calcification of the mitral annulus (CCMA) is a rare variant of mitral annular calcification with an estimated prevalence of 0.068 % [1–3]. It is characterized by an echodense outer shell and echolucent core [4]. The posterior mitral annulus is more often affected than the anterior. The inner core of the lesion represents the byproduct of liquefaction necrosis. Pathological examination reveals sterile, amorphous, acellular eosinophilic material with macrophage and lymphocyte infiltration [5].

The clinical course of CCMA is generally benign and often dynamic, with reports of spontaneous resolution of progression [3]. The complications of CCMA include hemodynamically significant mitral stenosis and regurgitation secondary to mass effect [5, 6], as well as erosion of the inner core into the left atrial chamber [7] and the left circumflex coronary artery [8].

Electronic supplementary material The online version of this chapter (doi:10.1007/978-1-4471-6672-6_3) contains supplementary material, which is available to authorized users.

T. Yingchoncharoen
Department of Cardiovascular Medicine, Cleveland Clinic,
9500 Euclid Avenue, Cleveland, OH 44195, USA
e-mail: teerapatmdcu@gmail.com

M. Desai et al. (eds.), *An Atlas of Mitral Valve Imaging*,
DOI 10.1007/978-1-4471-6672-6_3, © Springer-Verlag London 2015

Fig. 3.1 Transthoracic echocardiography (TTE), parasternal long-axis view showing a mass with round, smooth borders and a heterogeneous echo density located at the posterior mitral annulus (*arrows*). *Ao* aorta, *LA* left atrium, *LV* left ventricle, *RV* right ventricle

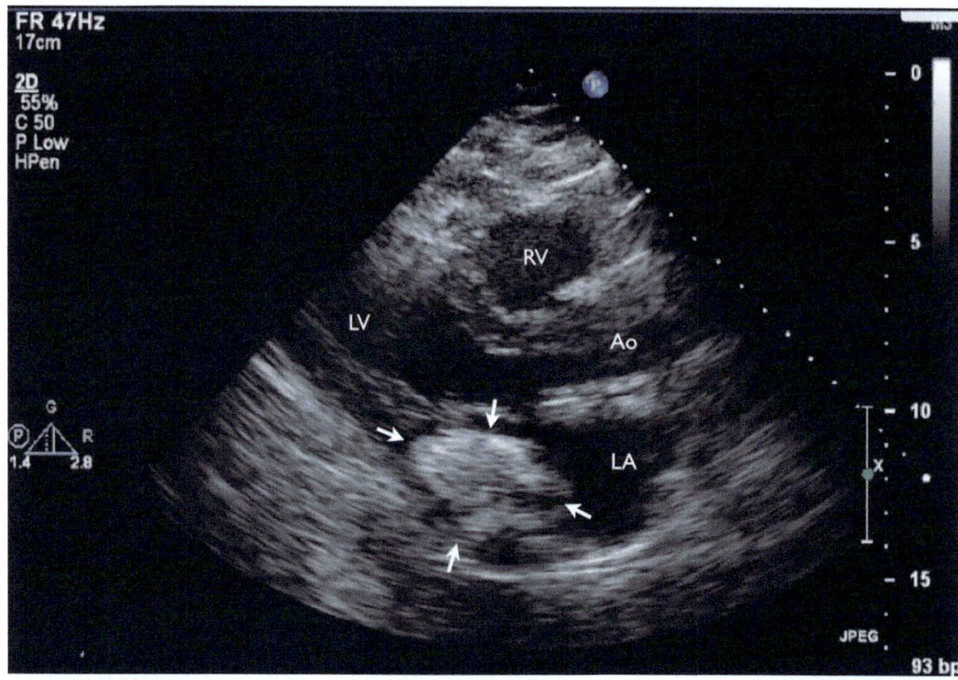

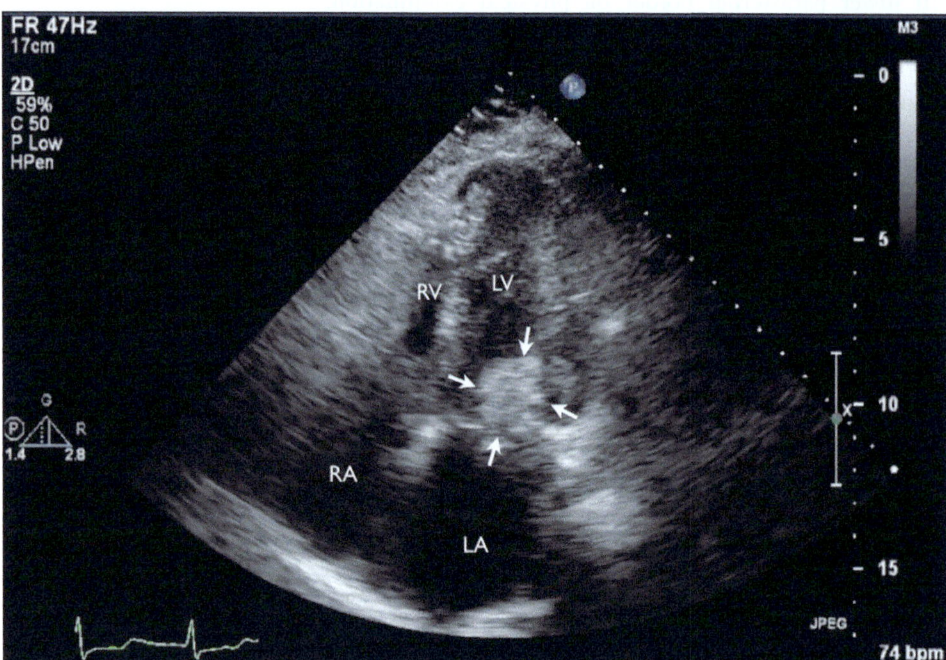

Fig. 3.2 TTE, apical four-chamber view showing a posterior mitral annulus mass (*arrows*). *RA* right atrium

Fig. 3.3 TTE, apical two-chamber view showing a posterior mitral annulus mass (*arrows*)

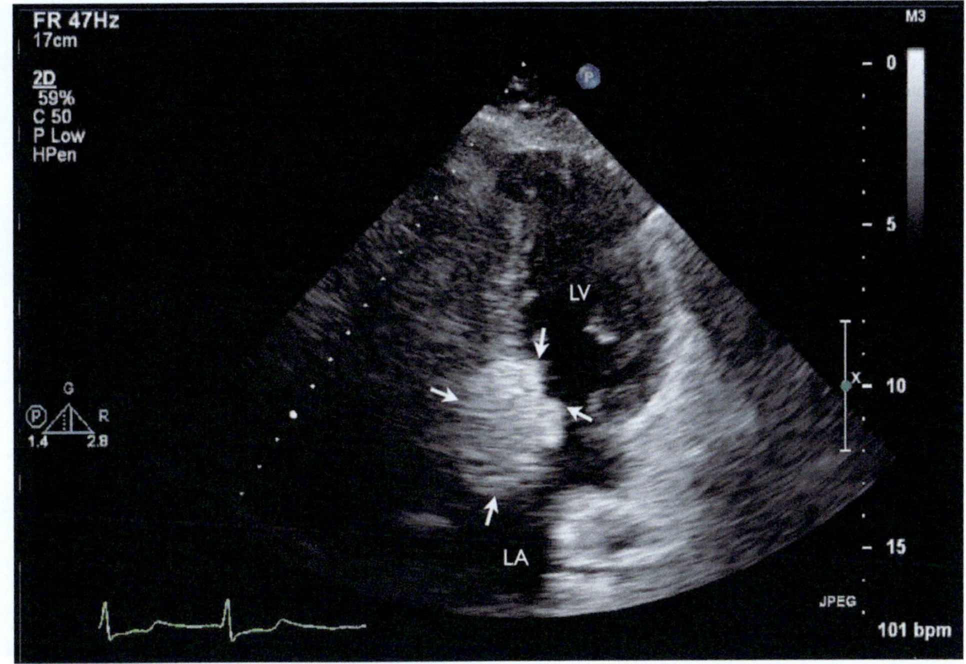

Fig. 3.4 Three-dimensional (3D) TTE, parasternal long-axis view again showing a mass with round, smooth borders and a heterogenous echo density located at the posterior mitral annulus (*arrows*)

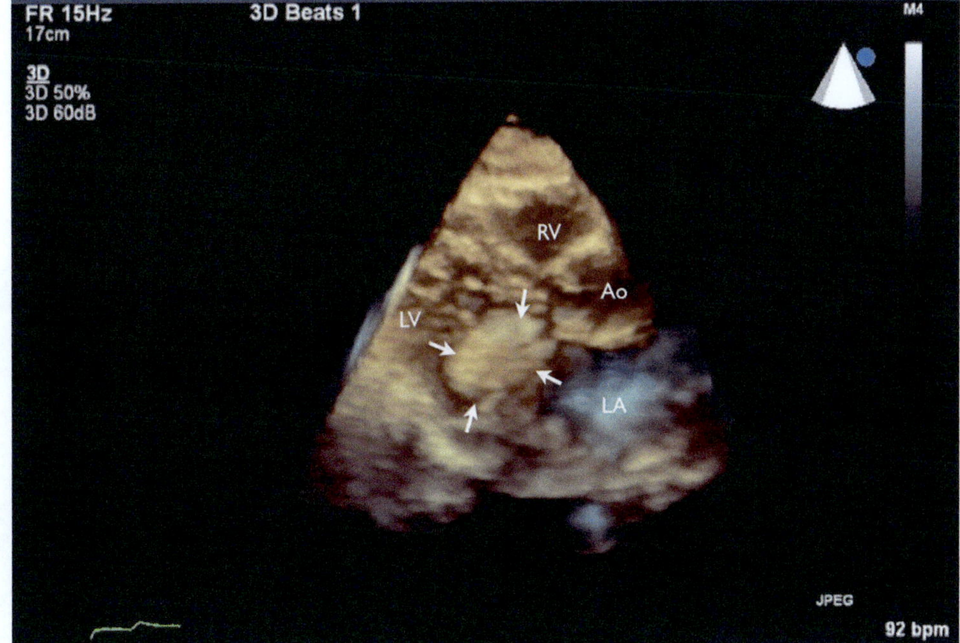

Fig. 3.5 3D TTE, mitral valve viewed from left atrium showing posterior mitral annulus prominence (*arrows*)

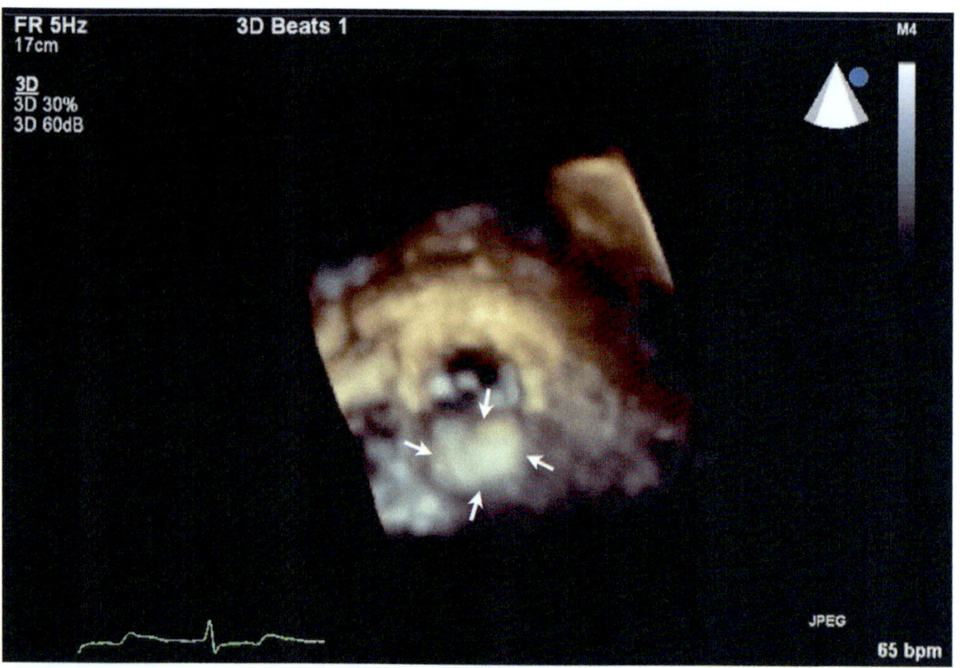

Fig. 3.6 Cardiac CT scans with multiplanar reconstruction confirmed the diagnosis and showed an intracardiac mass measuring 3.4×4.7 cm involving both anterior and posterior mitral annulus with extension into the left atrium (*LA*) wall (*arrow*). The periphery of this mass is densely calcified in spots, whereas the central portion has density of approximately 400 Hounsfield units, consistent with liquefaction of calcified mitral annulus

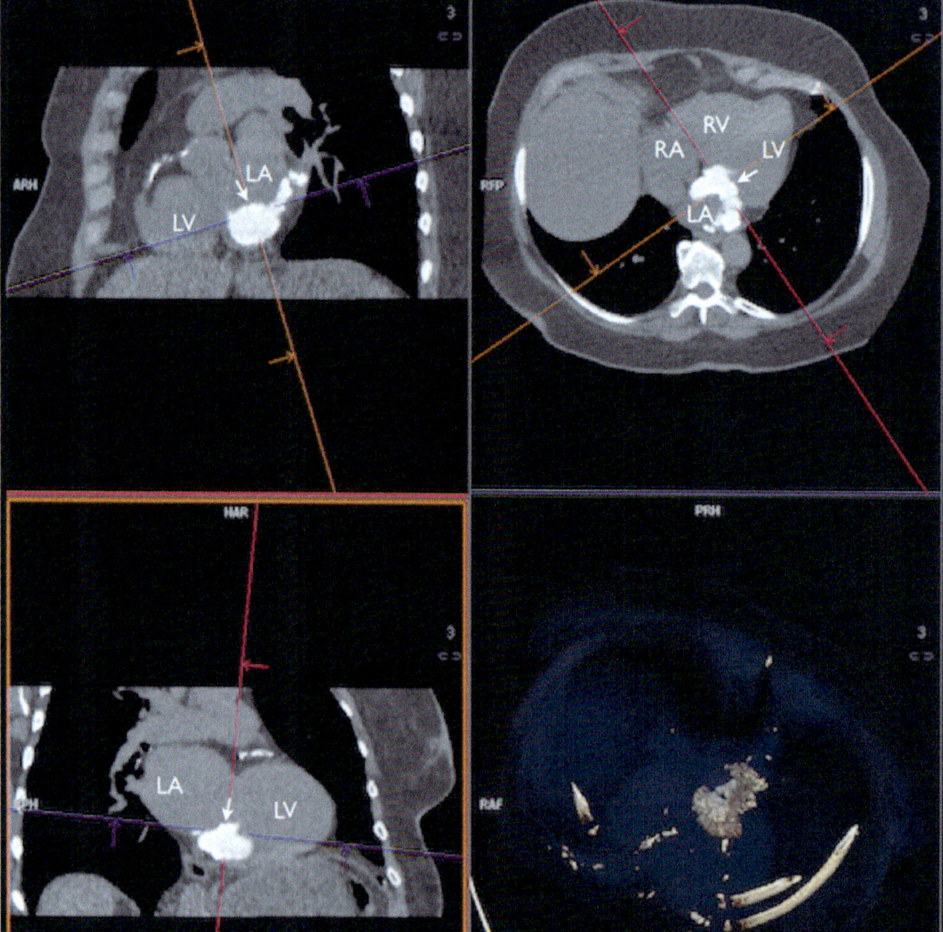

Fig. 3.7 3D CT reconstruction showing the extension of the mitral annular calcification mimicking a cardiac mass (*arrows*)

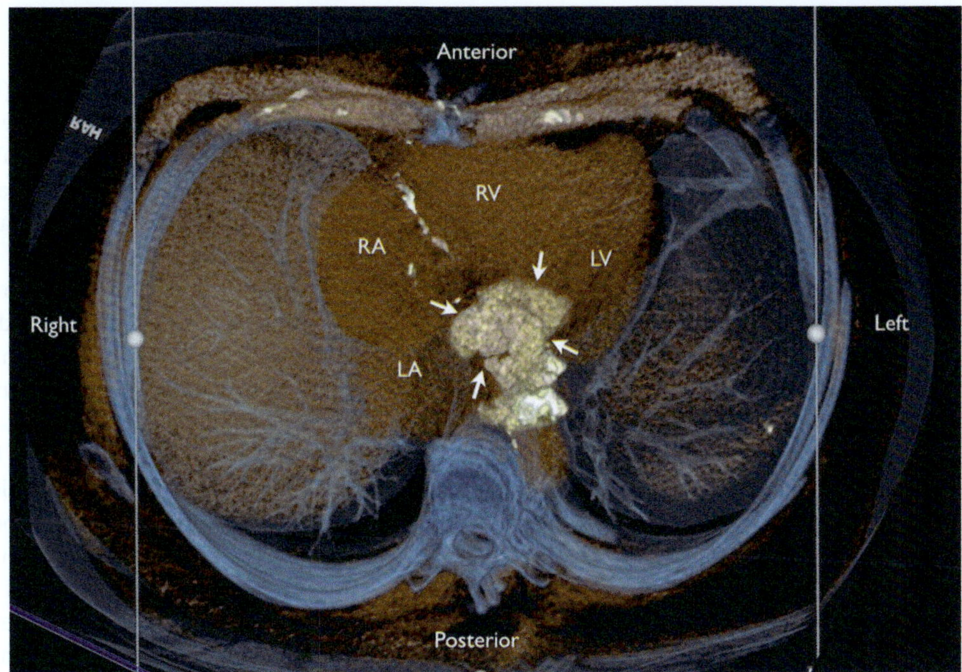

3.2 Case 2. Calcific Mitral Stenosis

A 55-year-old man with end-stage renal failure secondary to Alport's disease who is undergoing thrice-weekly hemodialysis reports increasing breathlessness with minimal exertion and palpitations. He was noted to have a murmur on auscultation (Figs. 3.8, 3.9, 3.10, 3.11, 3.12, 3.13, and 3.14).

Video 3.5 TTE, apical four- chamber view showed bright echodensities along the mitral annular plane involving both anterior and posterior aspects of the annulus, as well as calcified subvalvular apparatus

Video 3.6 TTE, apical four- chamber view with Doppler color flow imaging shows mild mitral regurgitation and turbulent flow across the mitral valve during diastole, consistent with mitral stenosis

Video 3.7 3D reconstruction of the mitral valve in short axis, demonstrating heavy leaflet and annular calcification, which restricts leaflet opening

3.2.1 Learning Points

Mitral annular calcification (MAC) occurs when calcium is deposited in the region between the posterior left ventricular wall and the posterior mitral leaflet [5]. Anterior involvement is less common but can be seen in advanced cases. Calcified aortic valve, papillary muscles, and chordae tendinae are frequent coexistent echocardiographic findings in patients with MAC. Key risk factors of MAC include advanced age, female sex, and end-stage renal disease. Mitral regurgitation is the most common form of valvular dysfunction from MAC because of impaired sphincter-like function of the mitral annulus and the posterior leaflet elevation from the calcium deposition at the base of the posterior leaflet [9]. Mitral stenosis (MS) is a less common complication of MAC. This form of MS can be differentiated from rheumatic MS by the absence of commissural fusion. The limiting orifice area of calcific MS is at the base of the mitral leaflets. These differences are well appreciated by real time three-dimensional echocardiography.

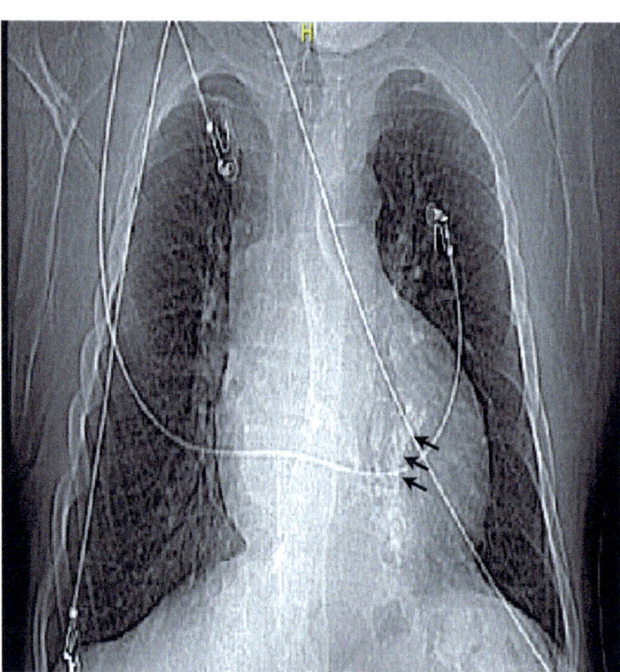

Fig. 3.8 Posteroanterior (PA) chest x-ray showed mitral annular calcification (*arrows*) and scoliotic curvature of the thoracolumbar spine, convex to the right

Fig. 3.9 TTE, apical four-chamber view showed bright echodensities along the mitral annular plane involving both anterior and posterior aspects of the annulus (*arrows*), as well as calcified subvalvular apparatus (*arrowhead*)

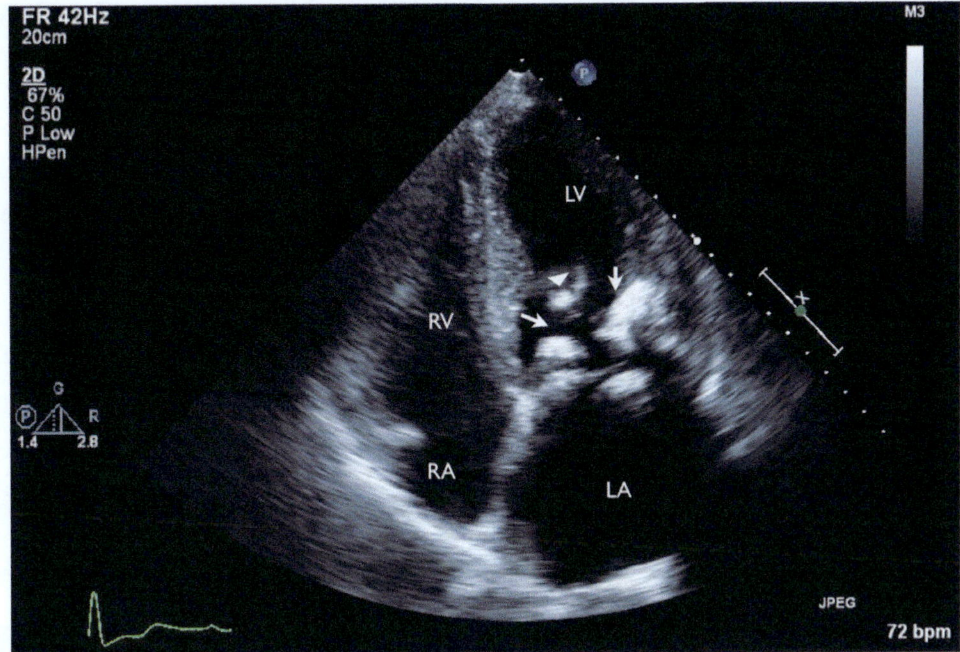

Fig. 3.10 TTE, apical four-chamber view with Doppler color flow imaging shows mild mitral regurgitation (*arrows*) and turbulent flow across the mitral valve during diastole, consistent with mitral stenosis

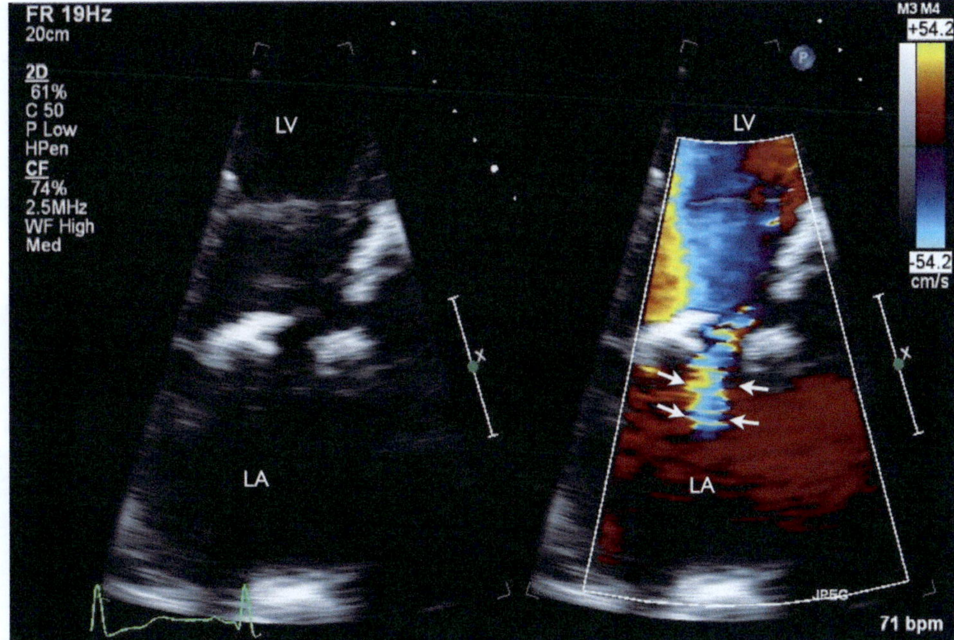

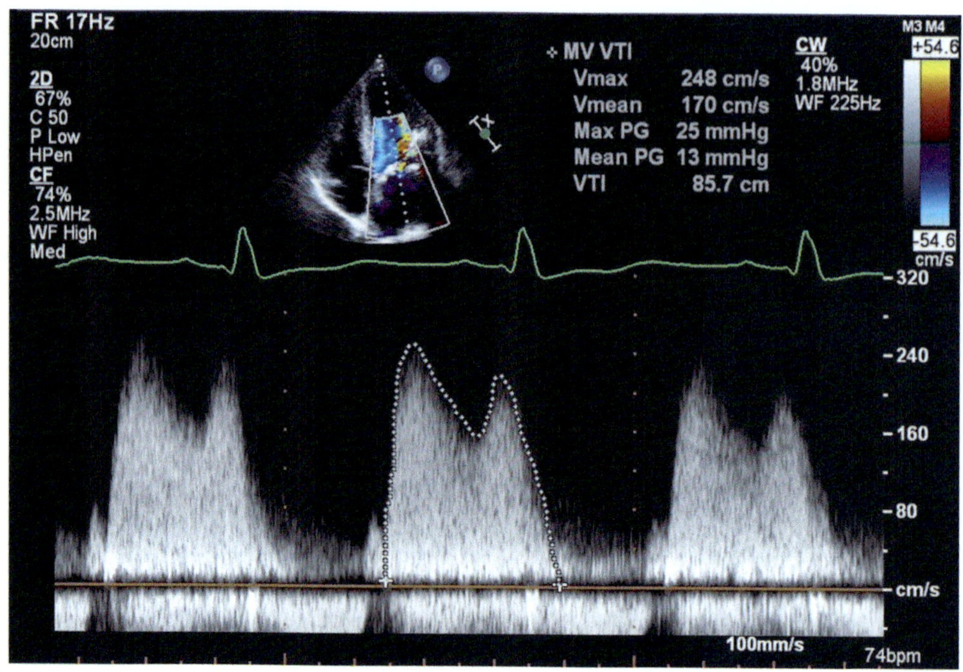

Fig. 3.11 Mitral inflow. Continuous-wave Doppler profile shows significant transmitral gradient (mean gradient 13 mmHg) consistent with severe mitral stenosis

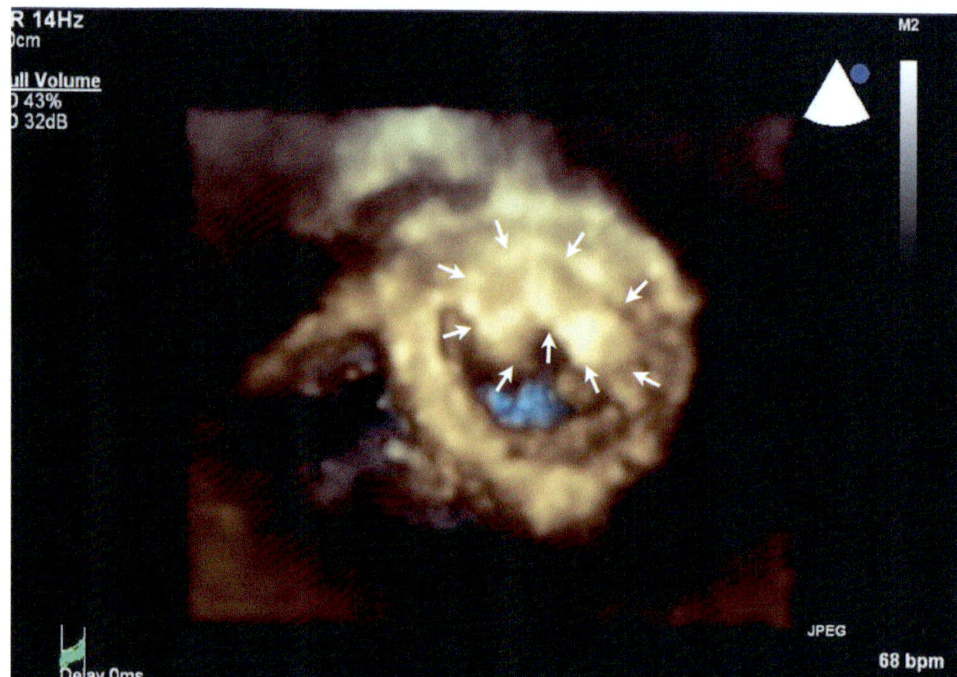

Fig. 3.12 3D reconstruction of the mitral valve in short axis, demonstrating heavy leaflet and annular calcification (*arrows*), which restricts leaflet opening

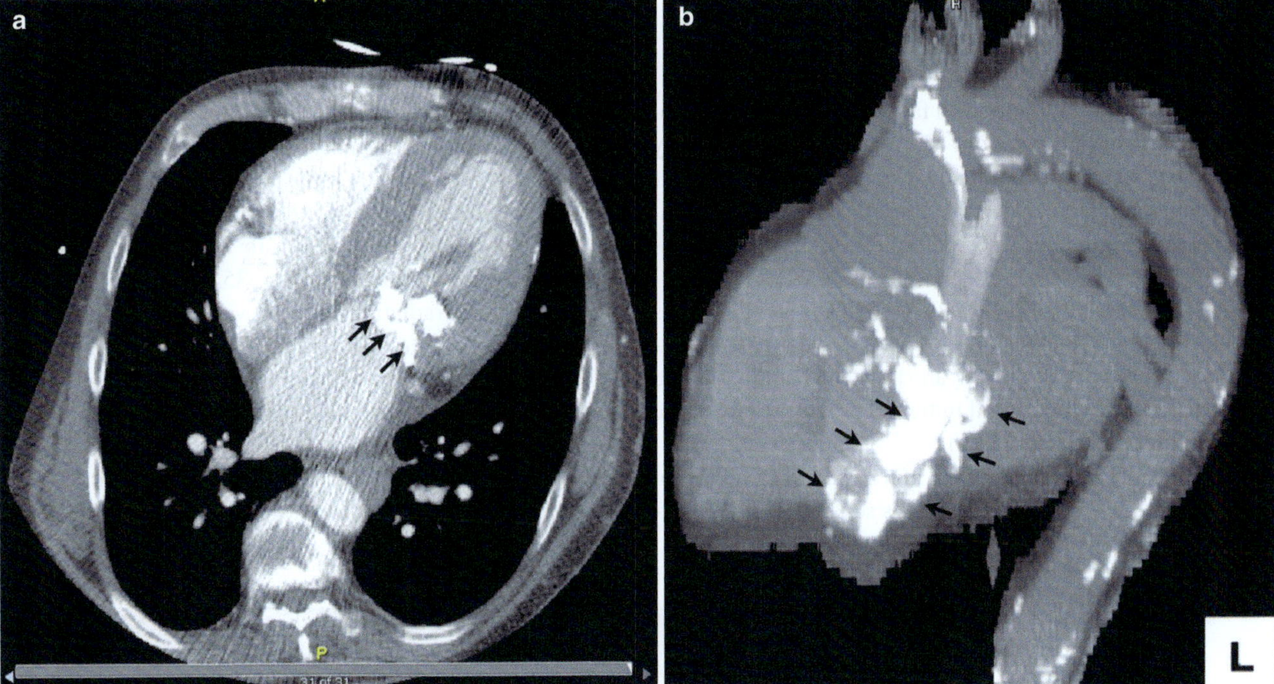

Fig. 3.13 Gated cardiac CT reconstructed in axial (**a**) and sagittal (**b**) orientations, shows almost circumferential mitral annular calcifications (*arrows*). There is particularly dense calcification in the lateral and inferior aspect of the annulus, with extension into the lateral myocardium. There is more dense wall calcification and less dense calcification in the central aspect, consistent with liquefied calcification

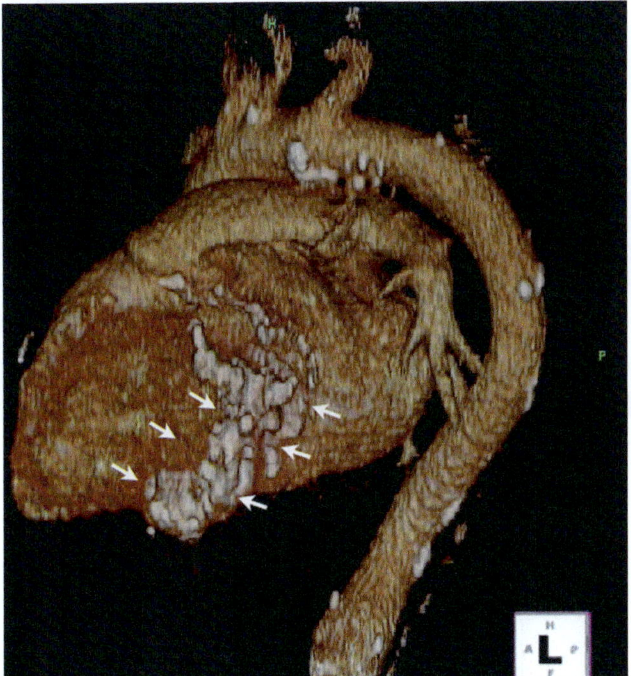

Fig. 3.14 3D reconstruction of the cardiac CT scans shows severe mitral annular calcification (*arrows*)

3.3   Case 3. Radiation-Associated Calcific Mitral Stenosis

A 53-year-old man presents with fatigue and an audible systolic murmur on auscultation. The patient was previously well except for Hodgkin's disease treated 30 years previously with chemotherapy and high-dose mediastinal radiation therapy (Figs. 3.15, 3.16, and 3.17).

Video 3.8 Parasternal long-axis view with simultaneous color Doppler imaging. Both mitral leaflets and mitral-aortic intervalvular fibrosa are thickened and calcified with moderate (2+) central mitral regurgitation and aortic regurgtitation (AVI 2172 kb)

Video 3.9 Biplane imaging of the mitral valve in parasternal and short-axis views (*right*), shows severe bileaflet thickening, with reduced leaflet excursion (AVI 3105 kb)

3.3.1   Learning Points

As the survival of patients with cancer has improved with advanced treatment, radiation heart disease is increasingly recognized. Thoracic malignancies that are commonly treated with radiation therapy include Hodgkin's disease and breast cancer. Autopsy studies have found the prevalence of valve fibrosis to be up to 80 % in patients who received chest radiation exceeding 35 Gy [9, 10], but clinically significant radiation-induced valve disease is present in only 6–15 % of treated patients [11]. Hallmark features of radiation-induced mitral stenosis include severe mitral annular calcification and thickening and calcification of the aorto-mitral curtain that extends along the anterior leaflet. In some cases, the posterior leaflet remains mobile, differentiating this entity from degenerative calcific mitral stenosis.

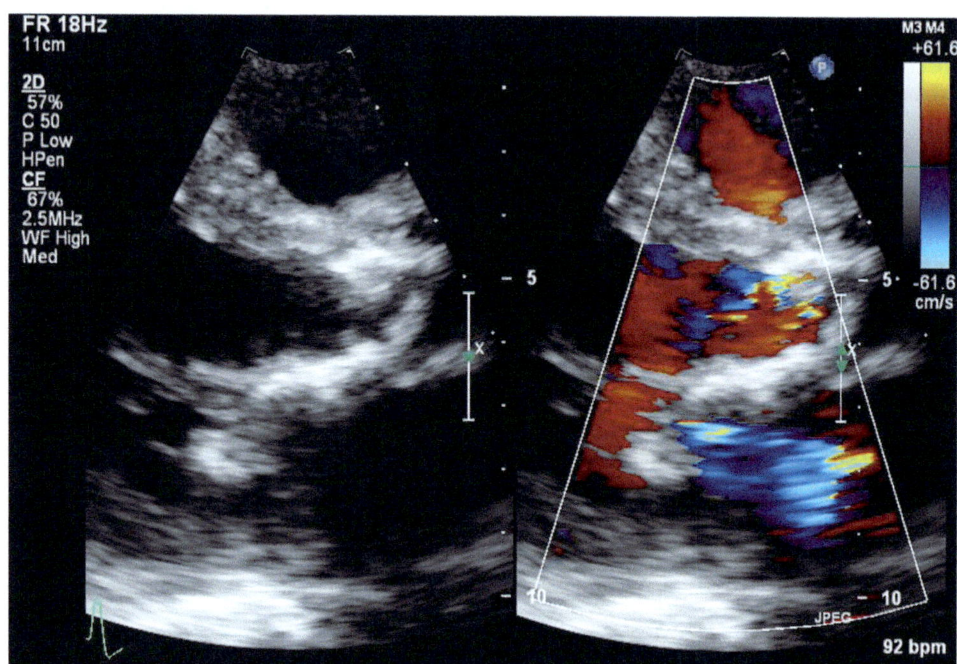

Fig. 3.15 Parasternal long-axis view 2D and with simultaneous color Doppler imaging. Both mitral leaflets are heavily thickened and calcified with moderate (2+) central mitral regurgitation. Mild mitral stenosis (mean gradient, 6 mmHg). The aortic also appears thickened with restriction of leaflet excursion

Fig. 3.16 Biplane imaging of the mitral valve in parasternal (*left*) and short-axis views (*right*), shows severe bileaflet thickening, with reduced leaflet excursion

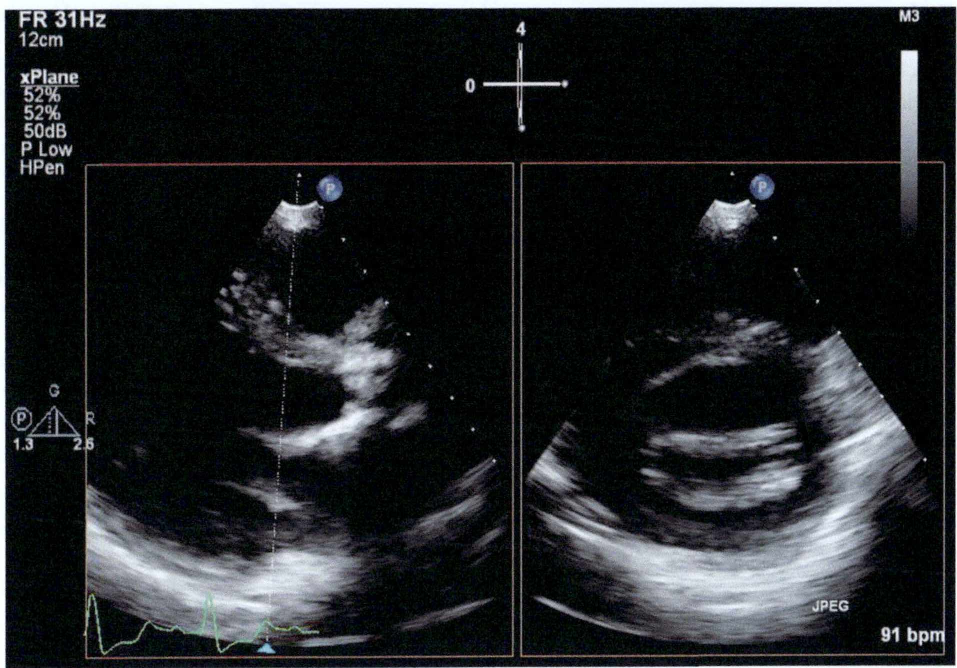

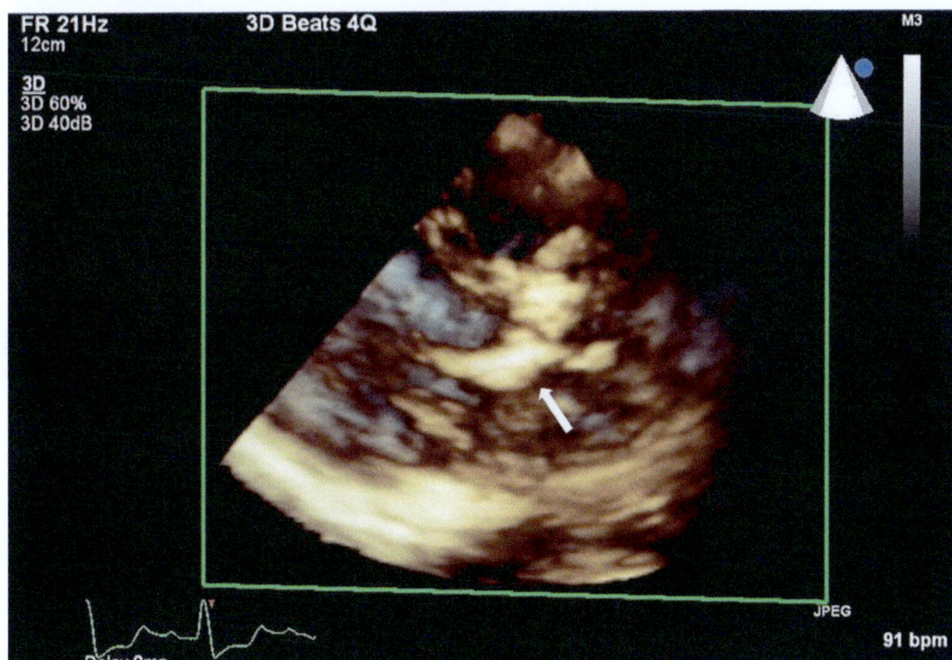

Fig. 3.17 Full-volume 3D reconstruction of the thickened mitral valve, aortic valve and aorto-mitral curtain (*arrow*) from a parasternal long-axis view

References

1. Marcu CB, Ghantous AE, Prokop EK. Caseous calcification of the mitral valve ring. Heart Lung Circ. 2006;15:187–8.
2. Chahal M, Temesy-Armos P, Stewart WJ. Big MAC: caseous calcification of the mitral annulus referred for possible cardiac tumor. Echocardiography. 2011;28:E76–8.
3. Deluca G, Correale M, Ieva R, Del Salvatore B, Gramenzi S, Di Biase M. The incidence and clinical course of caseous calcification of the mitral annulus: a prospective echocardiographic study. J Am Soc Echocardiogr. 2008;21:828–33.
4. Silbiger JJ. Anatomy, mechanics, and pathophysiology of the mitral annulus. Am Heart J. 2012;164:163–76.
5. Harpaz D, Auerbach I, Vered Z, Motro M, Tobar A, Rosenblatt S. Caseous calcification of the mitral annulus: a neglected, unrecognized diagnosis. J Am Soc Echocardiogr. 2001;14:825–31.
6. Pozsonyi Z, Toth A, Vago H, Adam Z, Apor A, Alotti N, et al. Severe mitral regurgitation and heart failure due to caseous calcification of the mitral annulus. Cardiology. 2011;118:79–82.
7. Teja K, Gibson RS, Nolan SP. Atrial extension of mitral annular calcification mimicking intracardiac tumor. Clin Cardiol. 1987;10:546–8.
8. Isotalo PA, Walley VM. Coronary artery erosion and dissection: an unusual complication of mitral annular calcification. Cardiovasc Pathol. 1999;8:141–4.
9. Payvandi LA, Rigolin VH. Calcific mitral stenosis. Cardiol Clin. 2013;31:193–202.
10. Adams MJ, Hardenbergh PH, Constine LS, Lipshultz SE. Radiation-associated cardiovascular disease. Crit Rev Oncol Hematol. 2003;45:55–75.
11. Hull MC, Morris CG, Pepine CJ, Mendenhall NP. Valvular dysfunction and carotid, subclavian, and coronary artery disease in survivors of Hodgkin lymphoma treated with radiation therapy. JAMA. 2003;290:2831–7.

Christine Jellis

4.1 Case 1. Posterior Leaflet Mitral Valve Prolapse

A 62-year-old man presented with a prominent systolic murmur and exertional dyspnea for several years. He also reported intermittent palpitations suggestive of paroxysmal atrial fibrillation. He was found to have posterior mitral valve leaflet prolapse with severe mitral regurgitation and underwent mitral valve repair (Figs. 4.1, 4.2, and 4.3).

Video 4.1 Transesophageal 3D reconstruction of the mitral valve demonstrating prolapse of the middle and lateral posterior leaflet scallops (P1 & P2) (AVI 950 kb)

Video 4.2 Transesophageal echo biplane (0 and 90°) view of the mitral valve demonstrating prolapse of P2 & P2 (AVI 5627 kb)

Video 4.3 The same views with color Doppler, demonstrating eccentric, anteriorly directed mitral regurgitation, which was classified as 3–4+ (AVI 1477 kb)

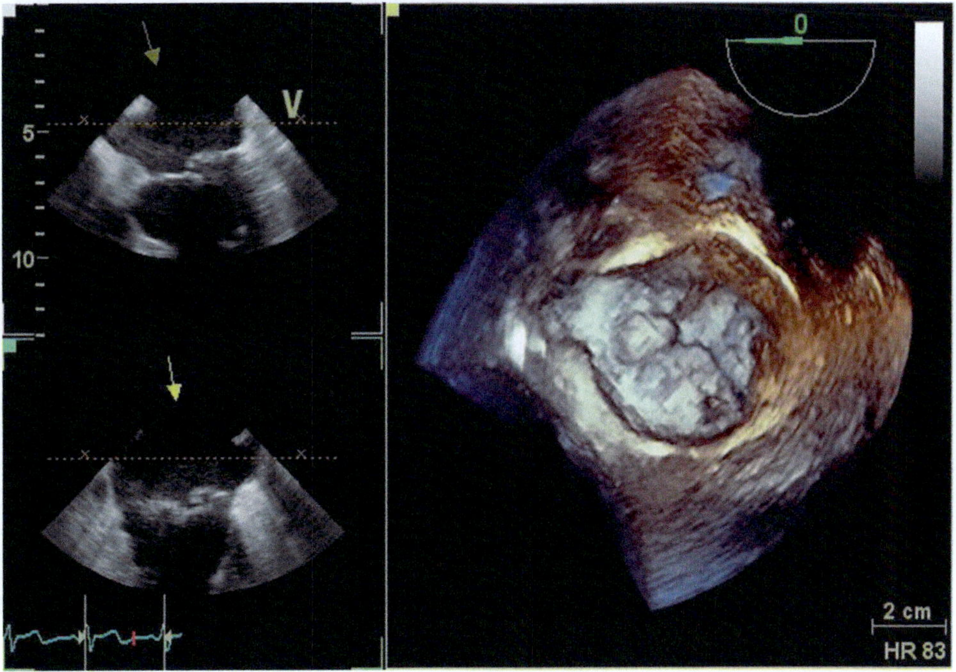

Fig. 4.1 Transesophageal 3D reconstruction of the mitral valve demonstrating prolapse of the middle and lateral posterior leaflet scallops (P1 & P2)

Electronic supplementary material The online version of this chapter (doi:10.1007/978-1-4471-6672-6_4) contains supplementary material, which is available to authorized users.

C. Jellis
Department of Cardiovascular Medicine, Cleveland Clinic, 9500 Euclid Avenue, Cleveland, OH 44195, USA
e-mail: jellisc@ccf.org

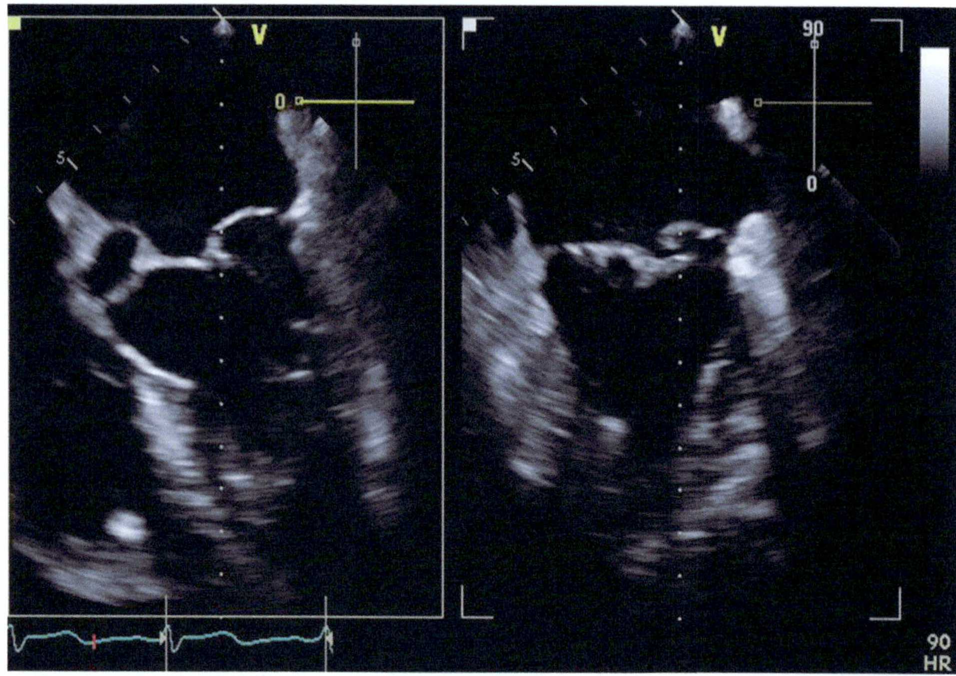

Fig. 4.2 Transesophageal echo biplane (0 and 90°) view of the mitral valve demonstrating prolapse of P2 & P2

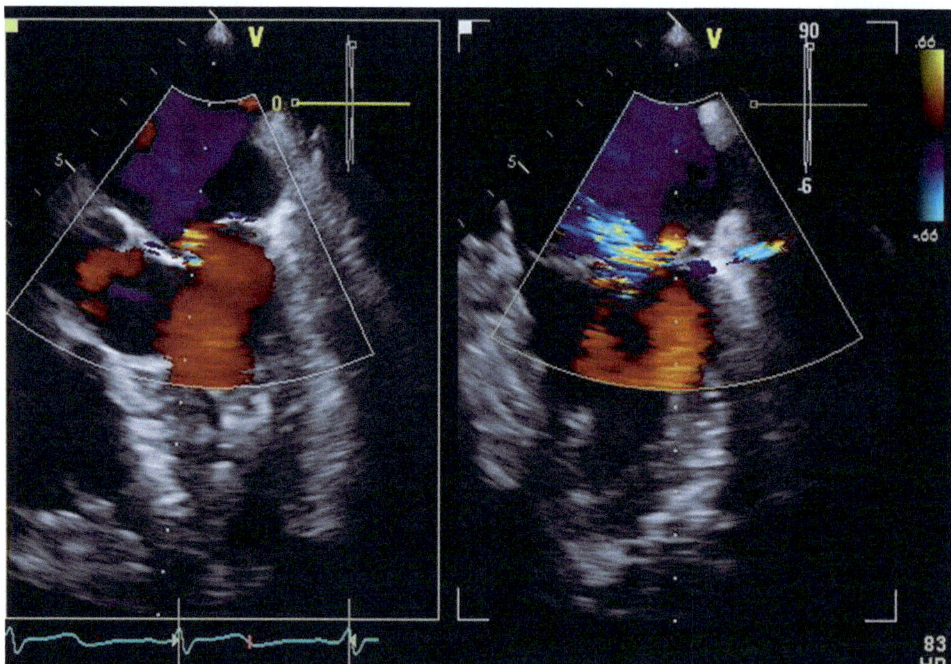

Fig. 4.3 The same views with color Doppler, demonstrating eccentric, anteriorly directed mitral regurgitation (MR), which was classified as 3–4+. Regurgitation can be difficult to quantitate on one view because of the eccentricity of the jet

4.2 Case 2. Mitral Valve Posterior Leaflet Flail

A 74-year-old man presented with increasing fatigue on a background history of inferior wall myocardial infarction, which had been medically managed 15 years earlier. Echocardiogram revealed a flail posterior mitral valve leaflet with severe mitral regurgitation and moderately elevated pulmonary pressures. He was referred for a mitral valve repair and a bypass graft to the right coronary artery (Figs. 4.4, 4.5, 4.6, 4.7, 4.8, and 4.9).

Video 4.4 Transesophageal 120° view confirms flail involving the middle posterior leaflet scallop (P2) (AVI 7312 kb)

Video 4.5 Transesophageal 120° view, zooming up on the flail middle posterior leaflet scallop (P2) (AVI 6013 kb)

Video 4.6 Color Doppler (transesophageal 120° view) demonstrating severe, anteriorly directed MR. Note wide vena contracta; proximal isovelocity surface area (PISA) measurements likely underestimate severity of MR owing to jet eccentricity (AVI 1247 kb)

Video 4.7 Three-dimensional (3D) reconstruction of the mitral valve demonstrating the flail middle posterior leaflet scallop (P2) (AVI 1144 kb)

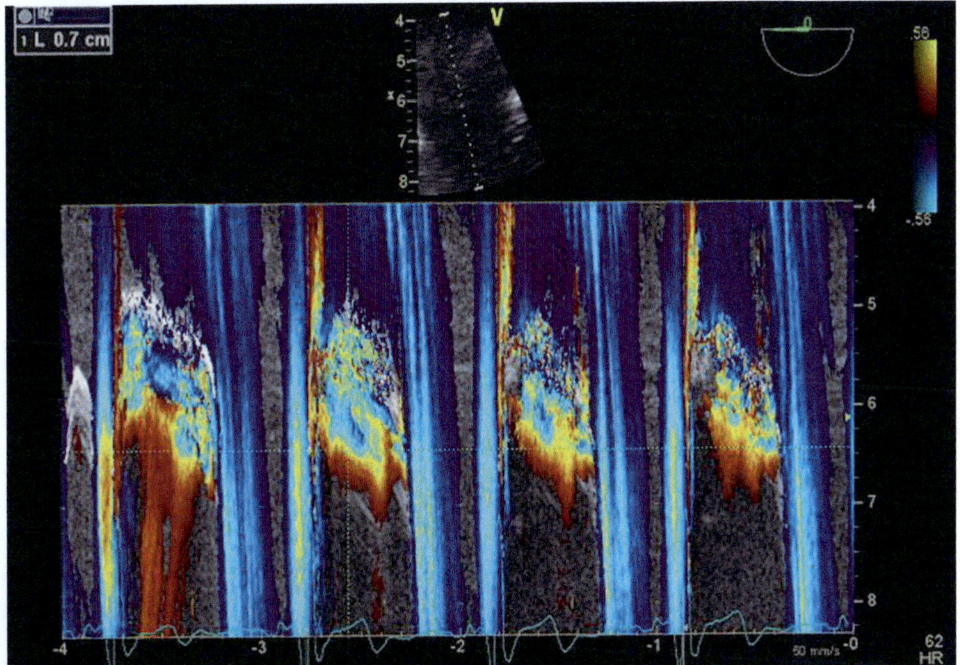

Fig. 4.4 Color M-mode through the mitral valve, demonstrating predominantly early-systolic and late-systolic MR

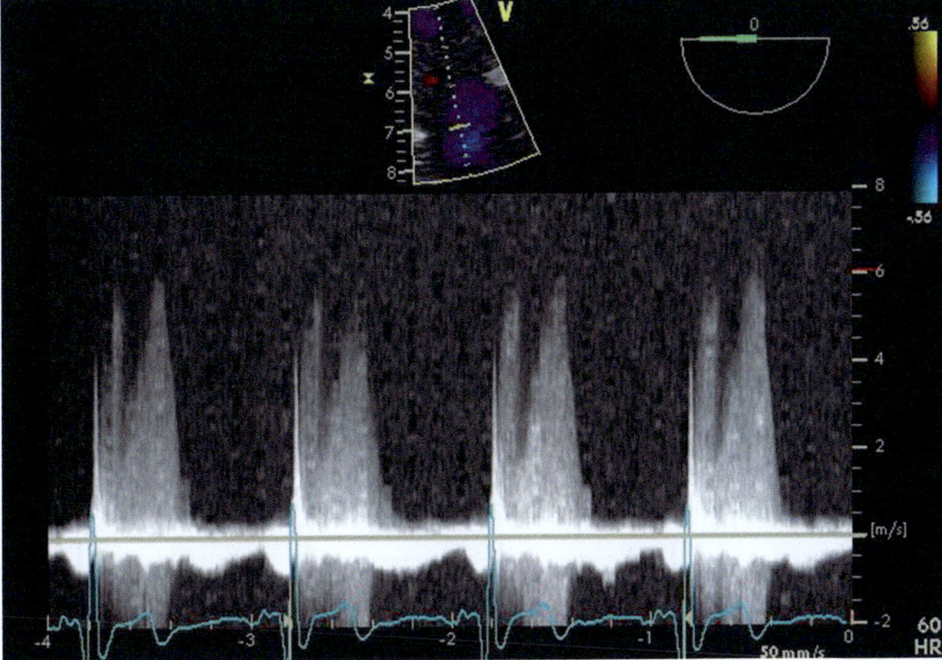

Fig. 4.5 Continuous-wave Doppler through the mitral valve, demonstrating predominantly early-systolic and late-systolic MR

Fig. 4.6 Transesophageal 120°
view confirms flail involving
the middle posterior leaflet
scallop (P2)

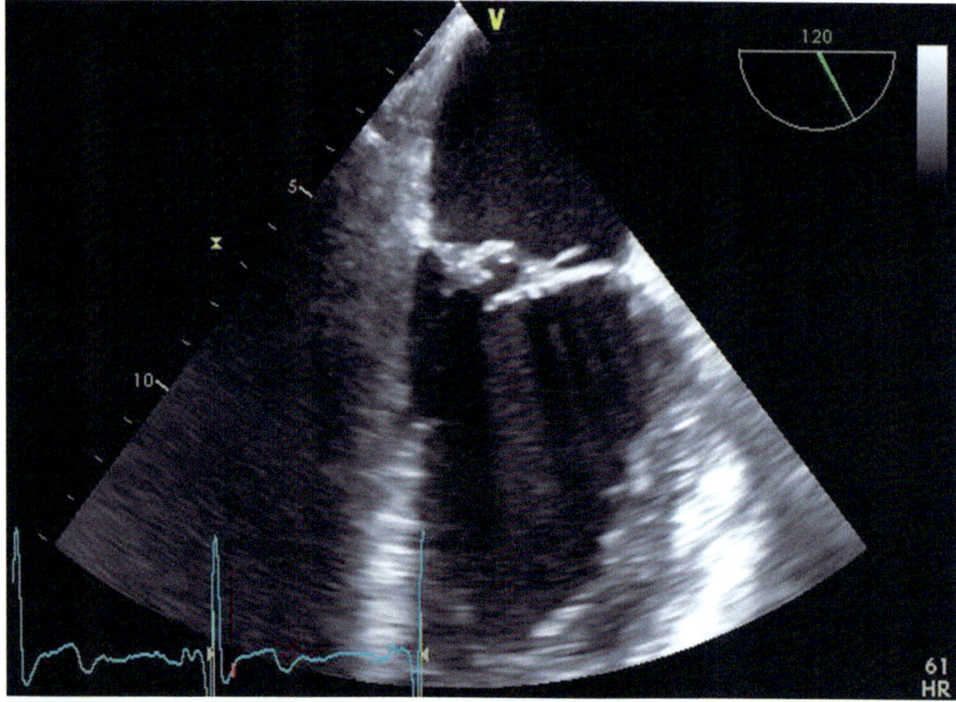

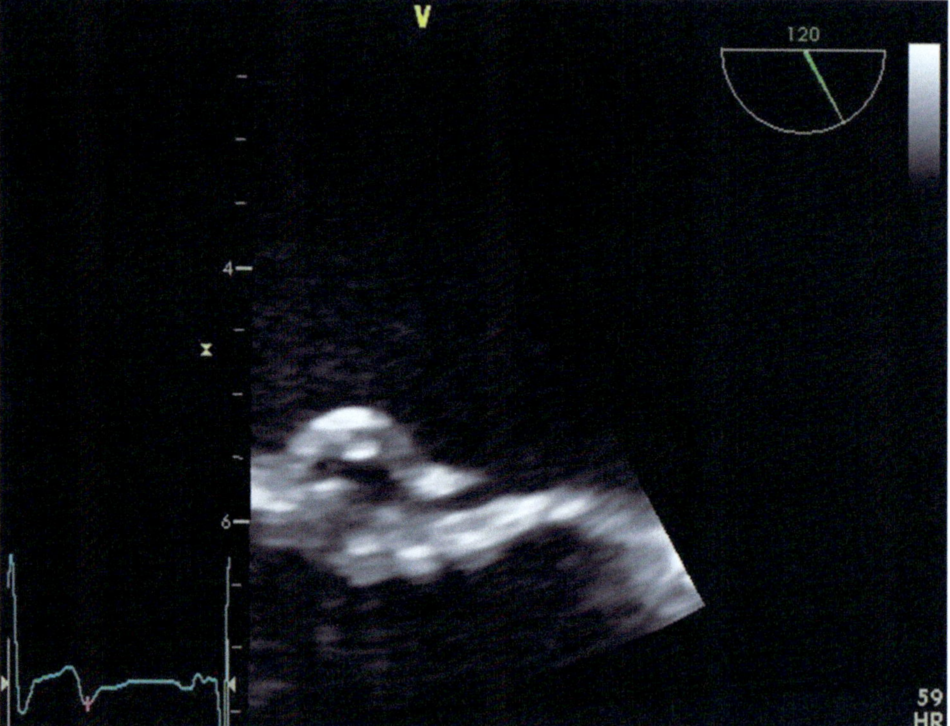

Fig. 4.7 Transesophageal 120°
view, zooming up on the flail
middle posterior leaflet scallop (P2)

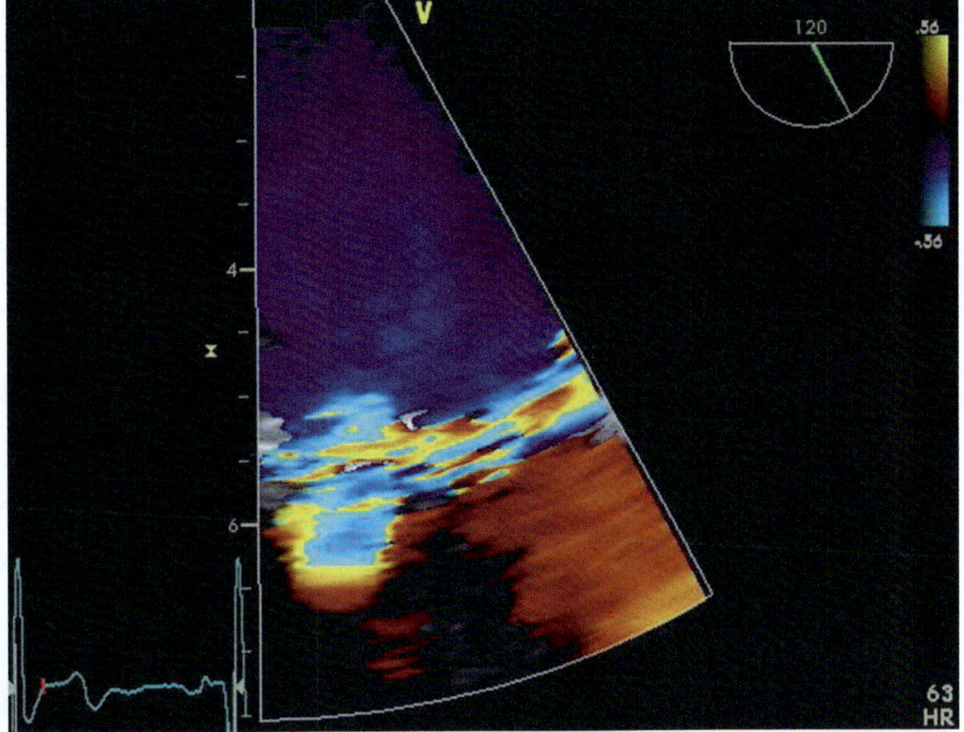

Fig. 4.8 Color Doppler (transesophageal 120° view) demonstrating severe, anteriorly directed MR. Note wide vena contracta; proximal isovelocity surface area (PISA) measurements likely underestimate severity of MR owing to jet eccentricity

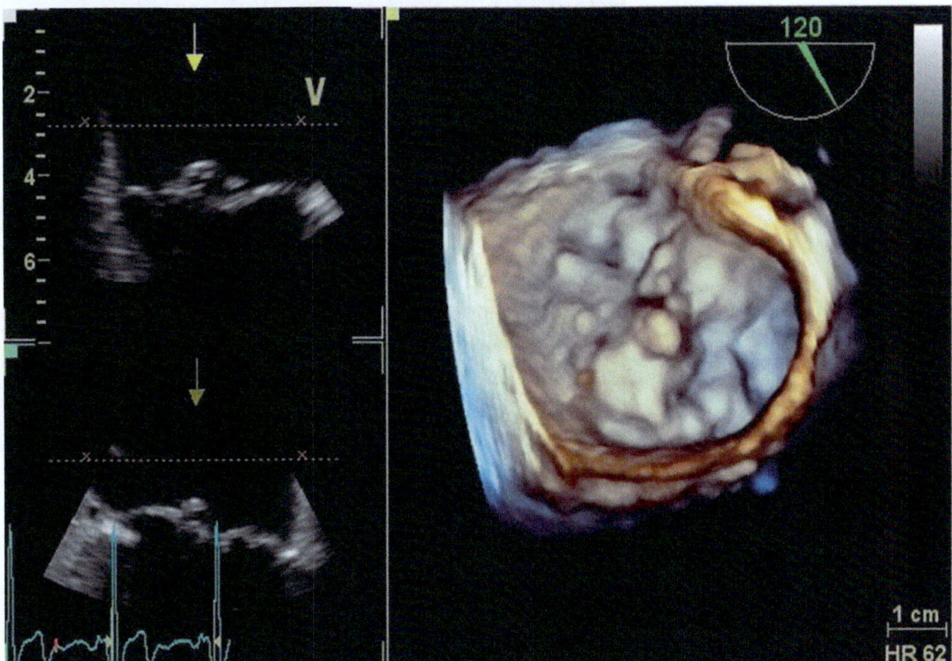

Fig. 4.9 Three-dimensional (3D) reconstruction of the mitral valve demonstrating the flail middle posterior leaflet scallop (P2)

4.3 Case 3. Posterior Mitral Valve Leaflet Prolapse After Previous Mitral Valve Repair

A 46-year-old male physician presented for surgical evaluation of mitral regurgitation (Carpentier type 2, severe mitral regurgitation secondary to posterior leaflet prolapse), on a background history of previous mitral valve repair several years earlier. He had remained essentially asymptomatic, but serial monitoring via echocardiography revealed an increasing effective regurgitant orifice area of 0.94 cm^2, regurgitant volume of 124 mL, severely dilated left and increasing pulmonary pressures (estimated right ventricular systolic pressure of 51 mmHg) (Figs. 4.10, 4.11, 4.12, and 4.13).

Video 4.8 Parasternal long-axis view in two-dimensional (2D) and color Doppler imaging demonstrating posterior leaflet prolapse with eccentric, anteriorly directed mitral regurgitation (AVI 2643 kb)

Video 4.9 Apical long-axis view demonstrating that the anterior mitral valve regurgitation is severe (AVI 3332 kb)

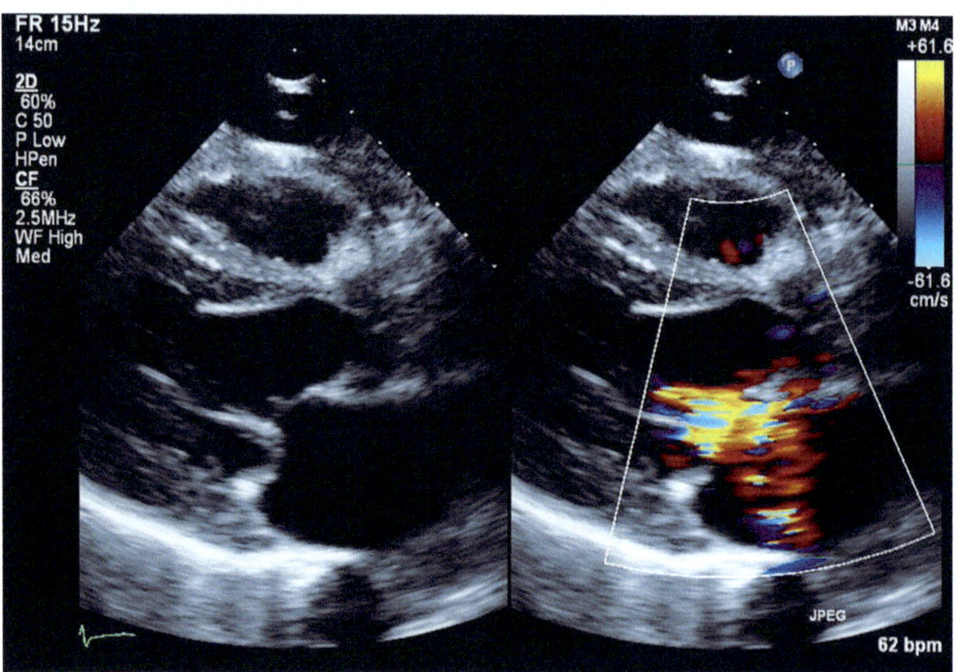

Fig. 4.10 Parasternal long-axis view in two-dimensional (2D) and color Doppler imaging demonstrating posterior leaflet prolapse with eccentric, anteriorly directed mitral regurgitation

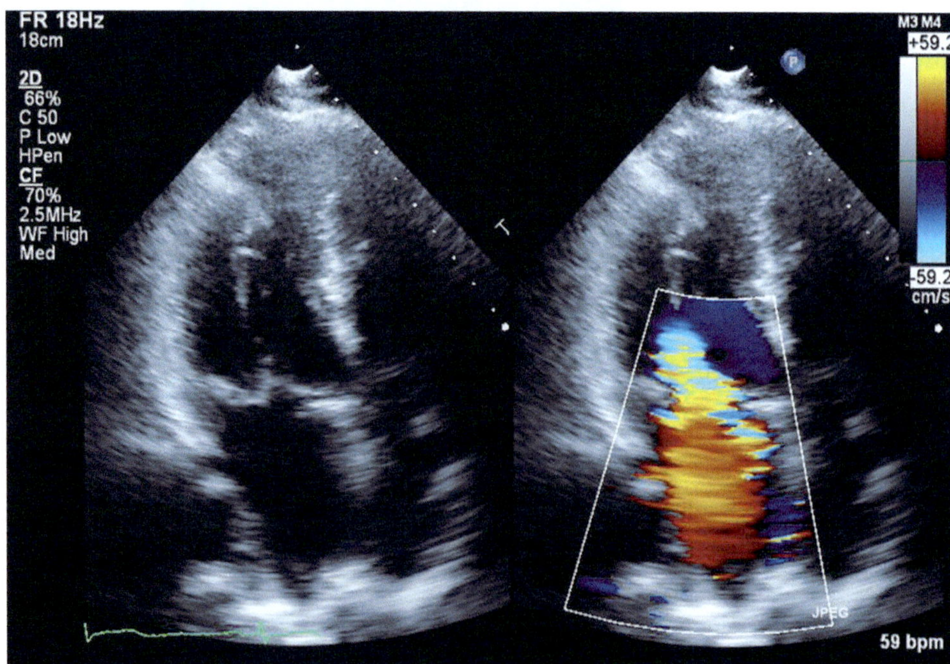

Fig. 4.11 Apical long-axis view demonstrating that the anterior mitral valve regurgitation is severe

Fig. 4.12 Continuous wave Doppler demonstrates the mitral regurgitant jet. Note the jet density and holosystolic profile, which supports the conclusion that the regurgitation is severe. The peak jet velocity may be underestimated because of the jet's eccentric nature; it is difficult to ensure that the transducer beam is parallel to the regurgitant jet

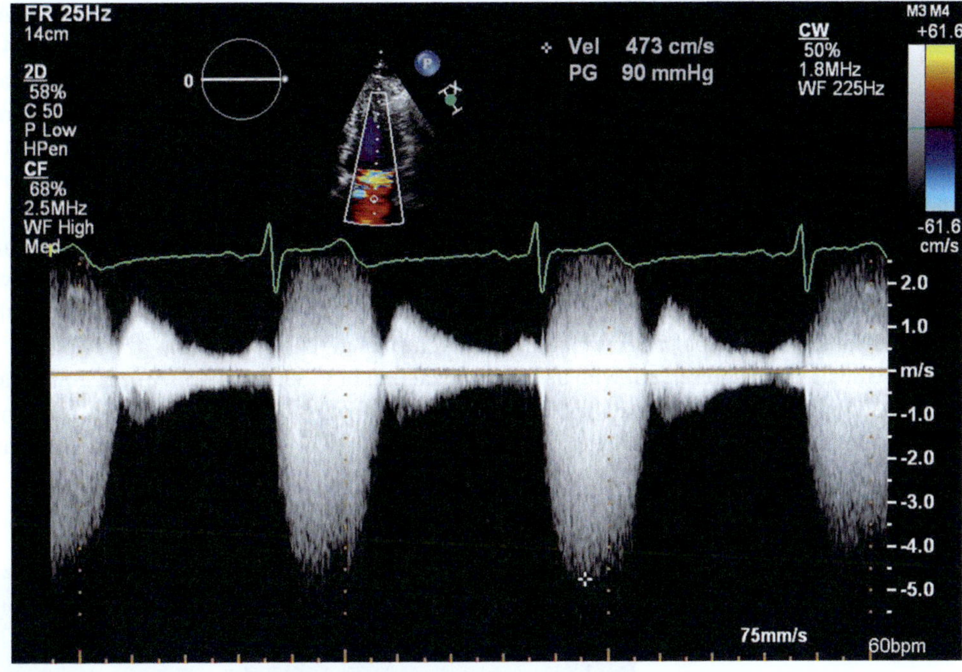

Fig. 4.13 From a PISA diameter of 1.27 cm, a mitral valve V_{max} of 473 cm/s, and an aliasing velocity of 61.6 cm/s (*see* Fig. 4.12), the estimated regurgitant orifice area is 1.3 cm^2, which is classified as severe

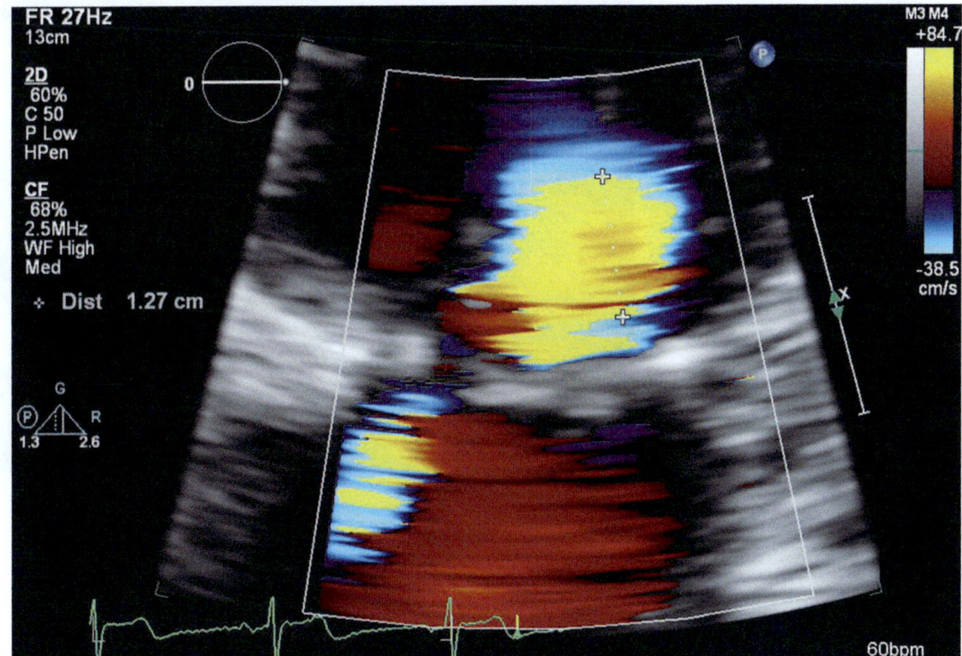

4.4   Case 4. Bileaflet Mitral Valve Prolapse and Flail

A 62-year-old man with known myxomatous mitral valve degeneration and secondary mitral insufficiency presented for consideration of minimally invasive mitral valve surgery. He had a longstanding history of heart murmur. Echocardiographic findings included severe mitral insufficiency, with an estimated regurgitant orifice area of 1.28 cm^2, mild pulmonary hypertension, and left ventricular dilatation (end-diastolic dimension of 5.9 cm), but his left ventricular systolic function was preserved, with an ejection fraction of 64 %. Although he was asymptomatic, his echocardiographic findings supported a recommendation for mitral valve surgery because of the regurgitation severity and the likelihood of a successful repair (AHA/ACC Class IIa) (Figs. 4.14, 4.15, 4.16, 4.17, 4.18, 4.19, 4.20, and 4.21).

Video 4.10 Parasternal long-axis imaging of the mitral valve demonstrates bileaflet mitral valve prolapse (AVI 7394 kb)

Video 4.11 Comparison with color Doppler imaging reveals severe central and anteriorly directed mitral regurgitation (AVI 2987 kb)

Video 4.12 Zooming in on imaging of the mitral valve in a parasternal long-axis view demonstrates anterior mitral valve leaflet prolapse with a flail posterior leaflet (AVI 10733 kb)

Video 4.13 Apical four-chamber 2D and color Doppler imaging demonstrates the posterior leaflet flail with severe, highly eccentric, anteriorly directed mitral regurgitation (AVI 3441 kb)

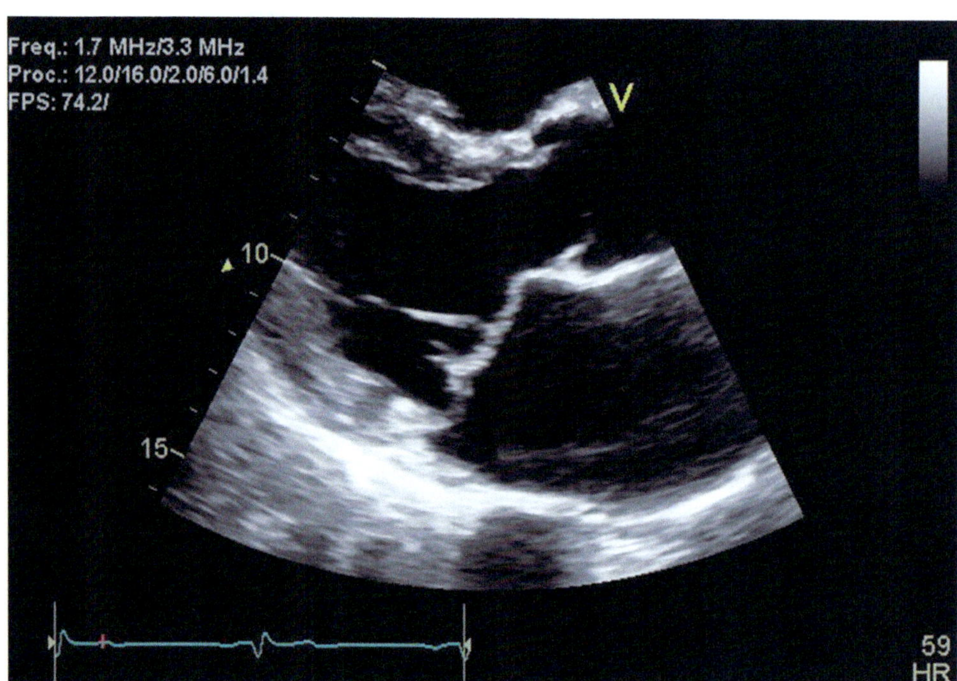

Fig. 4.14 Parasternal long-axis imaging of the mitral valve demonstrates bileaflet mitral valve prolapse

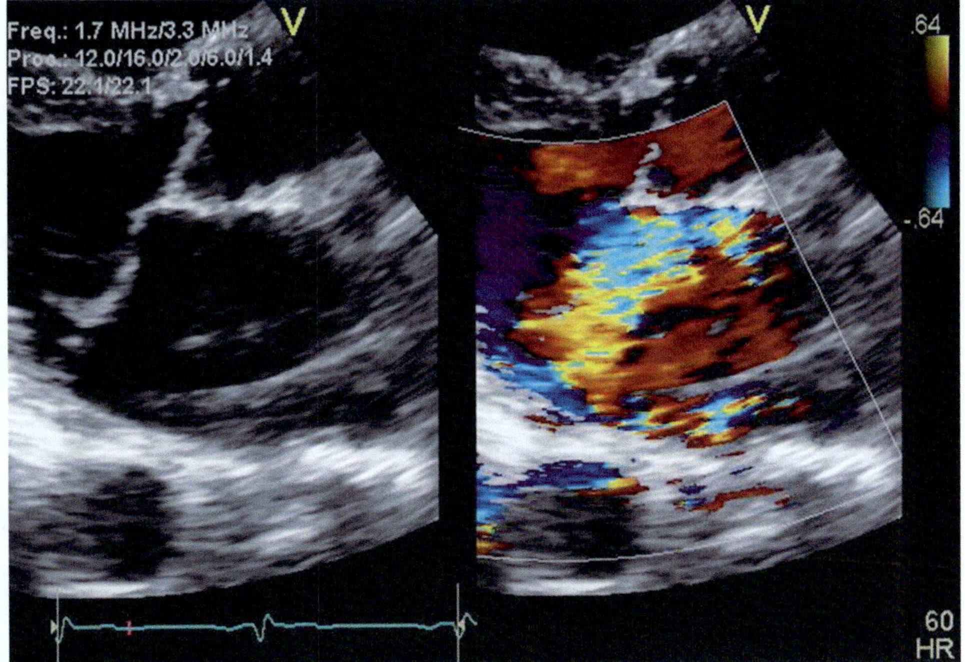

Fig. 4.15 Comparison with color Doppler imaging reveals severe central and anteriorly directed mitral regurgitation

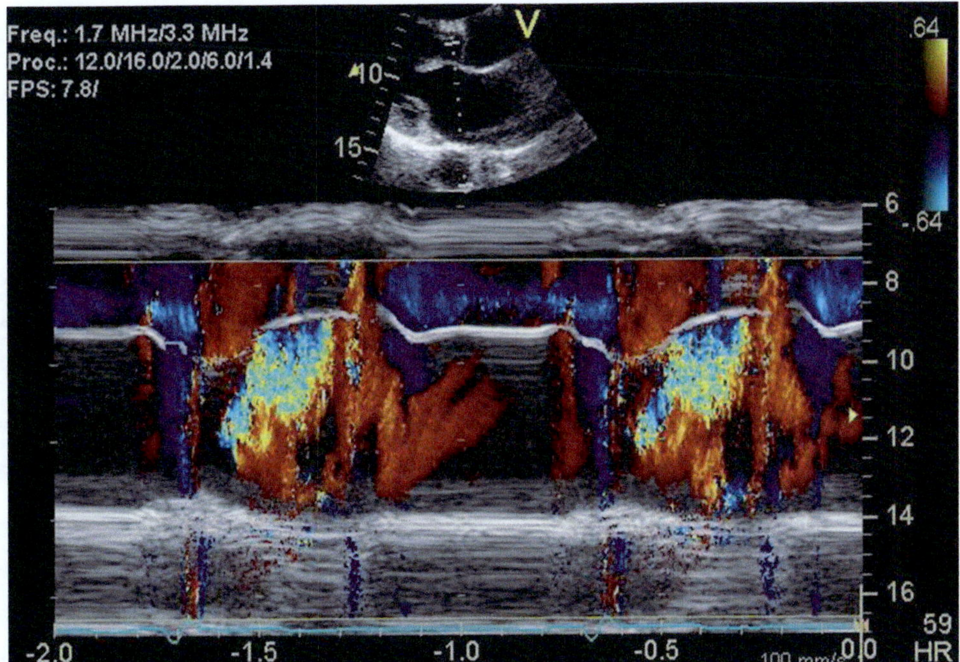

Fig. 4.16 Color M-mode reveals midsystolic mitral regurgitation consistent with prolapse

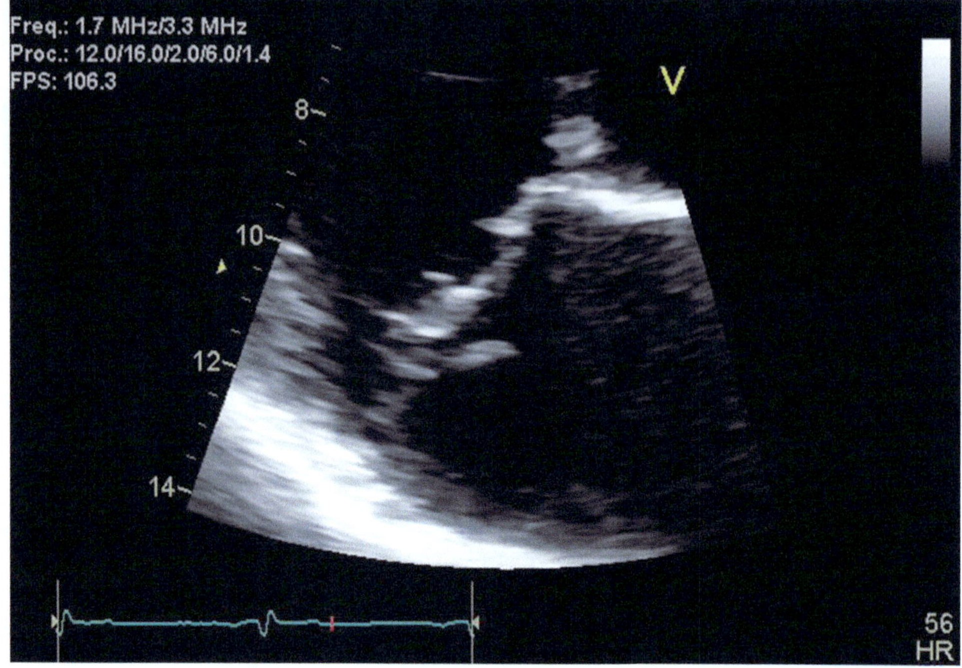

Fig. 4.17 Zooming in on imaging of the mitral valve in a parasternal long-axis view demonstrates anterior mitral valve leaflet prolapse with a flail posterior leaflet

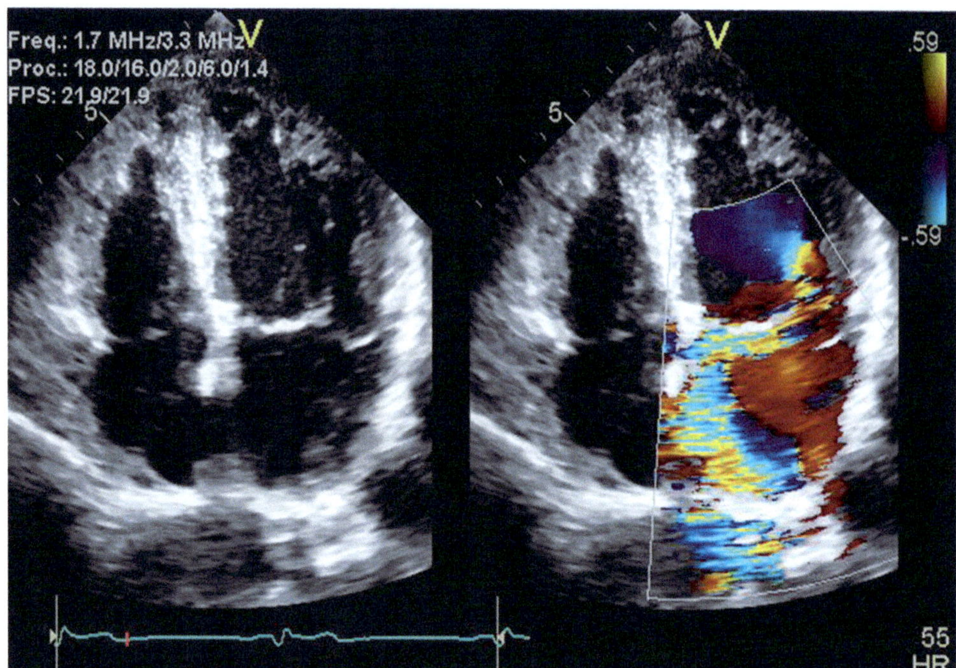

Fig. 4.18 Apical four-chamber 2D and color Doppler imaging demonstrates the posterior leaflet flail with severe, highly eccentric, anteriorly directed mitral regurgitation

Fig. 4.19 Pulse-wave spectral Doppler of pulmonary venous flow demonstrates systolic flow reversal consistent with severe mitral regurgitation

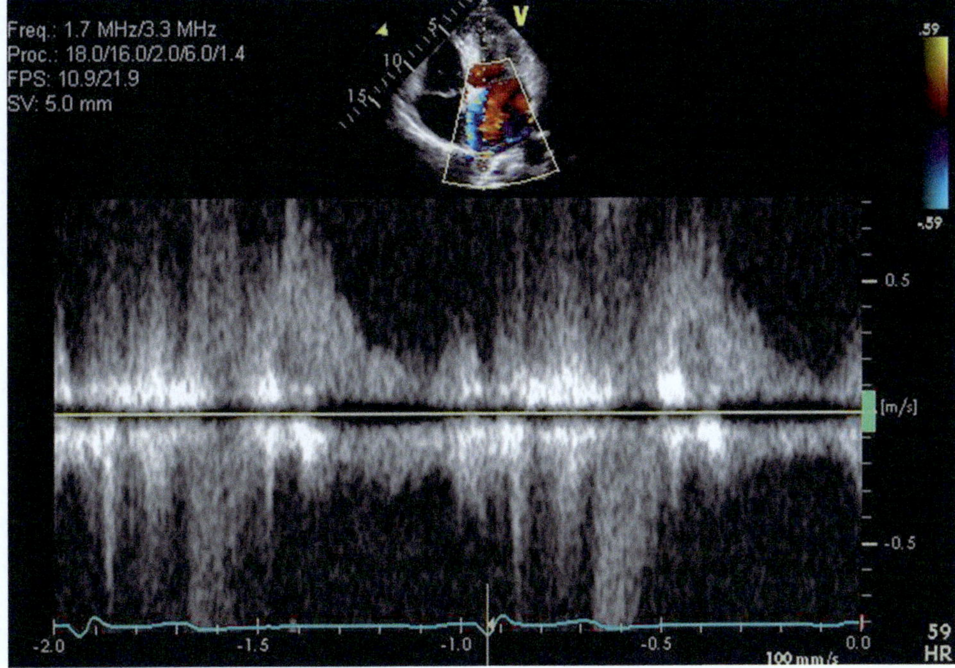

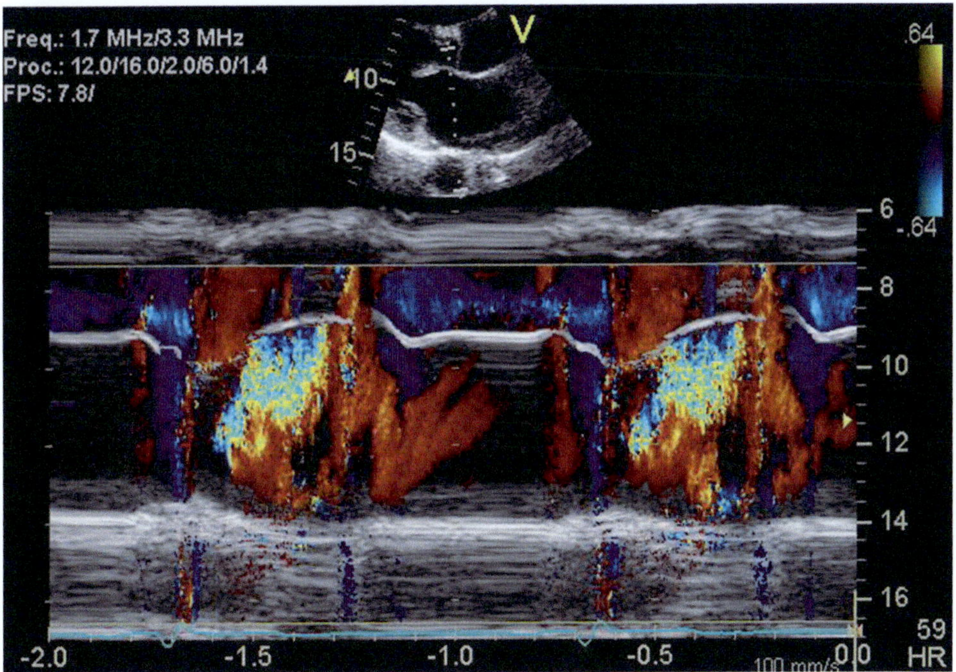

Fig. 4.20 Color M-mode in the left atrium demonstrates an anteriorly directed jet in mid to late systole

Fig. 4.21 Continuous wave Doppler trace through the mitral valve demonstrates flow predominantly in mid to late systole. The trace profile is limited by the eccentricity of the regurgitant jet

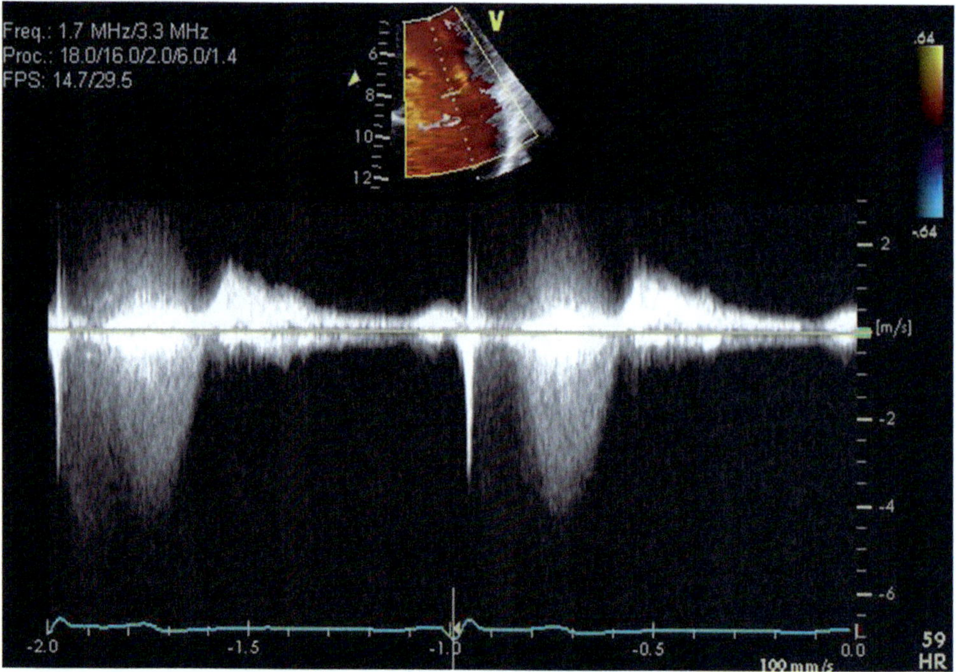

4.5   Case 5. Myxoid Degeneration in Barlow's Disease

A 78-year-old woman presented with chest pain, orthopnea, and peripheral edema. A non-ST elevation myocardial infarction was diagnosed based upon biomarker and EKG findings. She was noted to have severe mitral regurgitation associated with significant myxoid degeneration of both mitral valve leaflets. She was treated with a bioprosthetic mitral valve replacement and a saphenous vein bypass graft to the posterior descending artery, with resolution of symptoms.

Video 4.14 Transthoracic parasternal long-axis view demonstrating thickened and elongated mitral valve leaflets consistent with myxoid degeneration. There is bileaflet prolapse, with the bodies of the distended leaflet segments billowing beyond the plane of the annulus (posterior greater than anterior). The mitral annulus appears dilated. No calcification is noted (AVI 12935 kb)

Video 4.15 Apical two-chamber transthoracic view demonstrating prominent prolapse of the medial posterior leaflet (P3) with resultant anteriorly directed mitral regurgitation (AVI 2231 kb)

Video 4.16 Transesophageal 0° view of the mitral valve, demonstrating severe bileaflet prolapse (A2 and P2). The billowing medial scallop of the posterior leaflet (P3) is intermittently visible (AVI 8452 kb)

Video 4.17 Transesophageal 0° view of the mitral valve, demonstrating significant turbulence of transvalvular flow associated with the posterior leaflet. The jet of mitral regurgitation is not well appreciated because of its eccentric, anteriorly directed trajectory (AVI 2148 kb)

Video 4.18 Transesophageal 30° view of the mitral valve rotated medially to demonstrate prolapse and flail of the P3 scallop with severe, anteriorly directed mitral regurgitation on color Doppler imaging (AVI 2265 kb)

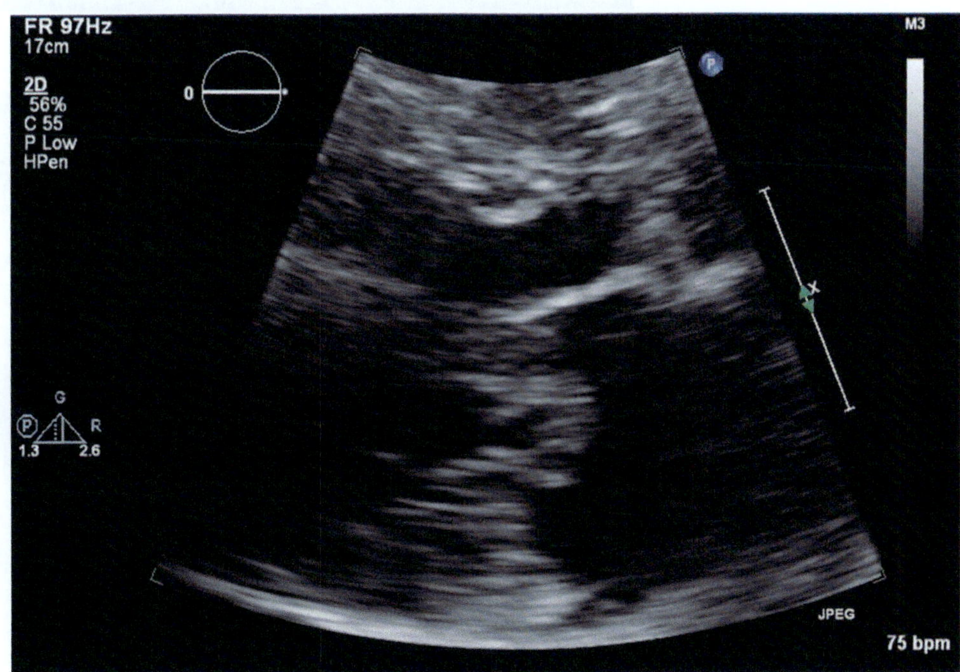

Fig. 4.22 Transthoracic parasternal long-axis view demonstrating thickened and elongated mitral valve leaflets consistent with myxoid degeneration. There is bileaflet prolapse, with the bodies of the distended leaflet segments billowing beyond the plane of the annulus (posterior greater than anterior). The mitral annulus appears dilated. No calcification is noted

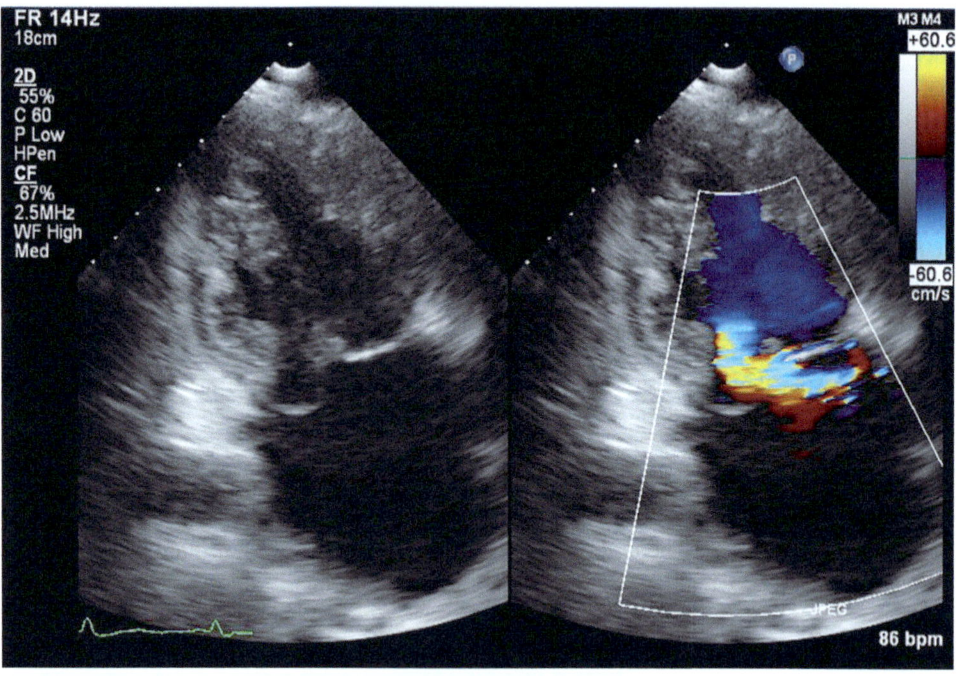

Fig. 4.23 Apical two-chamber transthoracic view demonstrating prominent prolapse of the medial posterior leaflet (P3) with resultant anteriorly directed mitral regurgitation

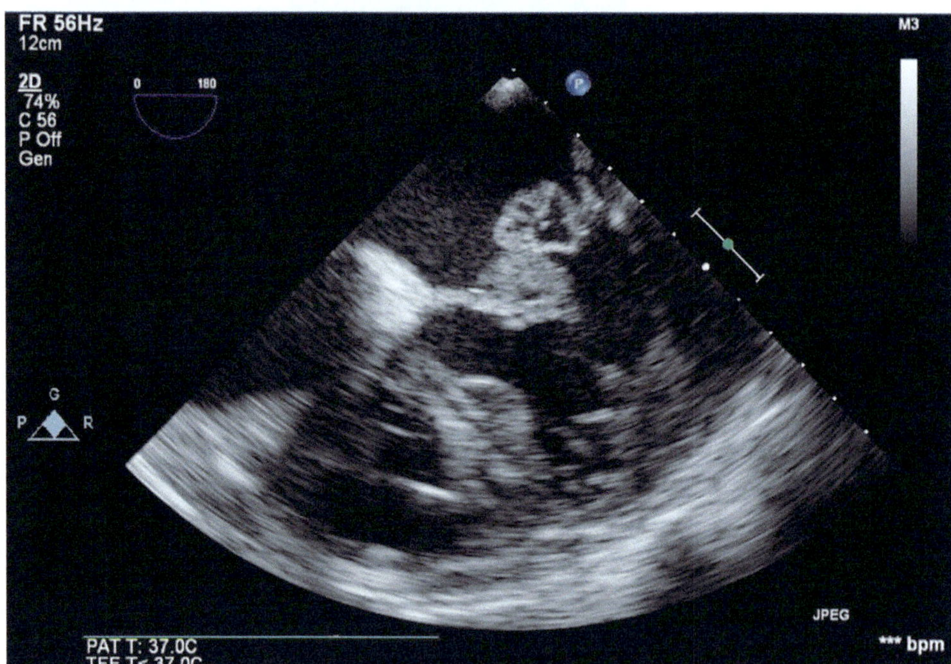

Fig. 4.24 Transesophageal 0° view of the mitral valve, demonstrating severe bileaflet prolapse (A2 and P2). The billowing medial scallop of the posterior leaflet (P3) is intermittently visible

Fig. 4.25 Transesophageal 0° view of the mitral valve, demonstrating significant turbulence of transvalvular flow associated with the posterior leaflet. The jet of mitral regurgitation is not well appreciated because of its eccentric, anteriorly directed trajectory

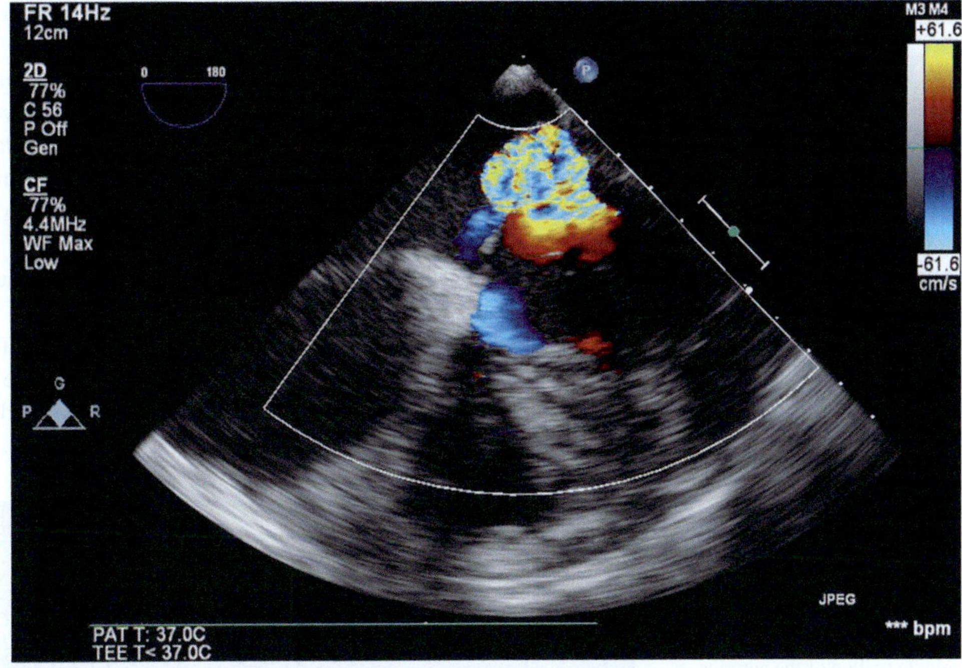

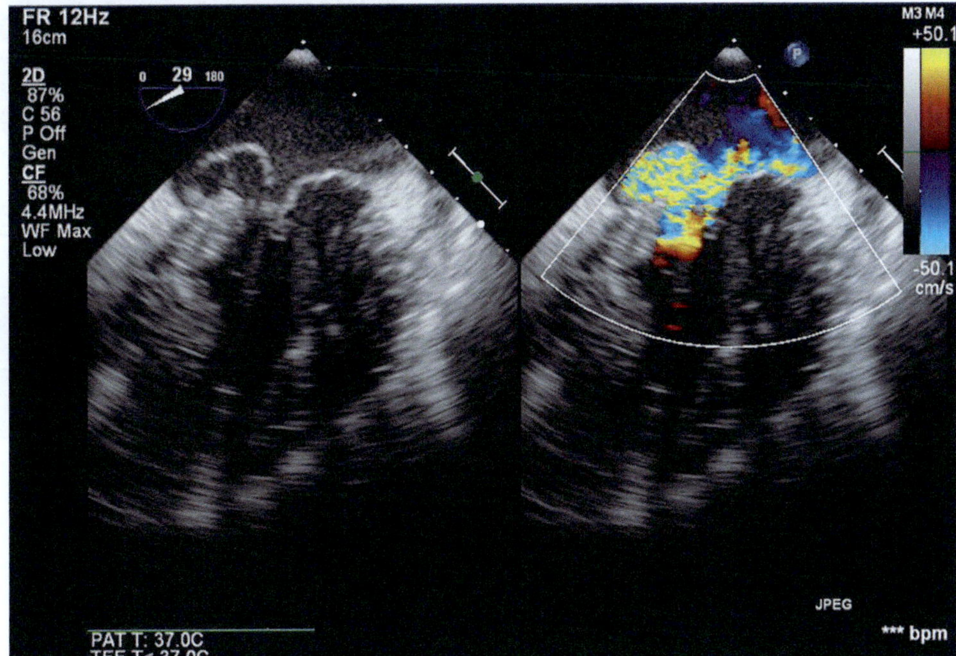

Fig. 4.26 Transesophageal 30° view of the mitral valve rotated medially to demonstrate prolapse and flail of the P3 scallop with severe, anteriorly directed mitral regurgitation on color Doppler imaging

4.6 Case 6. Anterior Mitral Valve Leaflet Flail

A 62-year-old man presented with exertional dyspnea increasing over 2 months. He also reported occasional dizziness associated with palpitations but no overt syncope. Echocardiography demonstrated severe (4+), posteriorly directed mitral regurgitation due to anterior leaflet prolapse with focal flail of the middle scallop of the anterior leaflet (A2). At the time of surgery, he was noted to have two ruptured chordae involving the mid and lateral A2 segments of the anterior leaflet. The flail chordae were resected, a Duran annuloplasty ring was implanted, and three neochordae were created with the use of Gore-Tex (Figs. 4.27, 4.28, 4.29, 4.30, 4.31, and 4.32).

Video 4.19 Preoperative simultaneous 2D and color Doppler imaging of the mitral valve viewed at 0° by transesophageal echocardiography. Flail of the middle scallop of the anterior leaflet (A2) is seen, with a resultant highly eccentric jet of severe, posteriorly directed mitral regurgitation (AVI 1179 kb)

Video 4.20 Postoperative simultaneous 2D and color Doppler imaging of the mitral valve viewed at 0° by transesophageal echocardiography. The mitral valvuloplasty is noted, with shortening and repair of the anterior leaflet. The mitral valve opens well and has no residual regurgitation (AVI 1076 kb)

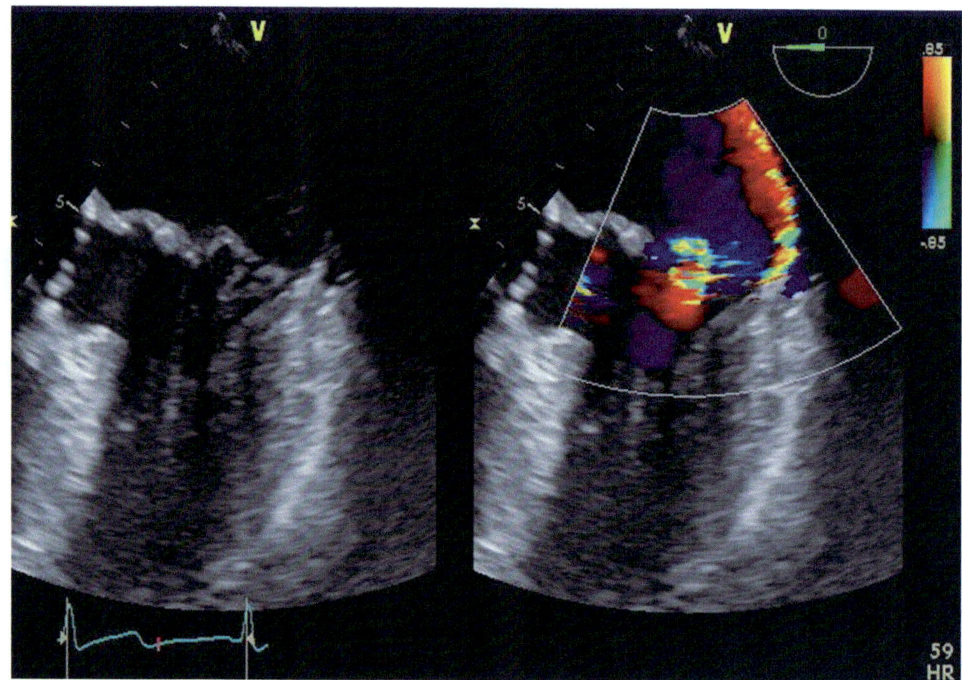

Fig. 4.27 Preoperative simultaneous 2D and color Doppler imaging of the mitral valve viewed at 0° by transesophageal echocardiography. Flail of the middle scallop of the anterior leaflet (A2) is seen, with a resultant highly eccentric jet of severe, posteriorly directed mitral regurgitation

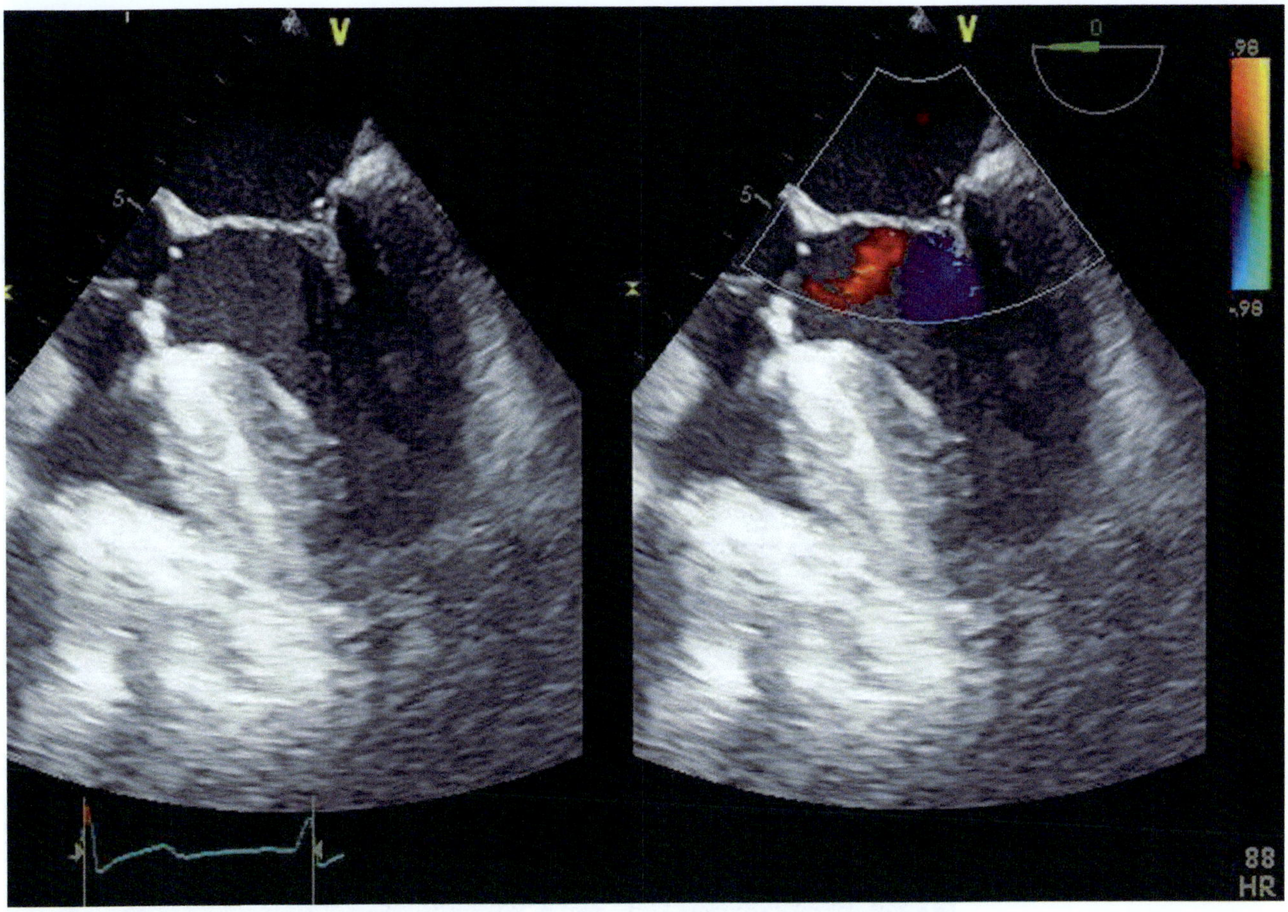

Fig. 4.28 Postoperative simultaneous 2D and color Doppler imaging of the mitral valve viewed at 0° by transesophageal echocardiography. The mitral valvuloplasty is noted, with shortening and repair of the anterior leaflet. The mitral valve opens well and has no residual regurgitation

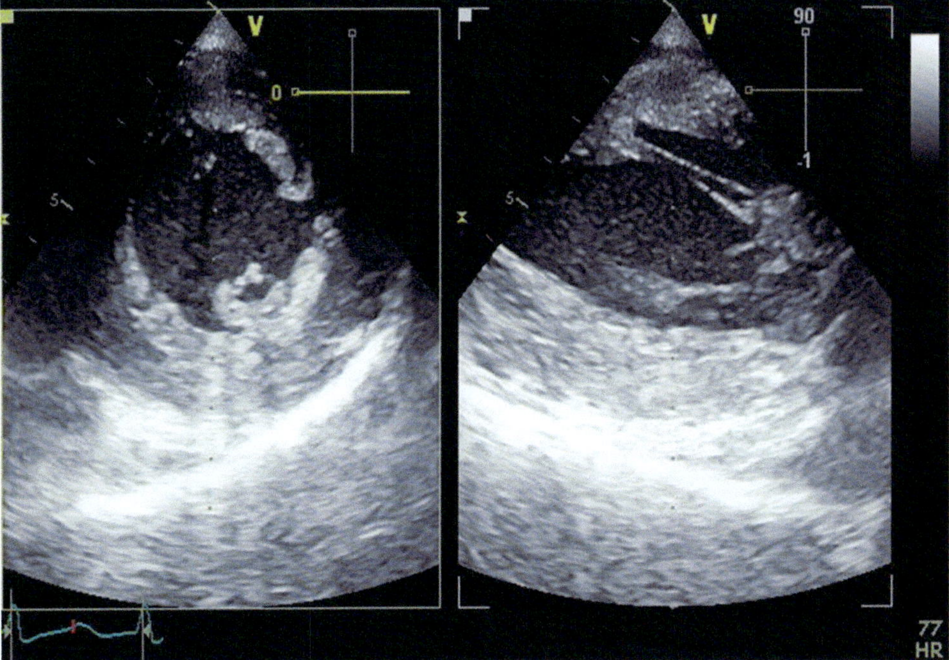

Fig. 4.29 Transgastric biplane view (short-axis and 90° views) on transesophageal echo. The right 90° image best demonstrates the neochordae attaching from the papillary muscles to the repaired mitral valve

Fig. 4.30 Continuous wave Doppler through the mitral valve demonstrates late-systolic mitral regurgitation

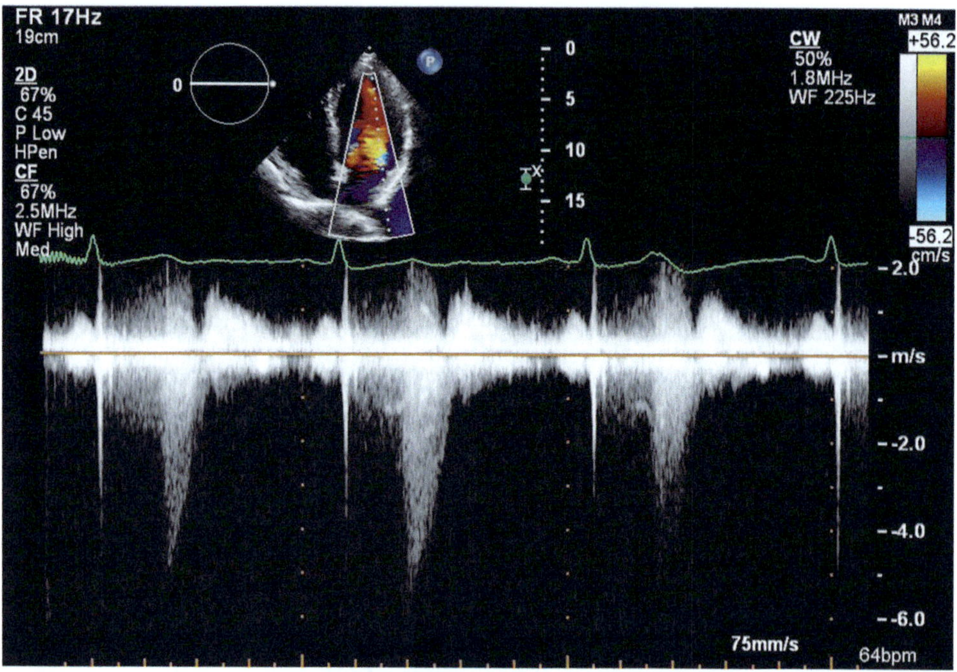

Fig. 4.31 Color M-mode through the mitral valve demonstrates late-systolic regurgitation and normal diastolic flow

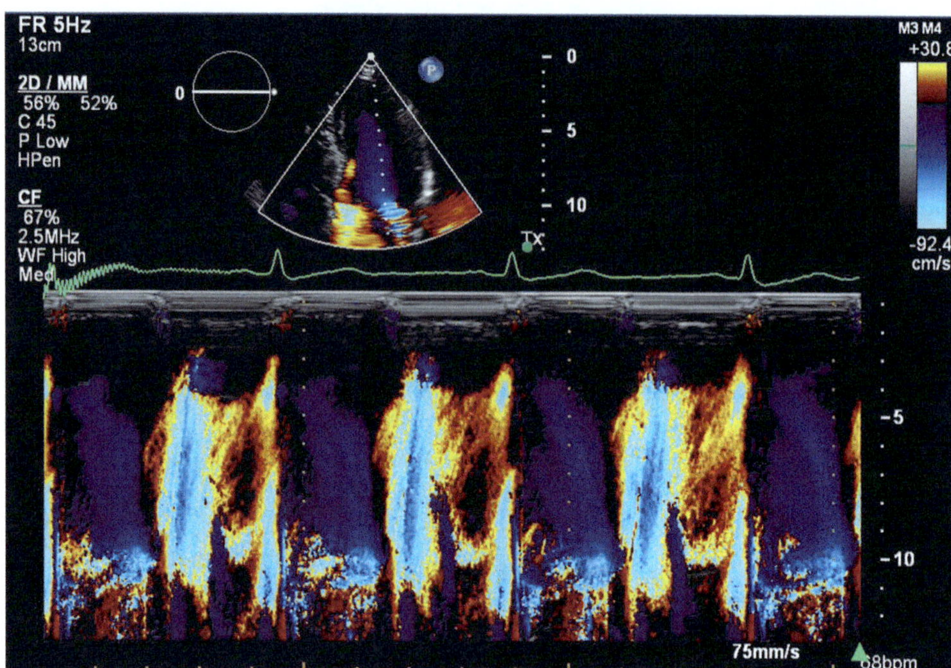

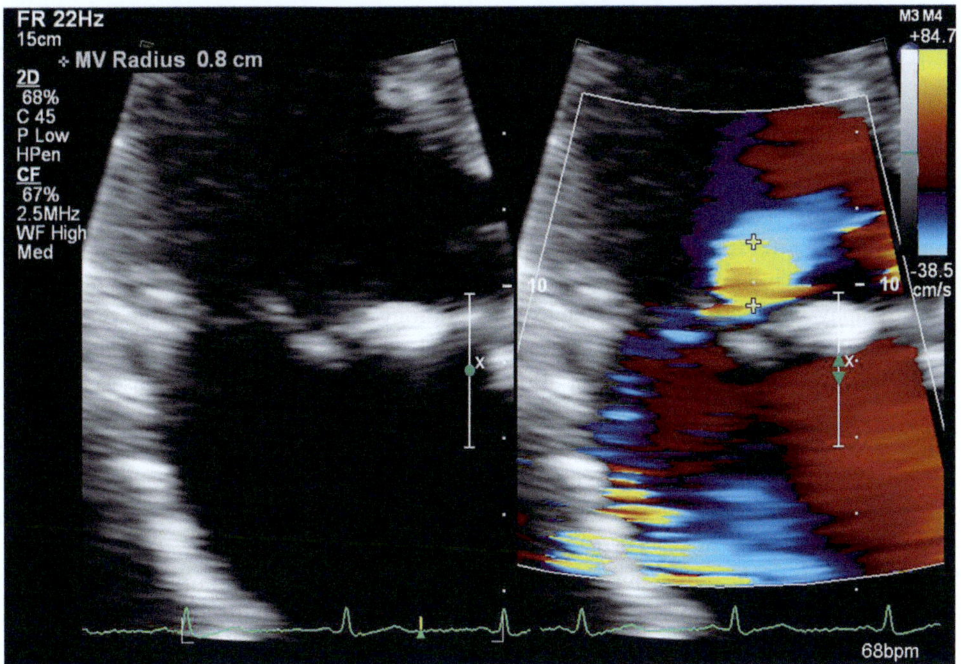

Fig. 4.32 The PISA of 0.8 cm on color Doppler may be underestimated because of the eccentricity of the jet

4.7 Case 7. Myxomatous Degenerative Disease with Posterior Leaflet Prolapse

An 88-year-old man was referred for consideration of MitraClip (Abbott Vascular). He had been previously diagnosed with severe (4+) mitral regurgitation due to leaflet prolapse and now reported increasing fatigue, but his left ventricular systolic function and size remained normal and he denied any symptoms of dyspnea. Transesophageal echocardiography was performed to establish the etiology and severity of his mitral regurgitation. He was noted to have flail of the central, medial (P2/P3) region of the posterior mitral valve leaflet, probably related to myxomatous degenerative disease. The regurgitant orifice area (ROA) was calculated as 0.44 cm^2, measured using the proximal isovelocity surface area (PISA) method, suggesting severe mitral regurgitation. Because the duration of the jet (seen on continuous wave spectral Doppler and color M-mode) was actually only from mid systole to late systole, however, the ROA was overestimating the severity of regurgitation, as it was assuming holosystolic regurgitation. The pulmonary venous flow profile was also noted to be normal, with no significant systolic flow reversal, also demonstrating that the mitral regurgitation was not severe. A final grading of moderate (3+) mitral regurgitation was reported based on these findings.

Video 4.21 Transesophageal 62° view demonstrating flail of the posterior mitral valve leaflet (P2/P3 region) (AVI 5729 kb)

Video 4.22 Transesophageal 62° view demonstrating significant associated mitral regurgitation due to leaflet coaptation, although the severity and direction of the jet are not well appreciated on this view (AVI 1361 kb)

Video 4.23 Transesophageal 87° view demonstrating that the flail segment primarily involves the region between the P2 and P3 scallops (AVI 5775 kb)

Video 4.24 Transesophageal 129° view demonstrates a significant jet of medially directed mitral regurgitation with a PISA radius of 0.94 cm, which gives an estimated regurgitant orifice area of 0.44 cm^2 (AVI 1373 kb)

Video 4.25 This 3D zoom view of the mitral valve from the left atrium demonstrates the flail posterior leaflet in the region between the P2 and P3 scallops (AVI 1015 kb)

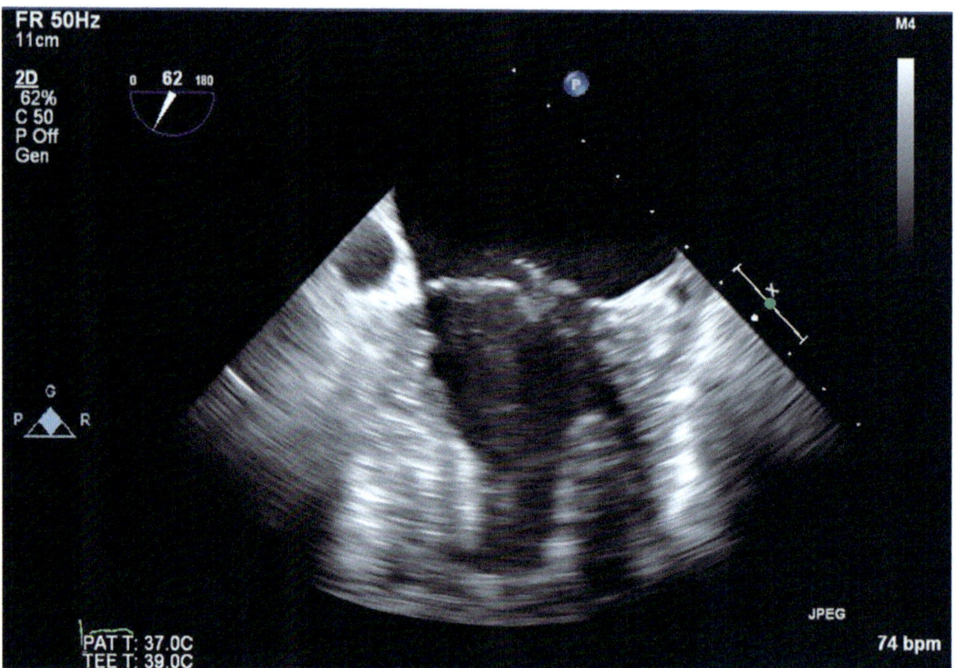

Fig. 4.33 Transesophageal 62° view demonstrating flail of the posterior mitral valve leaflet (P2/P3 region)

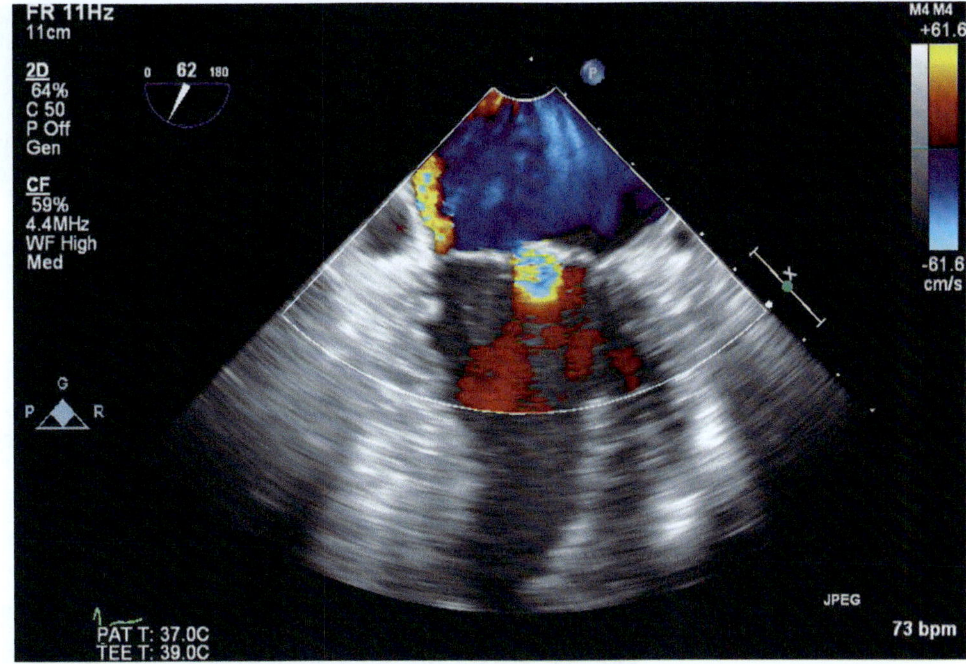

Fig. 4.34 Transesophageal 62° view demonstrating significant associated mitral regurgitation due to leaflet coaptation, although the severity and direction of the jet are not well appreciated on this view

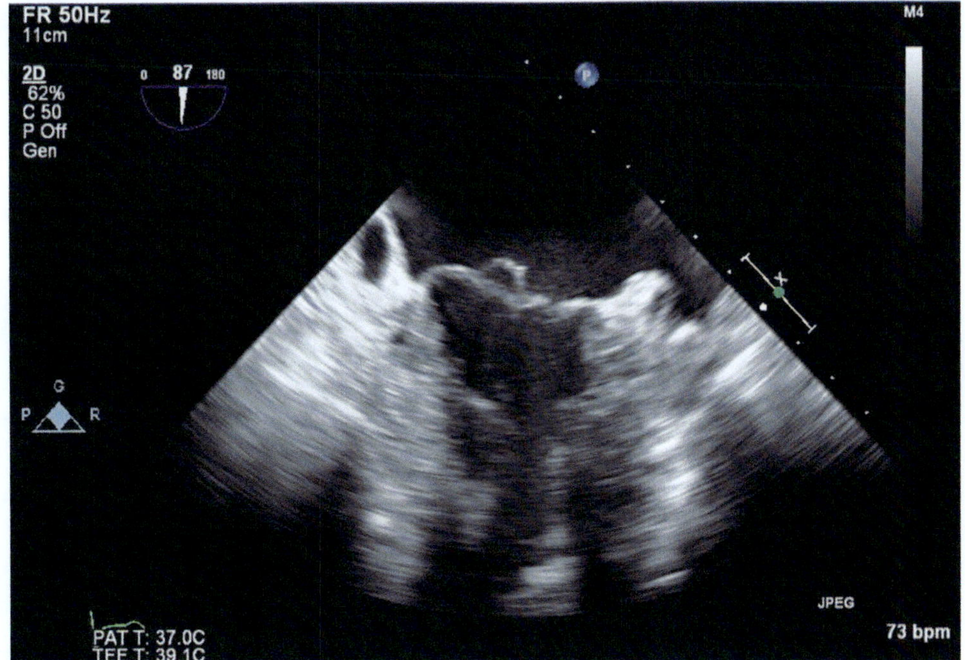

Fig. 4.35 Transesophageal 87° view demonstrating that the flail segment primarily involves the region between the P2 and P3 scallops

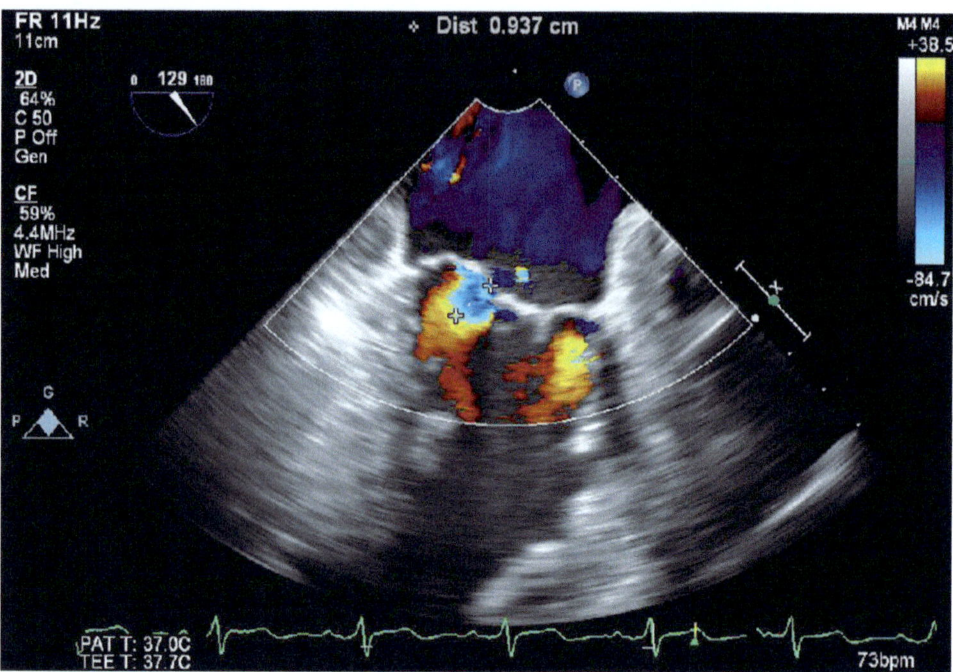

Fig. 4.36 Transesophageal 129° view demonstrates a significant jet of medially directed mitral regurgitation with a PISA radius of 0.94 cm, which gives an estimated regurgitant orifice area of 0.44 cm^2

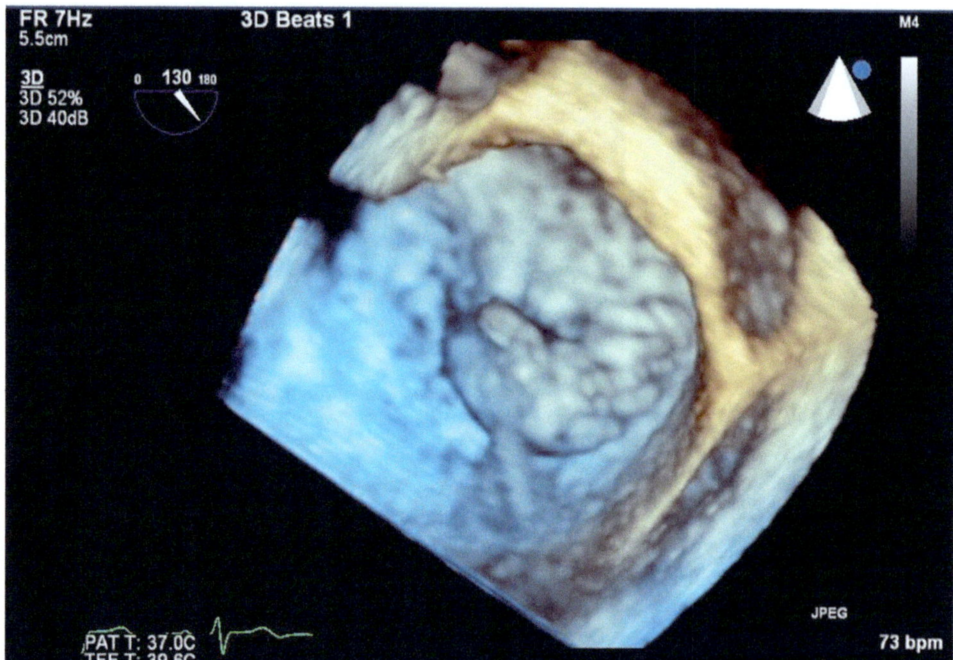

Fig. 4.37 This 3D zoom view of the mitral valve from the left atrium demonstrates the flail posterior leaflet in the region between the P2 and P3 scallops

Fig. 4.38 Pulse wave Doppler trace of the left upper pulmonary vein demonstrates a normal profile with no significant reversal of systolic flow

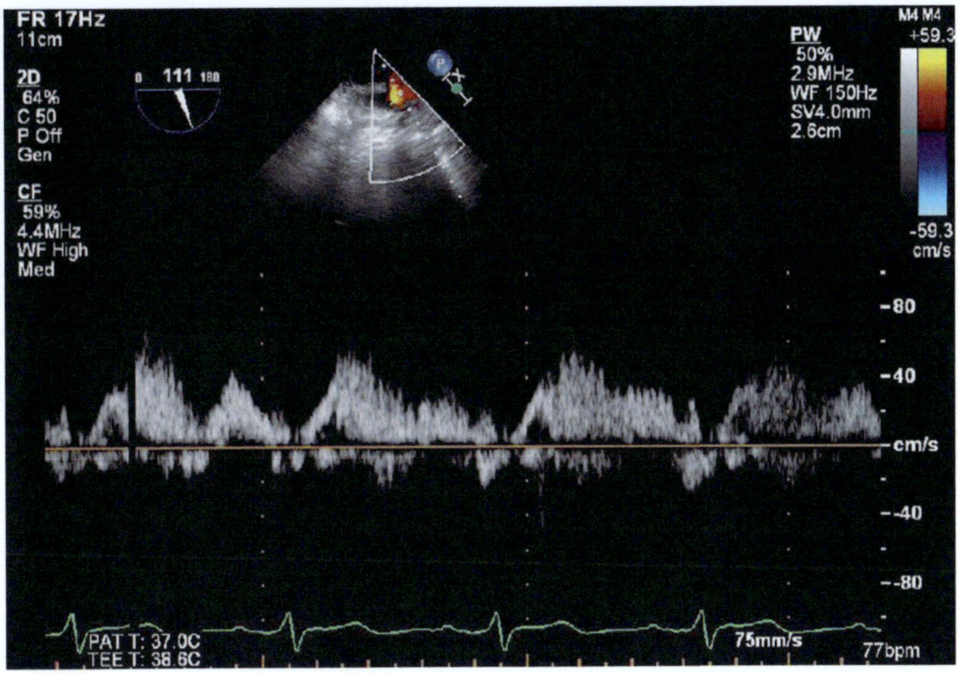

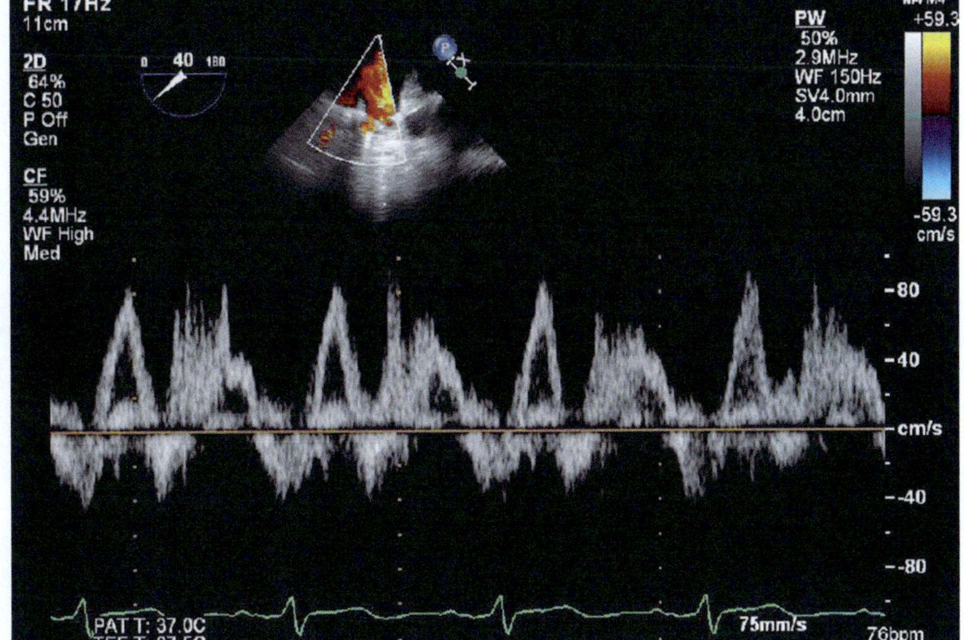

Fig. 4.39 Pulse wave Doppler trace of the right upper pulmonary vein demonstrates a normal profile with only a brief period of mid-systolic to late-systolic flow reversal, thereby supporting that the mitral regurgitation is not severe

Fig. 4.40 Color M-mode shows that the timing of mitral regurgitation is predominantly mid-systolic to late-systolic

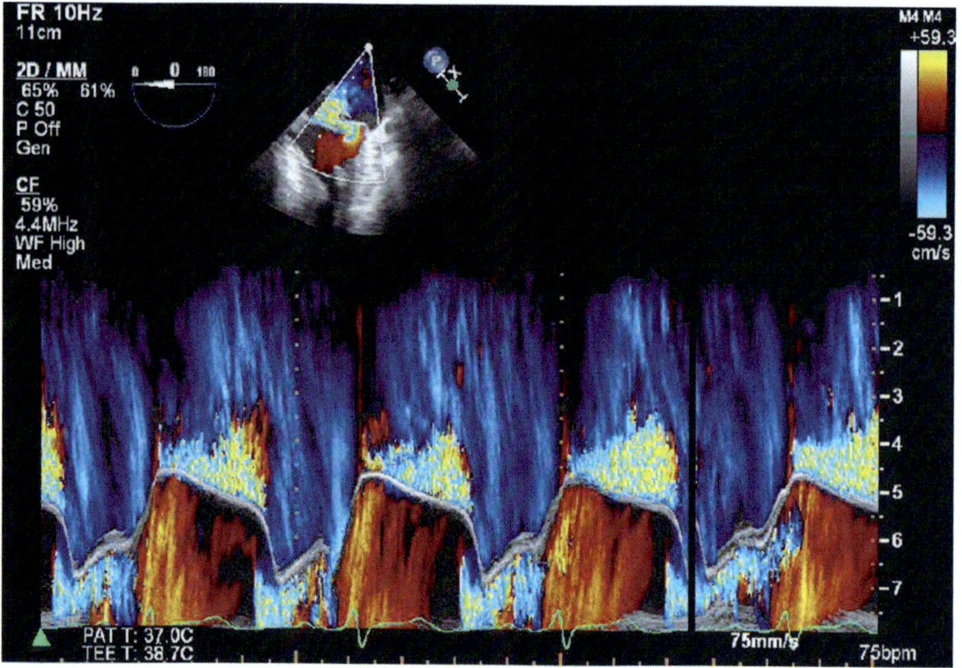

Fig. 4.41 Continuous wave Doppler through the mitral valve also demonstrates that regurgitant flow through the mitral valve is mid-systolic to late-systolic

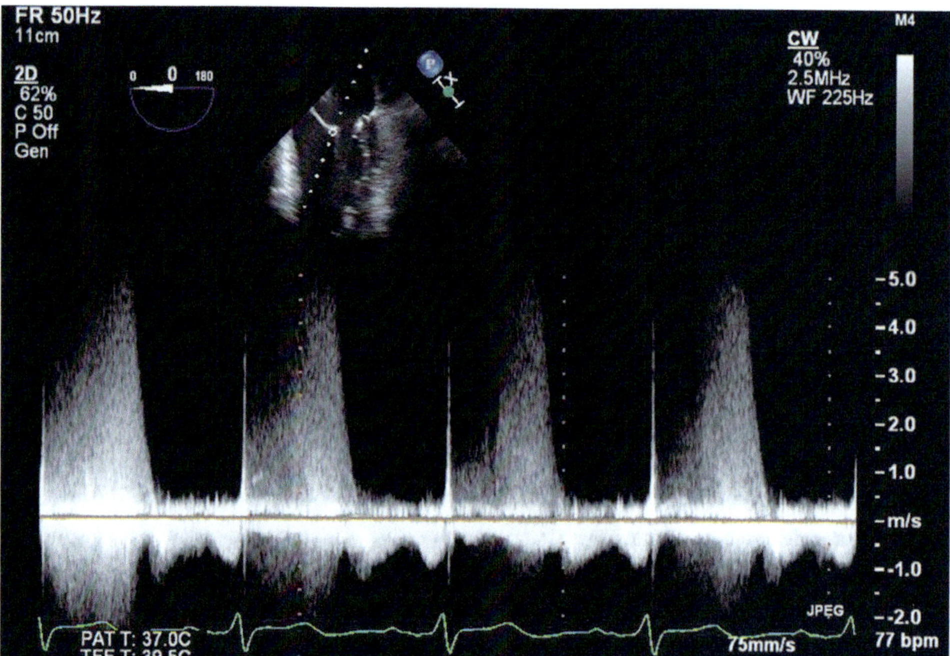

4.8   Learning Points

- Mitral valve prolapse is generally defined as displacement of one or both mitral valve leaflets by at least 2 mm above the annular plane on a parasternal long-axis view [1].
- Mitral valve prolapse was first described in 1966 by John Barlow [2]. Today, the term *Barlow's syndrome* or *Barlow's valve* is usually reserved for severe myxomatous valve degeneration with leaflet and chordal redundancy in younger patients, in contrast to older patients, who typically present with chordal rupture due to deficient fibroelasticity.
- Prolapse prevalence is approximated at 2–3 % within the general population [3].
- Progression from mitral valve prolapse to flail occurs when the leaflet becomes so mobile that the tip turns toward the left atrium rather than toward the left ventricle. Flail severity ranges from simple tip eversion to unrestricted leaflet motion due to complete chordal rupture. The degree of mitral regurgitation (MR) usually increases in proportion to the degree of flail.
- MR in the setting of mitral valve prolapse may not be holosystolic, but instead may predominate in mid to late systole. Hence, PISA-based calculations, which assume that the regurgitation is holosystolic, may overestimate the jet severity.
- Color M-mode and the continuous wave Doppler profile should be reviewed to examine the exact timing of the jet, which will influence the classification of MR severity.
- Conversely, the PISA method assumes proximal flow convergence to be hemispherical, which may not be accurate for the highly eccentric jets seen with leaflet prolapse or flail, when the shape is more hemi-elliptical and the valve is nonplanar. Depending on where the PISA dimension is measured, MR severity can thus be either underestimated or overestimated.
- Multiple views of the mitral valve are required to accurately identify the prolapsing or flail scallops and the severity and direction of associated MR. Transesophageal echocardiography typically provides the most accurate and consistent views.

References

1. Zoghbi WA, Enriquez-Sarano M, Foster E, Grayburn PA, Kraft CD, Levine RA, et al. Recommendations for evaluation of the severity of native valvular regurgitation with two-dimensional and Doppler echocardiography. J Am Soc Echocardiogr. 2003;16:777–802.
2. Barlow JB, Bosman CK. Aneurysmal protrusion of the posterior leaflet of the mitral valve. An auscultatory-electrocardiographic syndrome. Am Heart J. 1966;71:166–78.
3. Hayek E, Gring CN, Griffin BP. Mitral valve prolapse. Lancet. 2005;365:507–18.

Teerapat Yingchoncharoen

5.1 Case 1. Rheumatic Mitral Stenosis Undergoing Percutaneous Mitral Commissurotomy

A 21-year-old Caucasian college student was referred to our institution for management of severe mitral stenosis. His past medical history was significant for a history of acute rheumatic fever at age 12. He was then followed by his local cardiologist; yearly echocardiography found normal left ventricular (LV) ejection fraction without significant valvular abnormalities. He did not see a cardiologist for a few years, and his last echocardiogram was 5 years ago. He was doing well until 2 months ago, when he felt shortness of breath while playing volleyball. He went to see his cardiologist and was found to have moderate to severe mitral stenosis.

On physical examination, his vital signs are stable (BP 94/44, HR 66). Cardiac auscultation revealed normal S1 S2 with opening snap 3/6 diastolic rumbling murmur at the LV apex. He underwent successful status post balloon mitral valvuloplasty with reduction in mean mitral valve gradient from 16 to 4 mmHg and increase in mitral valve area from 0.9 to 3 cm^2 (Figs. 5.1, 5.2, 5.3, 5.4, 5.5, 5.6, 5.7, 5.8, 5.9, 5.10, 5.11, and 5.12).

Video 5.1 Transesophageal echocardiography (TEE) showed thickened mitral valve with restricted opening (AVI 2662 kb)

Video 5.2 Color flow imaging showed diastolic flow acceleration across the mitral valve during diastole (AVI 2135 kb)

Video 5.3 Three-dimensional imaging of the ventricular side of the mitral valve showed limited opening of the valve (AVI 2636 kb)

Video 5.4 X-plane imaging showing orthogonal imaging of the interatrial septum at the puncture site at the time of the percutaneous balloon mitral commissurotomy (PBMC) (AVI 2450 kb)

Video 5.5 The Inoue balloon inflated at the mitral valve (AVI 2191 kb)

Video 5.6 Post PBMC. Improved mitral valve opening (AVI 2952 kb)

Video 5.7 Post PBMC. Mitral valve area is increased (AVI 3022 kb)

Video 5.8 Post PBMC. Mild mitral regurgitation (AVI 1995 kb)

Electronic supplementary material The online version of this chapter (doi:10.1007/978-1-4471-6672-6_5) contains supplementary material, which is available to authorized users.

T. Yingchoncharoen
Department of Cardiovascular Medicine, Cleveland Clinic,
9500 Euclid Avenue, Cleveland, OH 44195, USA
e-mail: teerapatmdcu@gmail.com

M. Desai et al. (eds.), *An Atlas of Mitral Valve Imaging*,
DOI 10.1007/978-1-4471-6672-6_5, © Springer-Verlag London 2015

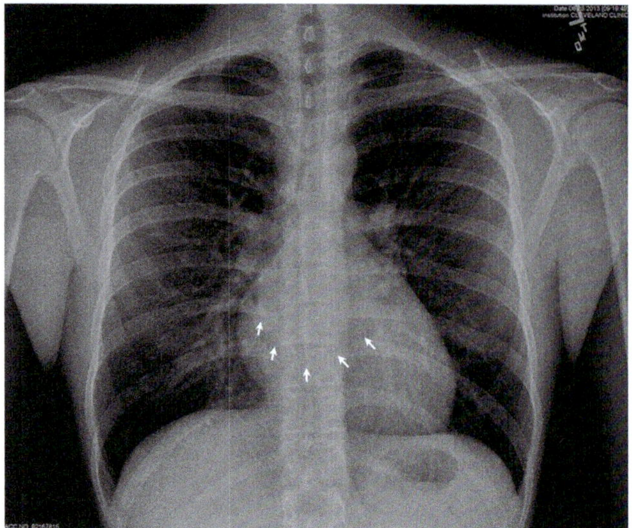

Fig. 5.1 Posteroanterior (PA) chest x-ray showed straightening of the left cardiac border with double contour sign (*arrows*) indicating left atrial enlargement as well as prominent pulmonary venous blood flow

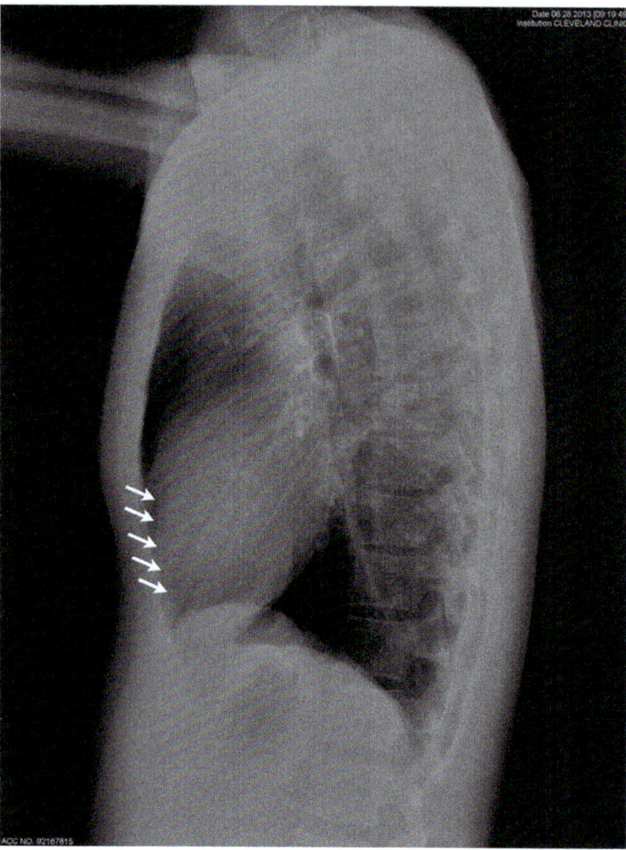

Fig. 5.2 Lateral chest x-ray showed obliteration of retrosternal space (*arrows*) consistent with right ventricular enlargement

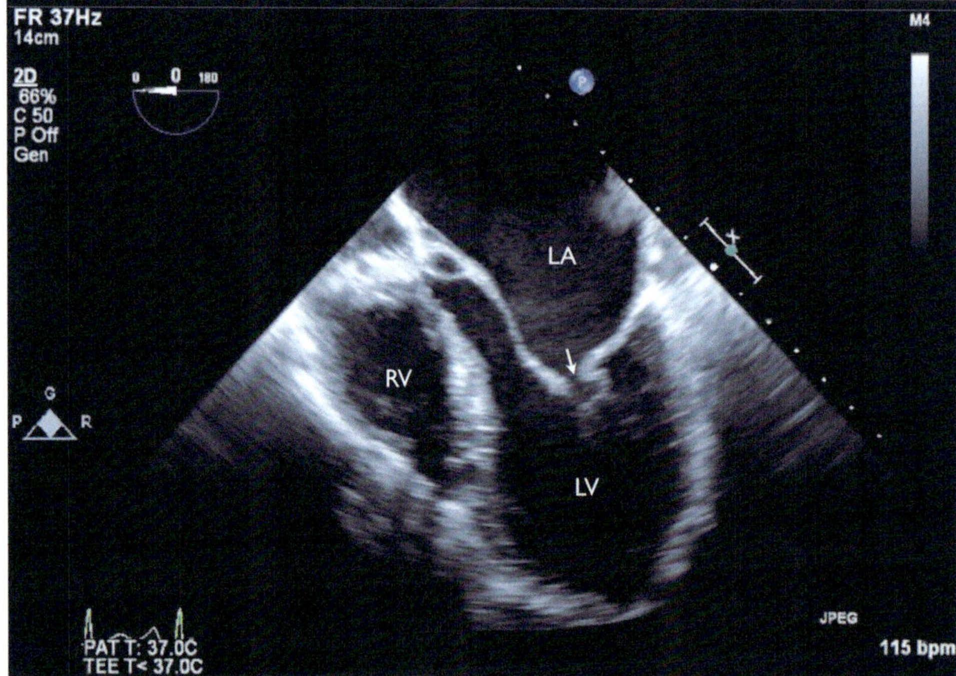

Fig. 5.3 Transesophageal echocardiography (*TEE*) showed thickened mitral valve with restricted opening (*arrow*). *LA* left atrium, *LV* left ventricle, *RV* right ventricle

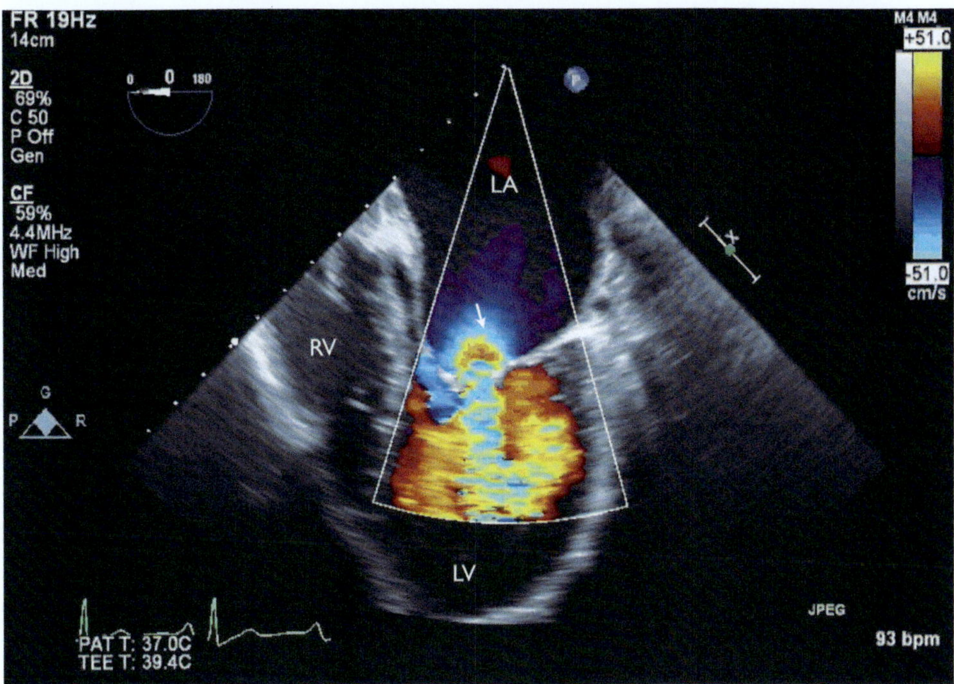

Fig. 5.4   Color flow imaging showed diastolic flow acceleration across the mitral valve during diastole (*arrow*)

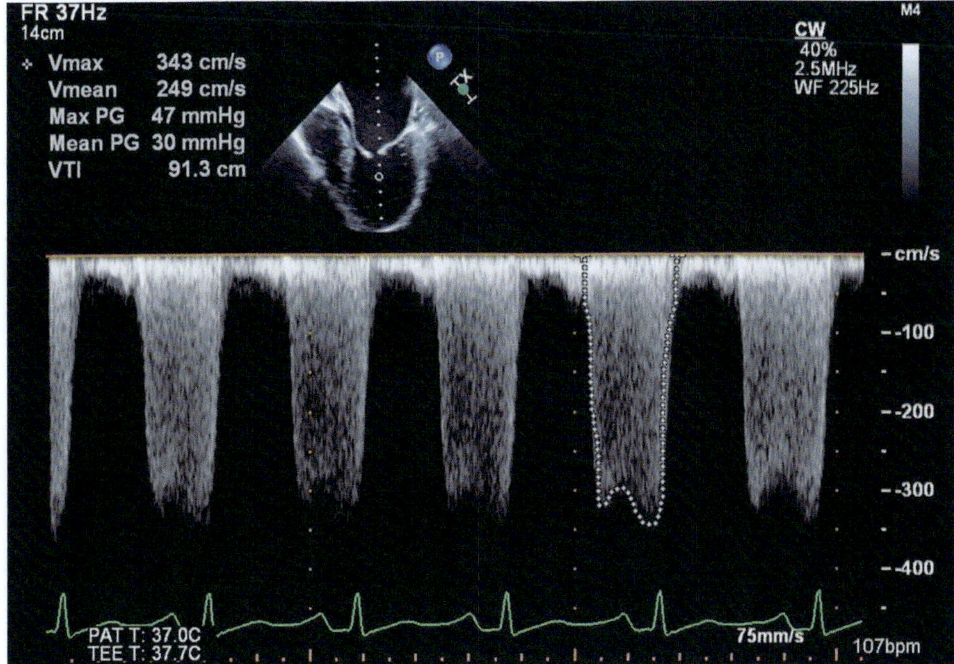

Fig. 5.5   Transmitral gradient across MV showed mean gradient of 30 mmHg, consistent with severe mitral stenosis

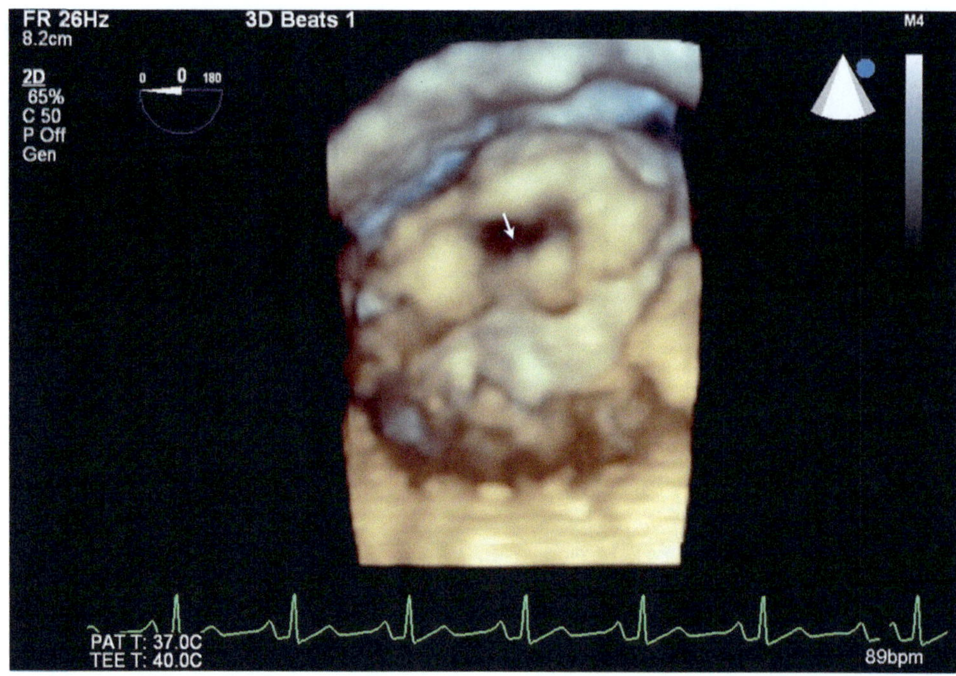

Fig. 5.6 Three-dimensional imaging of the ventricular side of the mitral valve showed limited opening of the valve (*arrow*)

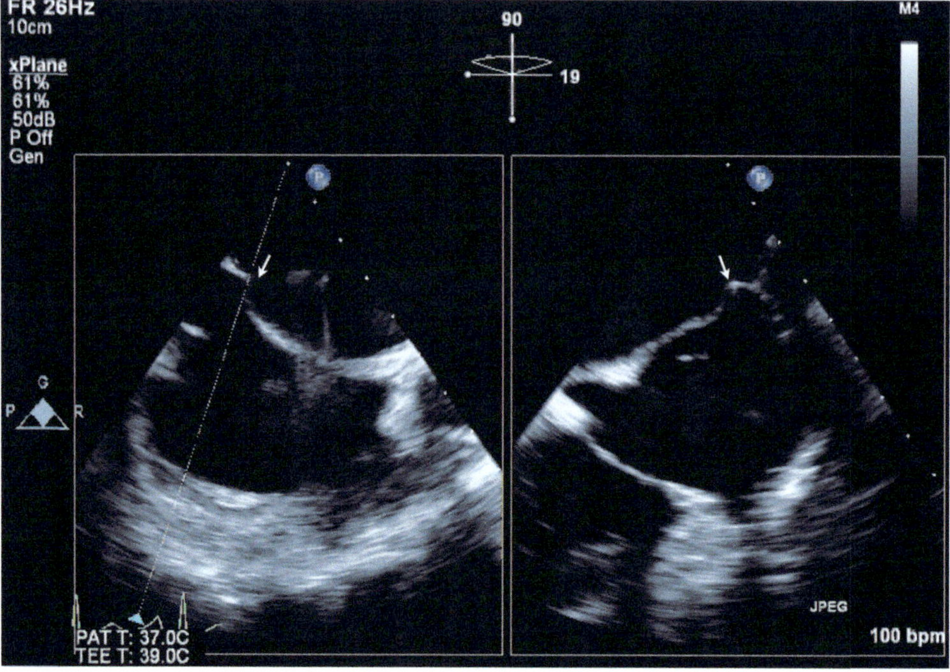

Fig. 5.7 X-plane imaging showing orthogonal imaging of the interatrial septum at the puncture site at the time of the percutaneous balloon mitral commissurotomy (PBMC) (*arrows*)

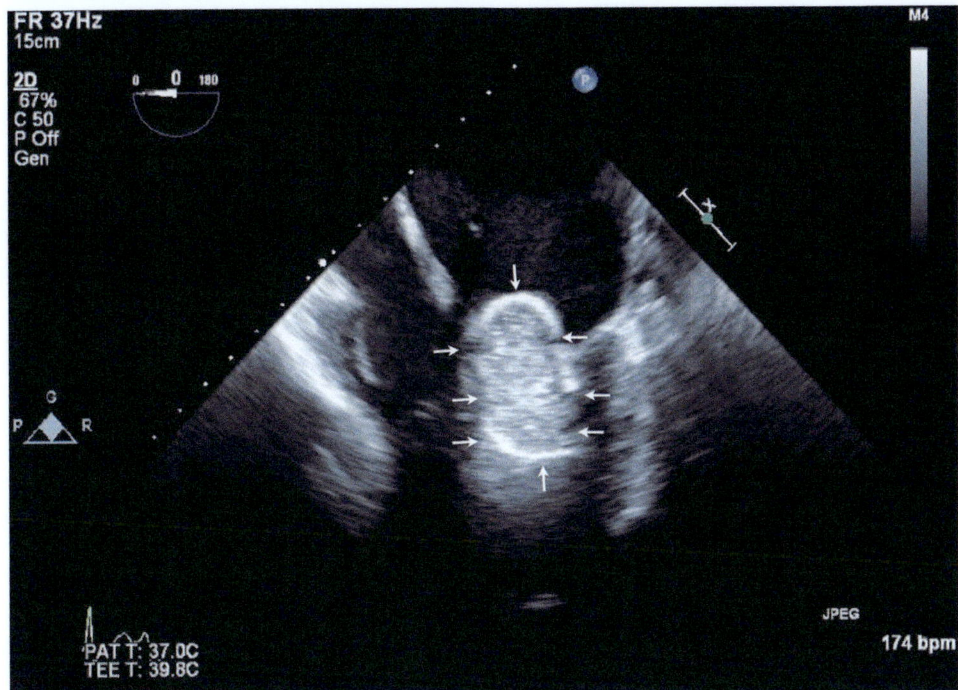

Fig. 5.8 The Inoue balloon (*arrows*) inflated at the mitral valve

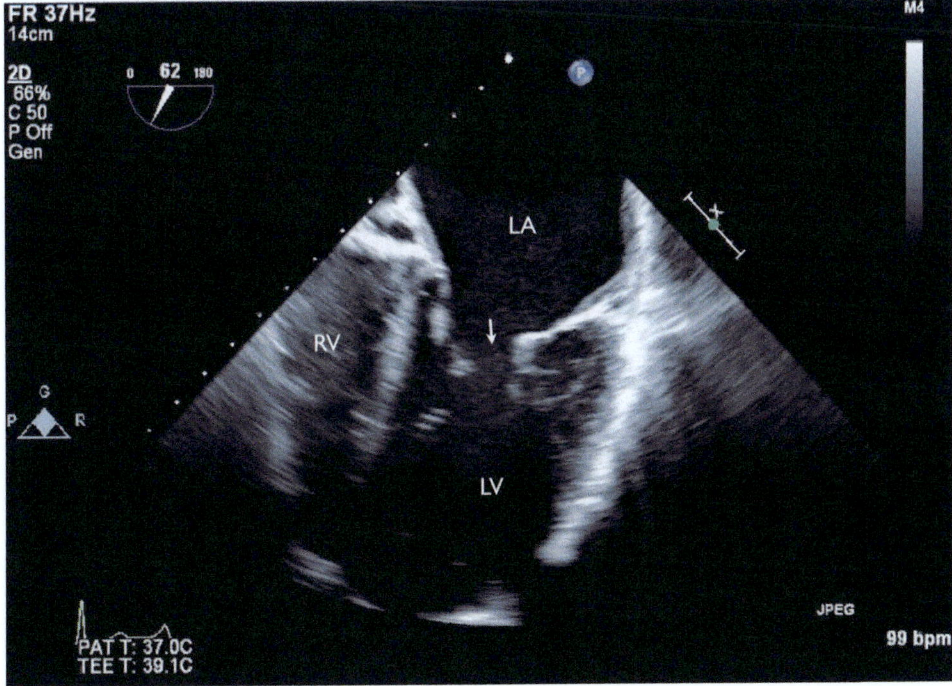

Fig. 5.9 Post PBMC. Improved mitral valve opening (*arrow*)

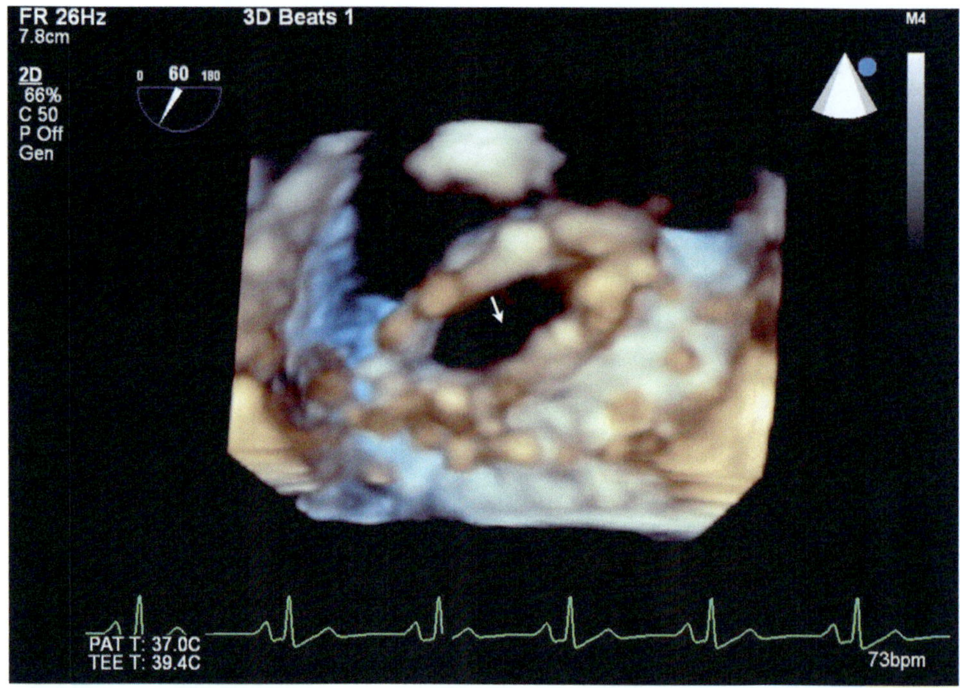

Fig. 5.10 Post PBMC. Mitral valve area (*arrow*) is increased

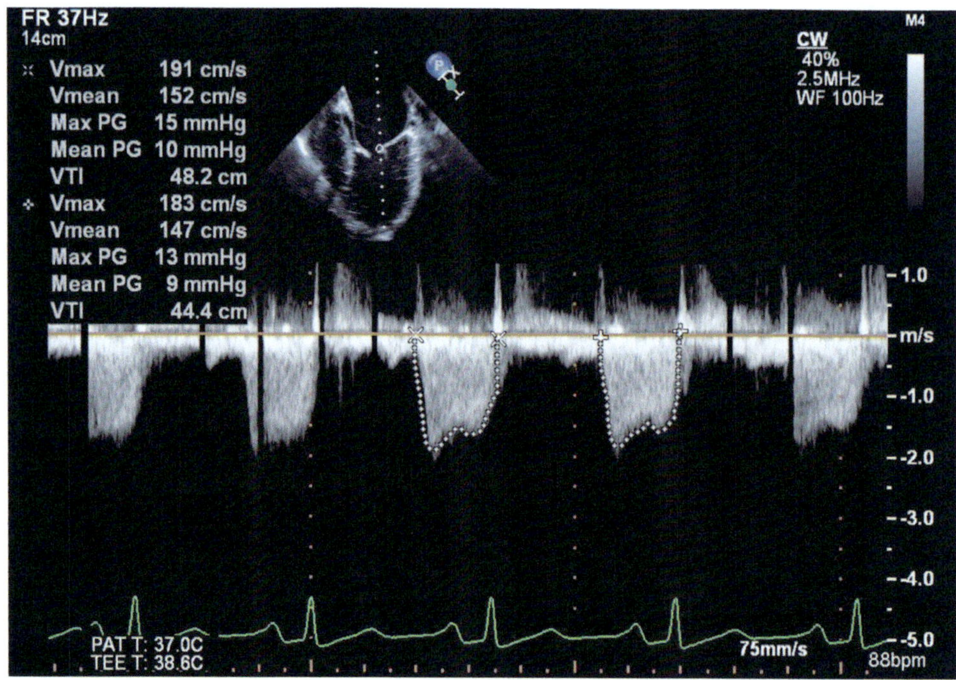

Fig. 5.11 Post PBMC. Decreased transmitral pressure gradient

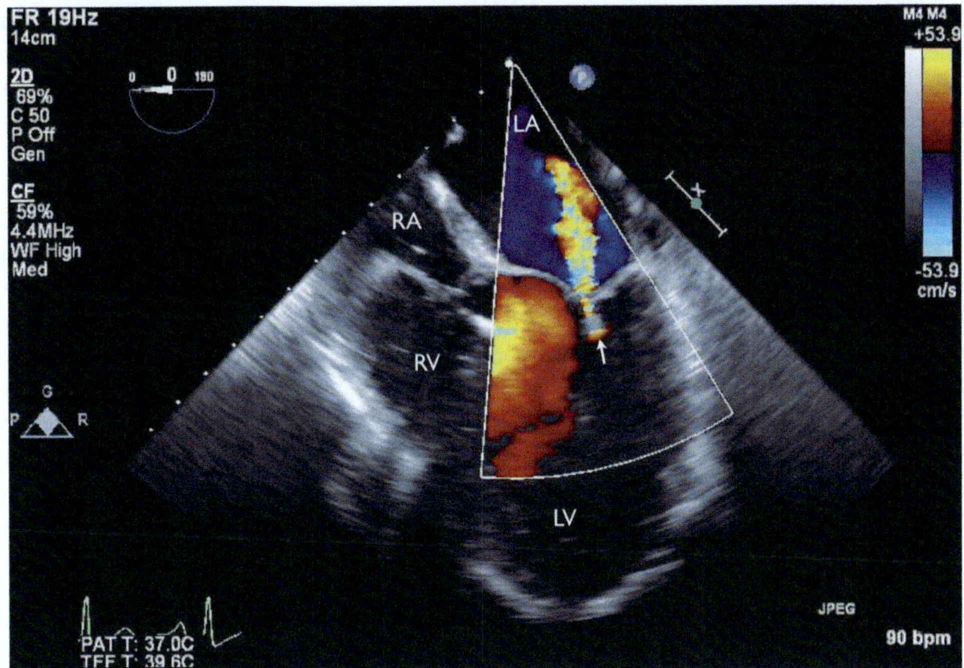

Fig. 5.12 Post PBMC. Mild mitral regurgitation (*arrow*). *RA* right atrium

5.1.1 Learning Points

Rheumatic mitral stenosis is a slowly progressive disease with a prolonged latent phase between the initial rheumatic illness and the development of valve stenosis. Currently, adequate assessment of mitral stenosis and associated lesions can be obtained in nearly all patients by transthoracic echocardiography (TTE), occasionally supplemented by transesophageal echocardiography (TEE). Several randomized controlled trials have established the safety and efficacy of percutaneous balloon mitral commissurotomy (PBMC), compared with surgical closed or open commissurotomy. The technique is generally performed by advancing one or more balloon catheters across the mitral valve and inflating them, thereby splitting the commissures. For the percutaneous approach to have an optimal outcome, it is essential that the valve morphology be predictive of success, generally being mobile, relatively thin, and free of calcium. This morphology is usually assessed by the Wilkins score, although other risk scores have also shown utility. Clinical factors such as age, NYHA class, and the presence or absence of atrial fibrillation are also predictive of outcome [1].

5.2 Case 2. Severe Rheumatic Mitral stenosis with Severe Pulmonary Hypertension and Severe Secondary Tricuspid Regurgitation

A 66-year-old woman presented with severe rheumatic mitral stenosis and moderate mitral regurgitation with severe pulmonary hypertension and severe secondary tricuspid regurgitation. She reports dyspnea, peripheral edema, and palpitations, which have been worsening over the past 6 months. She presents to her primary care physician with right-sided weakness and an expressive dysphasia and is found to be in atrial fibrillation. She underwent successful mitral valve replacement with tricuspid valve replacement and left atrial appendage ligation (Figs. 5.13, 5.14, 5.15, 5.16, 5.17, 5.18, 5.19, 5.20, 5.21, 5.22, 5.23, and 5.24).

Video 5.9 Transthoracic echocardiography (TTE), parasternal long-axis, showed severe mitral calcification with restricted opening. The aortic valve was also calcified, with restricted excursion, and the right ventricle is enlarged (AVI 3307 kb)

Video 5.10 TTE, parasternal with color Doppler flow imaging, showed mitral regurgitation (AVI 1480 kb)

Video 5.11 TTE (four-chamber view) demonstrating severe calcification of the mitral valve resulting in severe pulmonary hypertension (estimated right ventricular systolic pressure of 91 mmHg) and severe right ventricular dilatation with resultant failure of tricuspid valve leaflet coaptation. Severe atrial enlargement and a pericardial effusion are noted (AVI 3907 kb)

Video 5.12 Color Doppler imaging across the tricuspid valve confirms the presence of associated severe tricuspid regurgitation (AVI 2575 kb)

Video 5.13 TTE (five-chamber view) showing calcified and thickened aortic valve with restricted opening (AVI 3033 kb)

Video 5.14 TTE (five-chamber view) with color Doppler flow showing mild aortic insufficiency (AVI 2135 kb)

Video 5.15 TEE (four-chamber view) confirms severely calcified mitral valve with malcoapted tricuspid valve (AVI 5443 kb)

Video 5.16 TEE (four-chamber view) with color Doppler flow imaging confirms moderate mitral regurgitation and enlarged right-sided cardiac chambers (AVI 2091 kb)

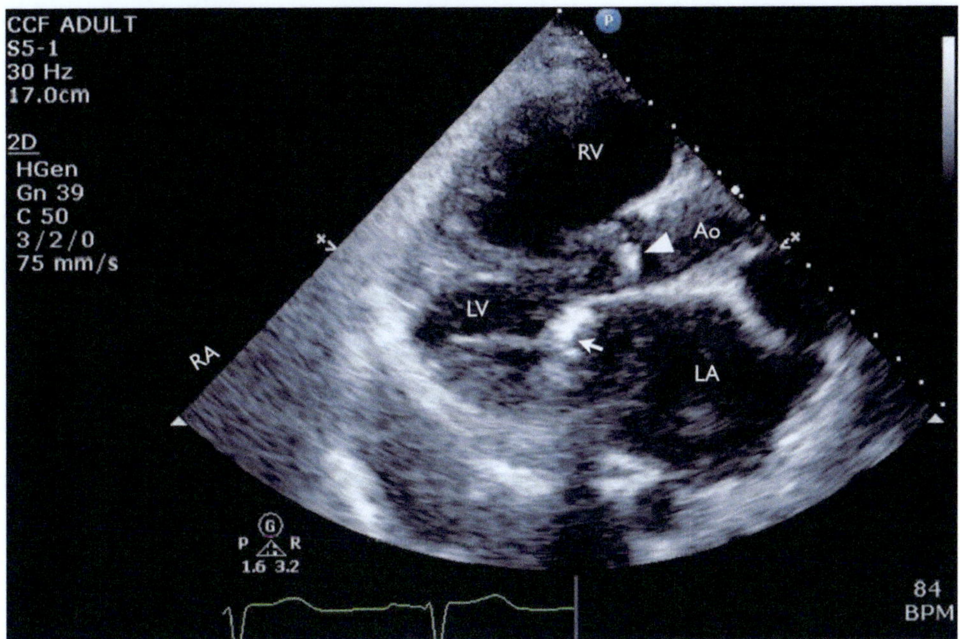

Fig. 5.13 Transthoracic echocardiography (TTE), parasternal long-axis, showed severe mitral calcification with restricted opening (*arrow*). The aortic valve was also calcified, with restricted excursion (*arrowhead*), and the right ventricle is enlarged. *Ao* aorta

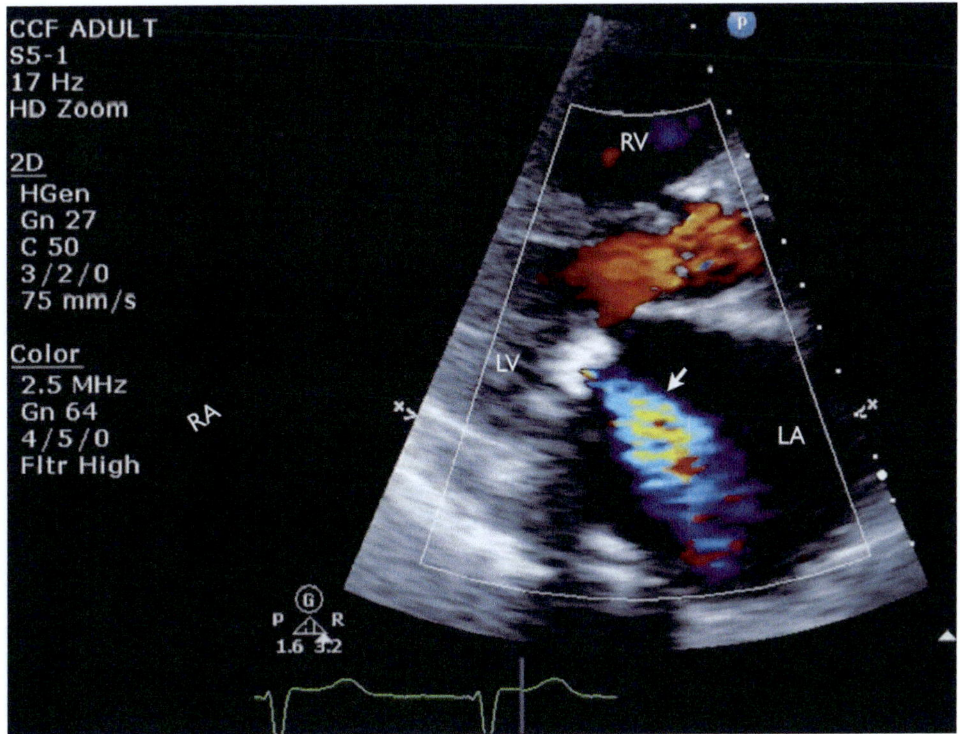

Fig. 5.14 TTE, parasternal with color Doppler flow imaging, showed mitral regurgitation (*arrow*)

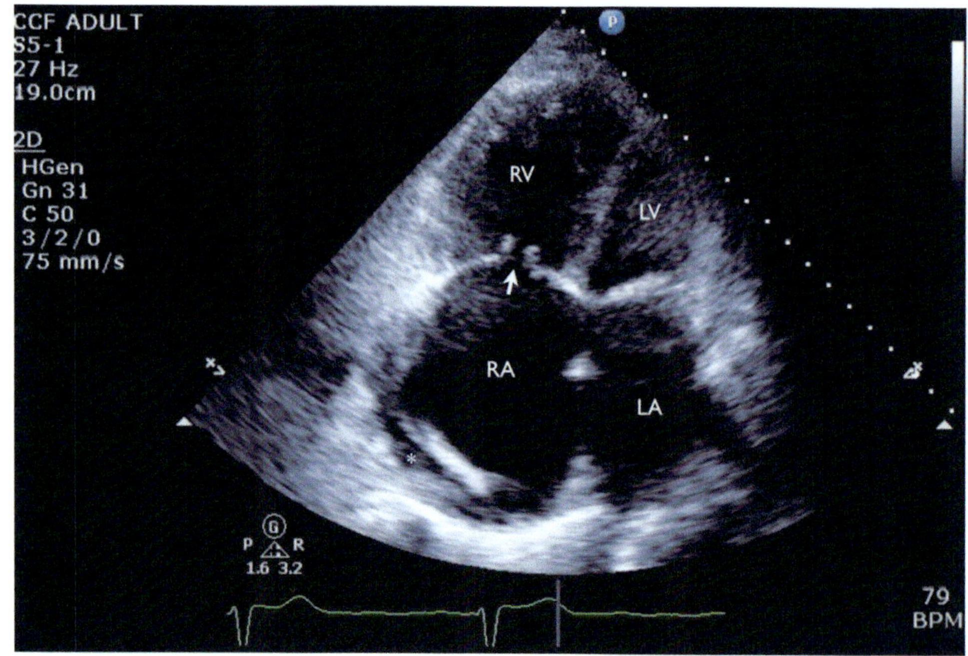

Fig. 5.15 TTE (four-chamber view) demonstrating severe calcification of the mitral valve resulting in severe pulmonary hypertension (estimated right ventricular systolic pressure of 91 mmHg) and severe right ventricular dilatation with resultant failure of tricuspid valve leaflet coaptation (*arrow*). Severe atrial enlargement and a pericardial effusion (*asterisk*) are noted

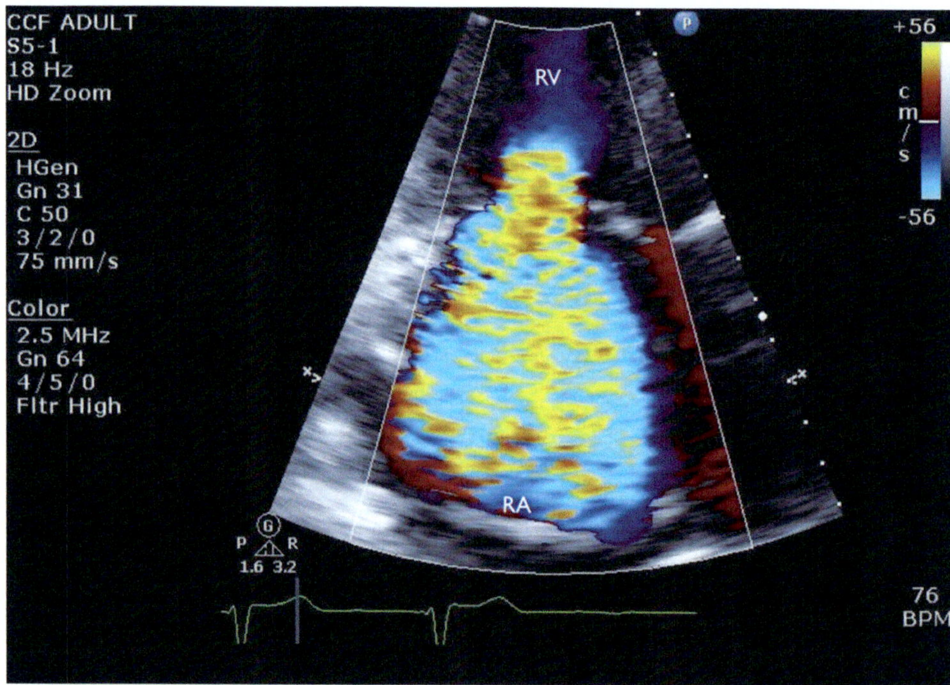

Fig. 5.16 Color Doppler imaging across the tricuspid valve confirms the presence of associated severe tricuspid regurgitation

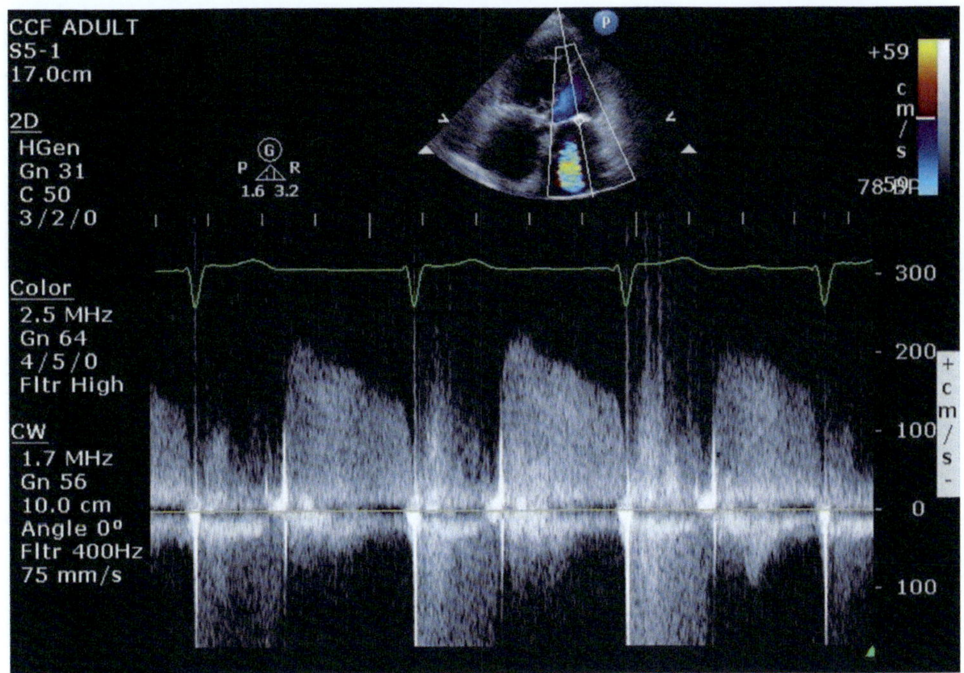

Fig. 5.17 Continuous wave Doppler imaging through the mitral valve confirms severe mitral stenosis (mean gradient 12 mmHg)

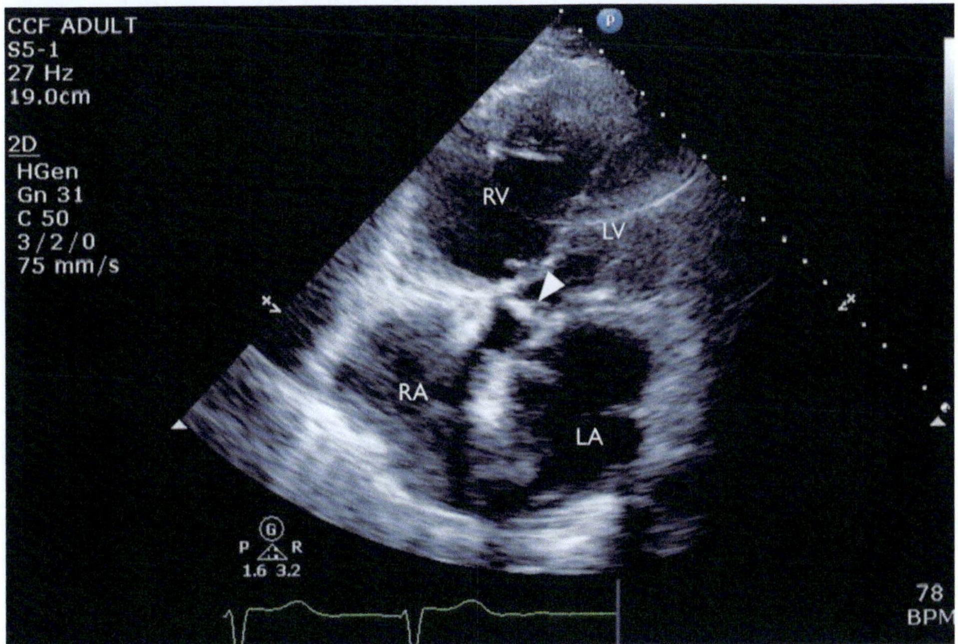

Fig. 5.18 TTE (five-chamber view) showing calcified and thickened aortic valve with restricted opening (*arrowhead*)

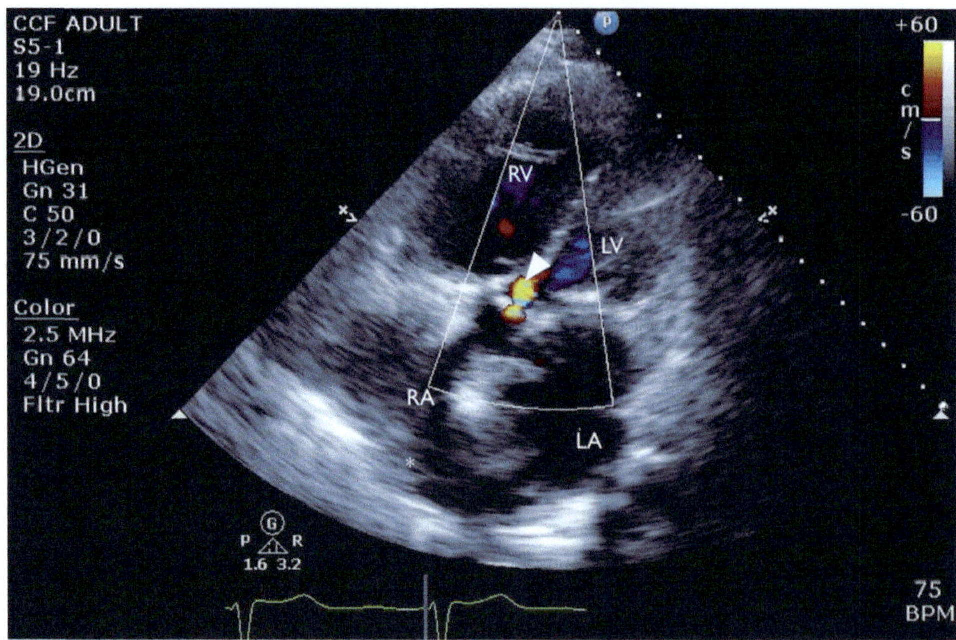

Fig. 5.19 TTE (five-chamber view) with color Doppler flow showing mild aortic insufficiency (*arrowhead*)

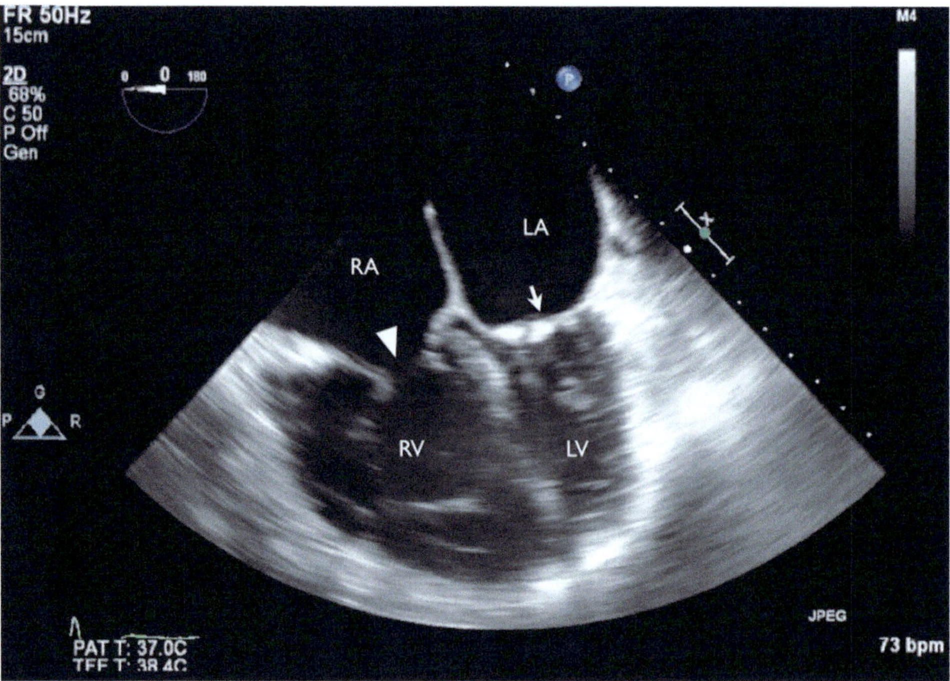

Fig. 5.20 TEE (four-chamber view) confirmed severely calcified mitral valve (*arrow*) with malcoapted tricuspid valve (*arrowhead*)

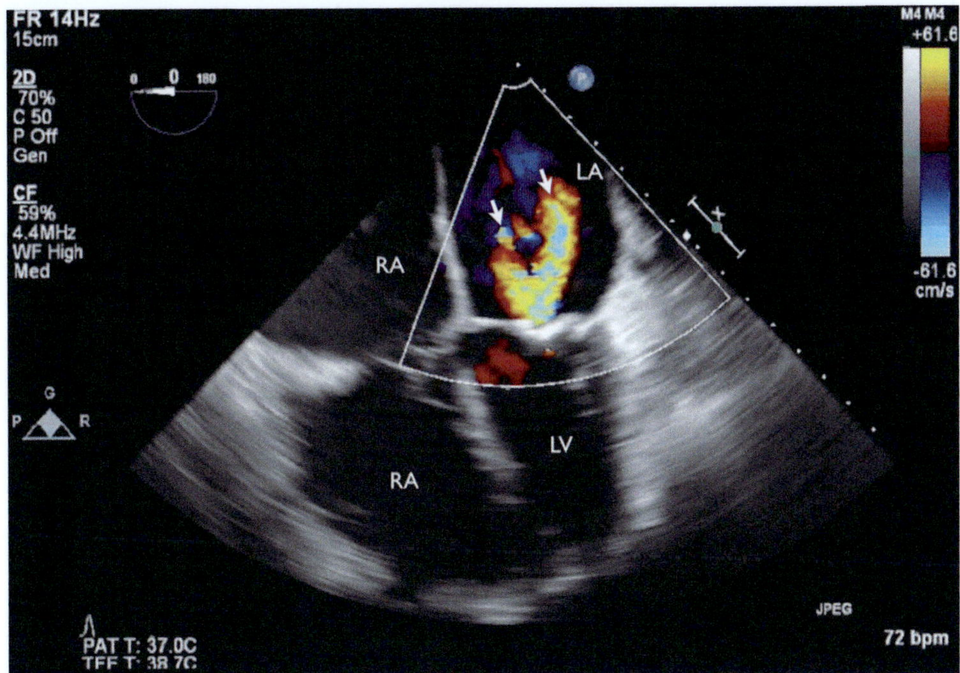

Fig. 5.21 TEE (four-chamber view) with color Doppler flow imaging confirmed moderate mitral regurgitation (*arrows*) and enlarged right-sided cardiac chambers

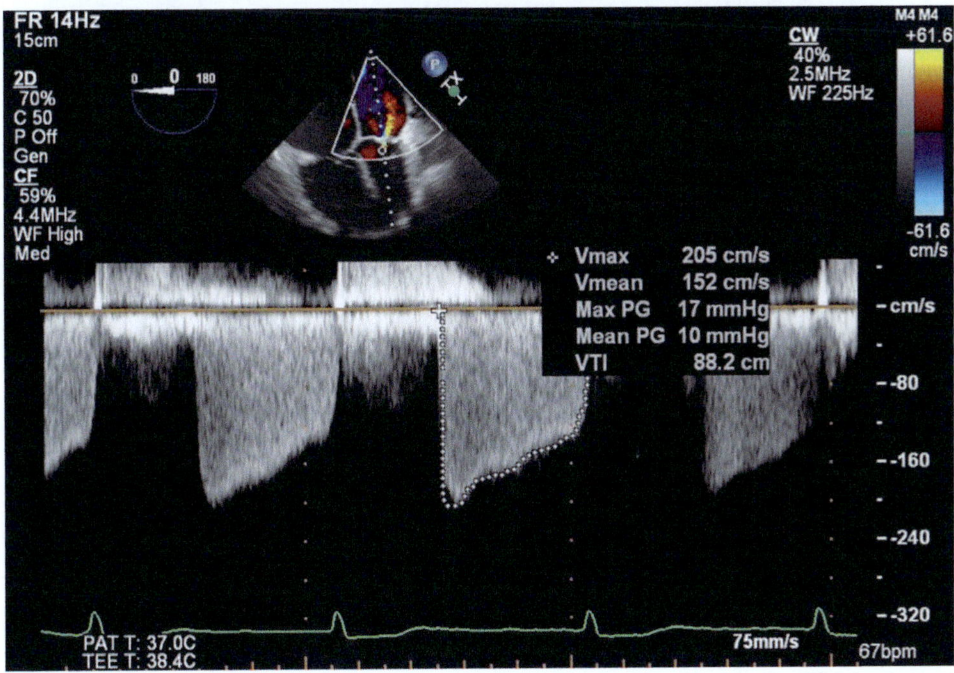

Fig. 5.22 Continuous wave Doppler imaging through the mitral valve confirms severe mitral stenosis (mean gradient 10 mmHg)

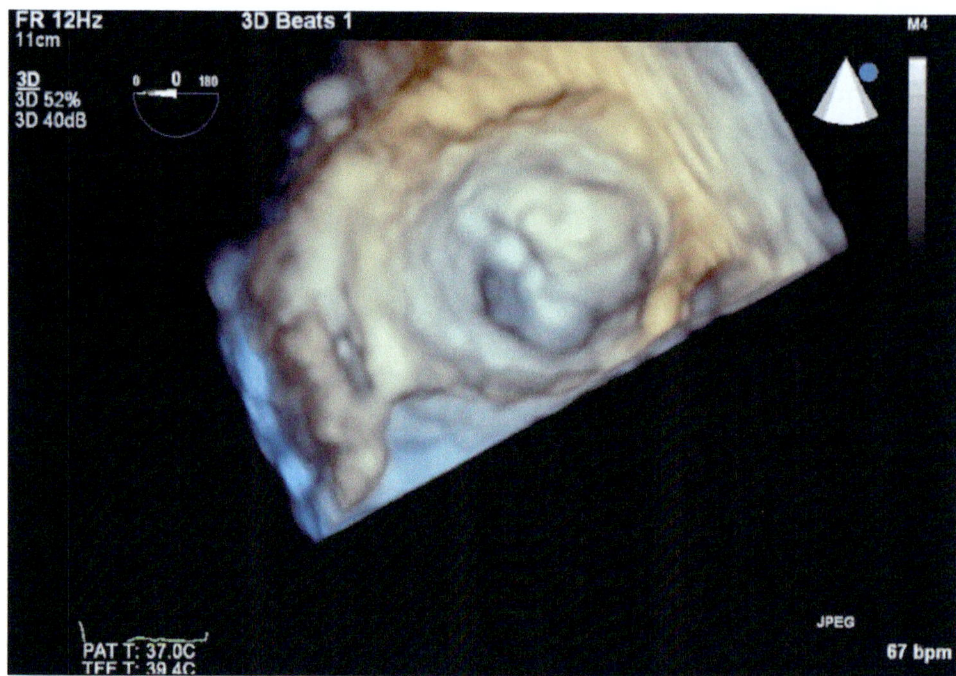

Fig. 5.23 Three-dimensional TEE of the mitral valve (surgical view) showed severe valve thickening with restricted opening

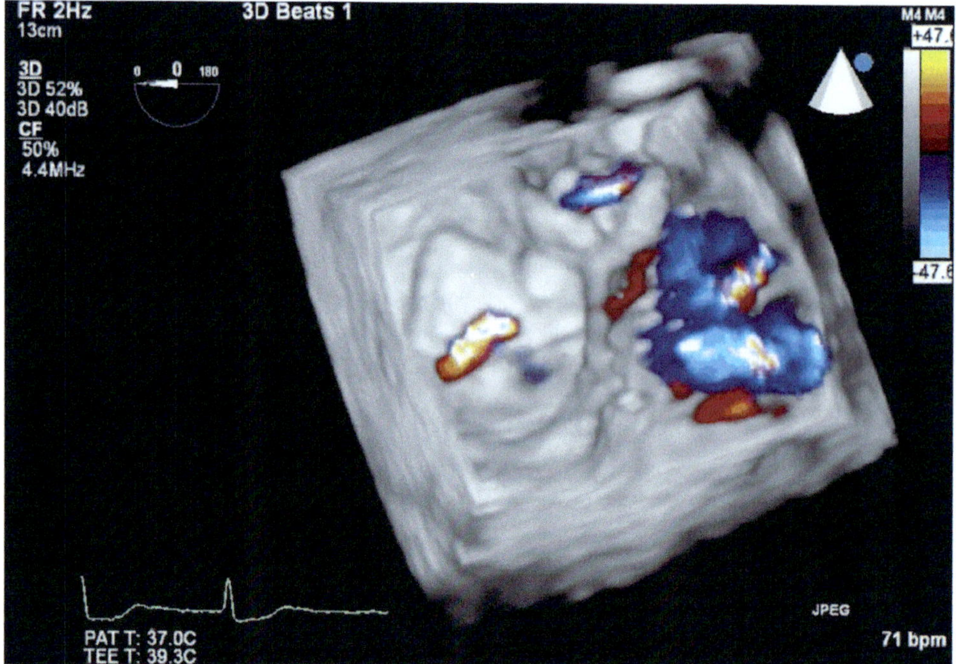

Fig. 5.24 Three-dimensional TEE with color Doppler imaging showed restricted opening and a turbulent jet through the mitral valve during diastole

5.2.1 Learning Points

Surgical options involving the mitral valve include (1) closed commissurotomy, where the valve is opened blindly through the left atrium or left ventricle; (2) open commissurotomy, which allows more extensive surgery under direct visualization; and (3) mitral valve replacement, which is preferred in the presence of severe valvular thickening and subvalvular fibrosis with leaflet tethering. In addition to patients with suboptimal valve anatomy (or those in whom percutaneous mitral balloon commissurotomy has failed), patients with moderate or severe tricuspid regurgitation also may have a better outcome with a surgical approach that includes tricuspid valve repair [1]. This patient's severely calcified mitral valve was not suitable for PBMC, and her severe tricuspid regurgitation would benefit from tricuspid valve surgery.

5.3 Case 3. Rheumatic Mitral Regurgitation

A 44-year-old man with a history of progressive shortness of breath was admitted to the hospital owing to decompensated heart failure. He reported a 1-year history of orthopnea, as well as palpitations and dizziness, but denied syncope. Echocardiography showed severe mitral regurgitation (mean gradient 9 mmHg, ejection fraction 60 %) and mild mitral stenosis (valve area 1.9 cm^2). Catheterization revealed severe disease of the left main and left anterior descending arteries. The patient underwent successful mitral valve replacement and coronary artery bypass grafting (Figs. 5.25, 5.26, 5.27, 5.28, 5.29, and 5.30).

Video 5.17 TTE (parasternal long-axis view) showed a thickened mitral valve with diastolic doming and restricted opening, findings consistent with rheumatic mitral valve disease (AVI 3378 kb)

Video 5.18 TTE (parasternal long-axis view) with color Doppler imaging showed severe mitral regurgitation (AVI 4245 kb)

Video 5.19 TTE (four-chamber view) showed dilated left atrium with severe mitral valve thickening with restricted opening and closure (AVI 3318 kb)

Video 5.20 TTE (four-chamber view) zoomed at mitral valve and left atrium showed severe mitral regurgitation (AVI 3582 kb)

Video 5.21 TEE (four-chamber view) showed malcoapted mitral valve due to severe restriction of the leaflets (AVI 3196 kb)

Video 5.22 TEE (long-axis view) again showed malcoapted mitral valve due to severe restriction of the leaflets (AVI 3215 kb)

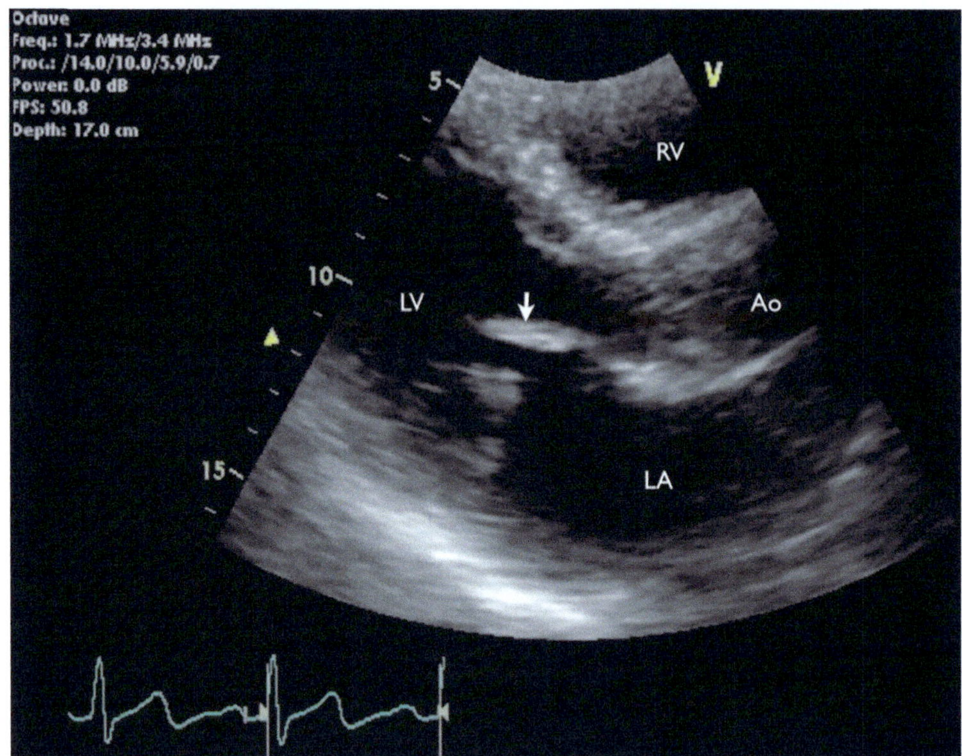

Fig. 5.25 TTE (parasternal long-axis view) showed a thickened mitral valve with diastolic doming and restricted opening, findings consistent with rheumatic mitral valve disease (*arrow*)

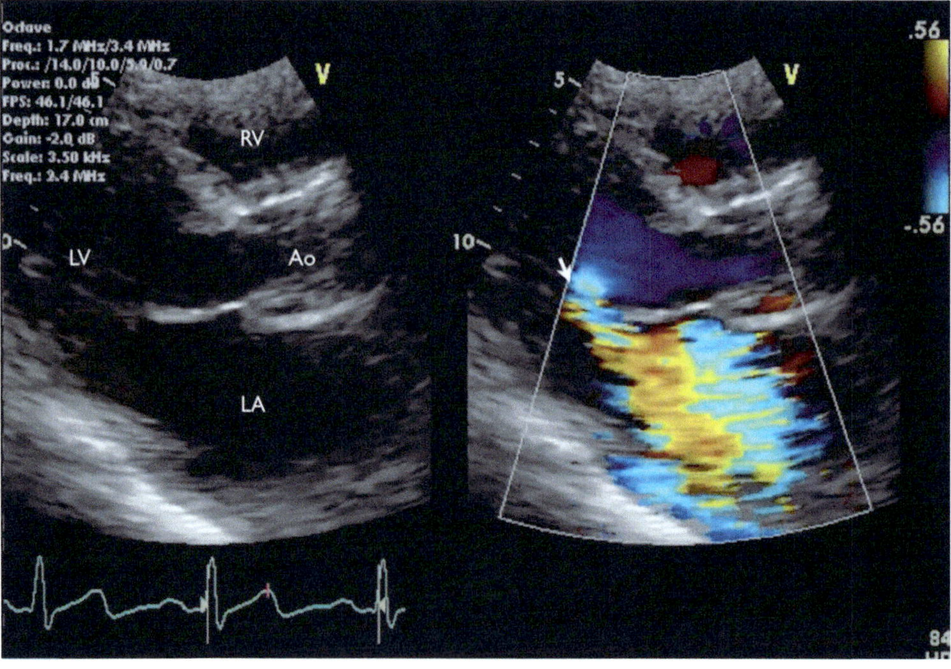

Fig. 5.26 TTE (parasternal long-axis view) with color Doppler imaging showed severe mitral regurgitation (*arrow*)

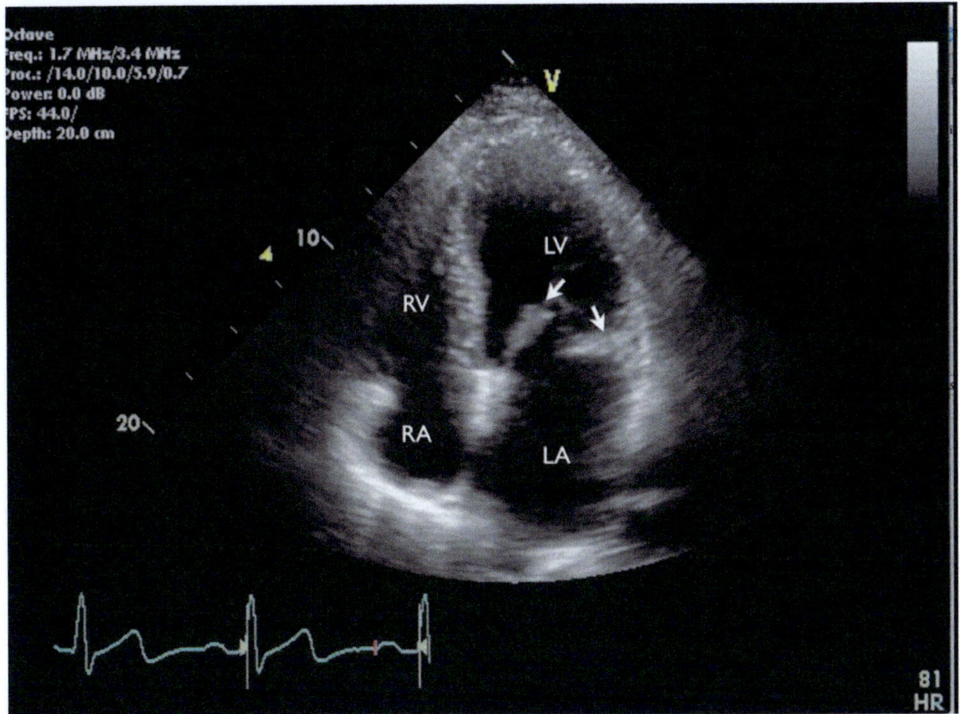

Fig. 5.27 TTE (four-chamber view) showed dilated left atrium with severe mitral valve thickening with restricted opening and closure (*arrows*)

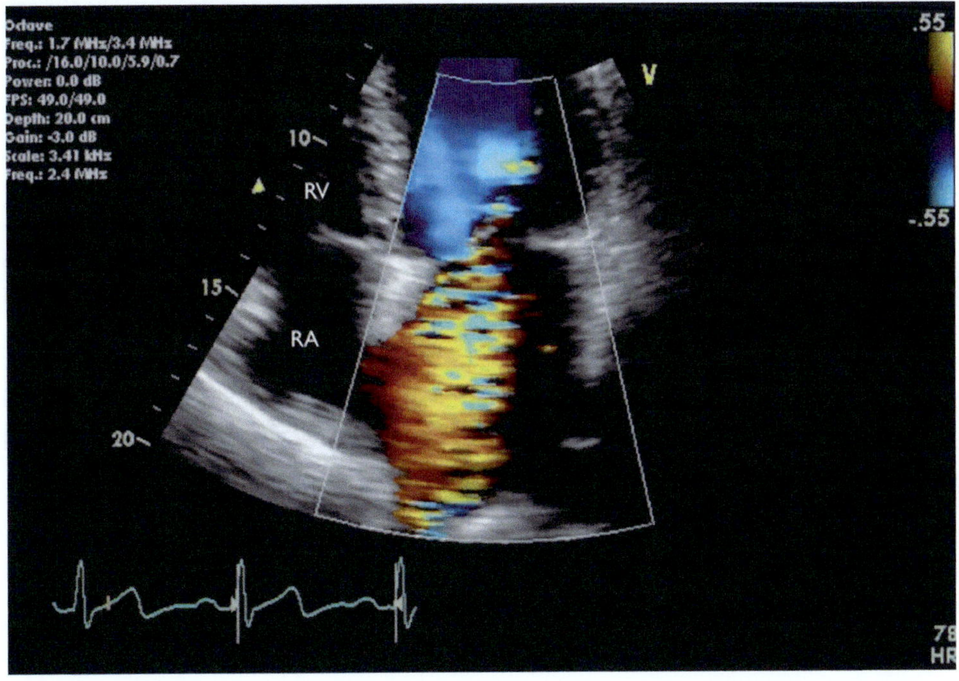

Fig. 5.28 TTE (four-chamber view) zoomed at mitral valve and left atrium showed severe mitral regurgitation

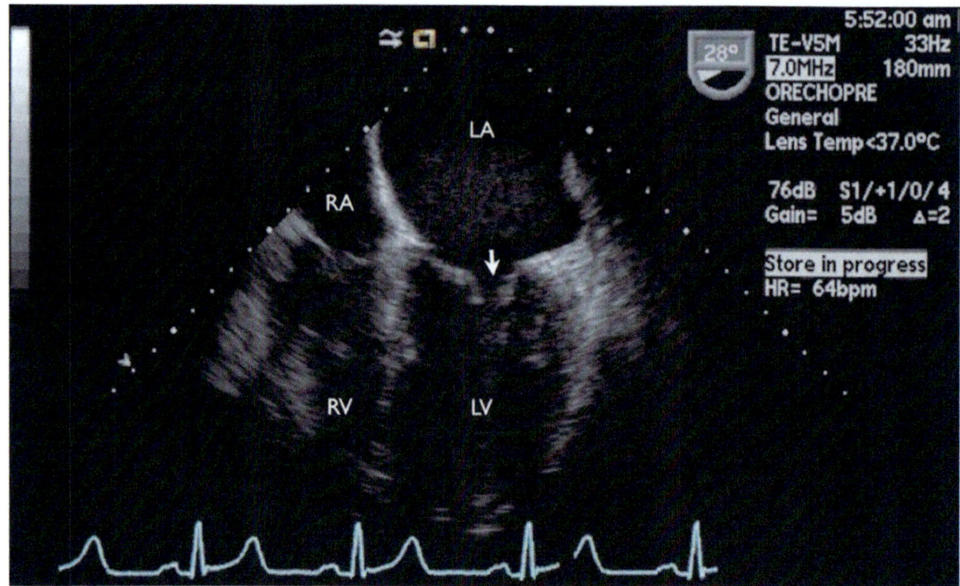

Fig. 5.29 TEE (four-chamber view) showed malcoapted mitral valve due to severe restriction of the leaflets (*arrow*)

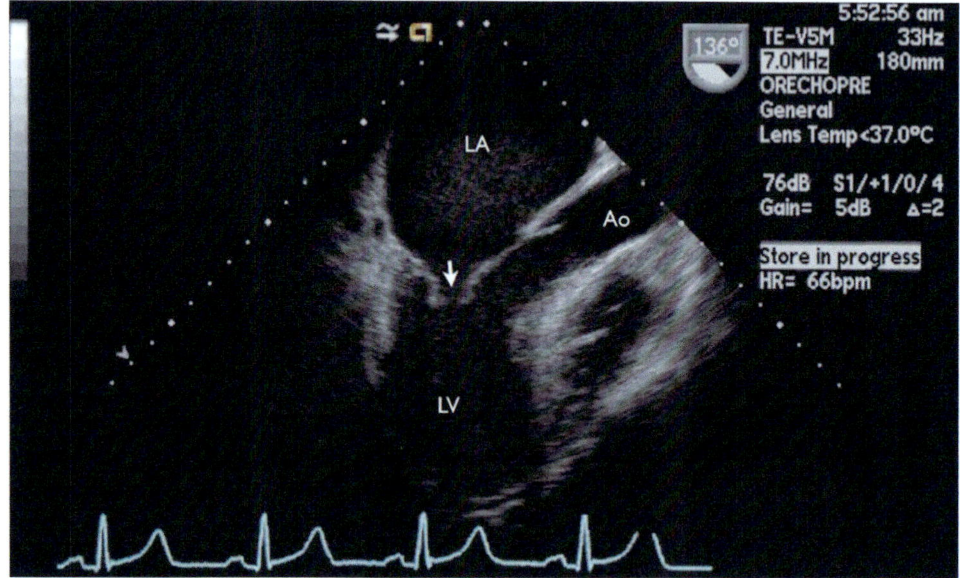

Fig. 5.30 TEE (long-axis view) again showed malcoapted mitral valve due to severe restriction of the leaflets (*arrow*)

5.3.1   Learning Points

Rheumatic mitral regurgitation causes retraction of tendinous chords and leaflets, as well as annular dilation, thus compromising coaptation between the two leaflets and was classified as Type IIIa mitral regurgitation according to Carpentier's classification. Similar changes are observed in postinflammatory and postradiotherapy MR. Morphological features of rheumatic mitral valve disease include anterior mitral valve leaflet thickening, chordal thickening, restricted leaflet motion, and excessive leaflet tip motion during systole. Excessive leaflet tip motion is the result of elongation of the primary chords, and is defined as displacement of the tip or edge of an involved leaflet towards the left atrium resulting in abnormal coaptation and regurgitation. It is the predominant mechanism of mitral regurgitation in the setting of acute rheumatic carditis. Excessive leaflet tip motion does not need to meet the standard echocardiographic definition of the mitral valve prolapse disease, as that refers to a different disease process.

Reference

1. Nishimura RA, Otto CM, Bonow RO, Carabello BA, Erwin 3rd JP, Guyton RA, et al. ACC/AHA Task Force Members. 2014 AHA/ACC guideline for the management of patients with valvular heart disease: a report of the American College of Cardiology/American Heart Association Task Force on Practice Guidelines. Circulation. 2014;129:e521–643.

Christine Jellis

6.1 Devices

6.1.1 MitraClip

The MitraClip (Fig. 6.1) is a percutaneous mitral valve repair system from Abbott Vascular. The device incorporates a steerable guide catheter that traverses the interatrial septum and enables accurate positioning and trajectory of the clip (Fig. 6.2).

The clip itself consists of two arms and two grippers. Using catheter guidance, the leaflets are positioned in the base of the V shape created between the gripper and clip arm. Once there is appropriate leaflet stability, the device is deployed from the catheter with the leaflet tips sandwiched between the gripper and clip arm on either side (Fig. 6.3). The goal is to deploy the clip perpendicular to the valve leaflets with complete leaflet insertion bilaterally and stable leaflet tissue medial and lateral to the clip (Fig. 6.4).

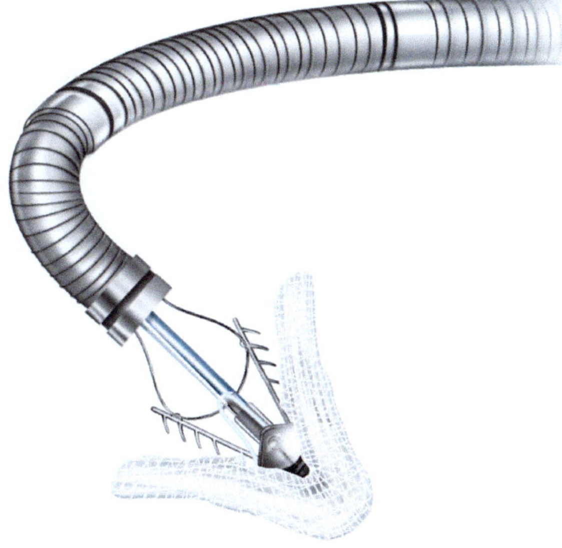

Fig. 6.1 MitraClip device (Abbott Vascular)

Electronic supplementary material The online version of this chapter (doi:10.1007/978-1-4471-6672-6_6) contains supplementary material, which is available to authorized users.

C. Jellis
Department of Cardiovascular Medicine, Cleveland Clinic,
9500 Euclid Avenue, Cleveland, OH 44195, USA
e-mail: jellisc@ccf.org

M. Desai et al. (eds.), *An Atlas of Mitral Valve Imaging*,
DOI 10.1007/978-1-4471-6672-6_6, © Springer-Verlag London 2015

Fig. 6.2 (**a**) Mechanism of MitraClip. (**b**) Clip and guide catheter

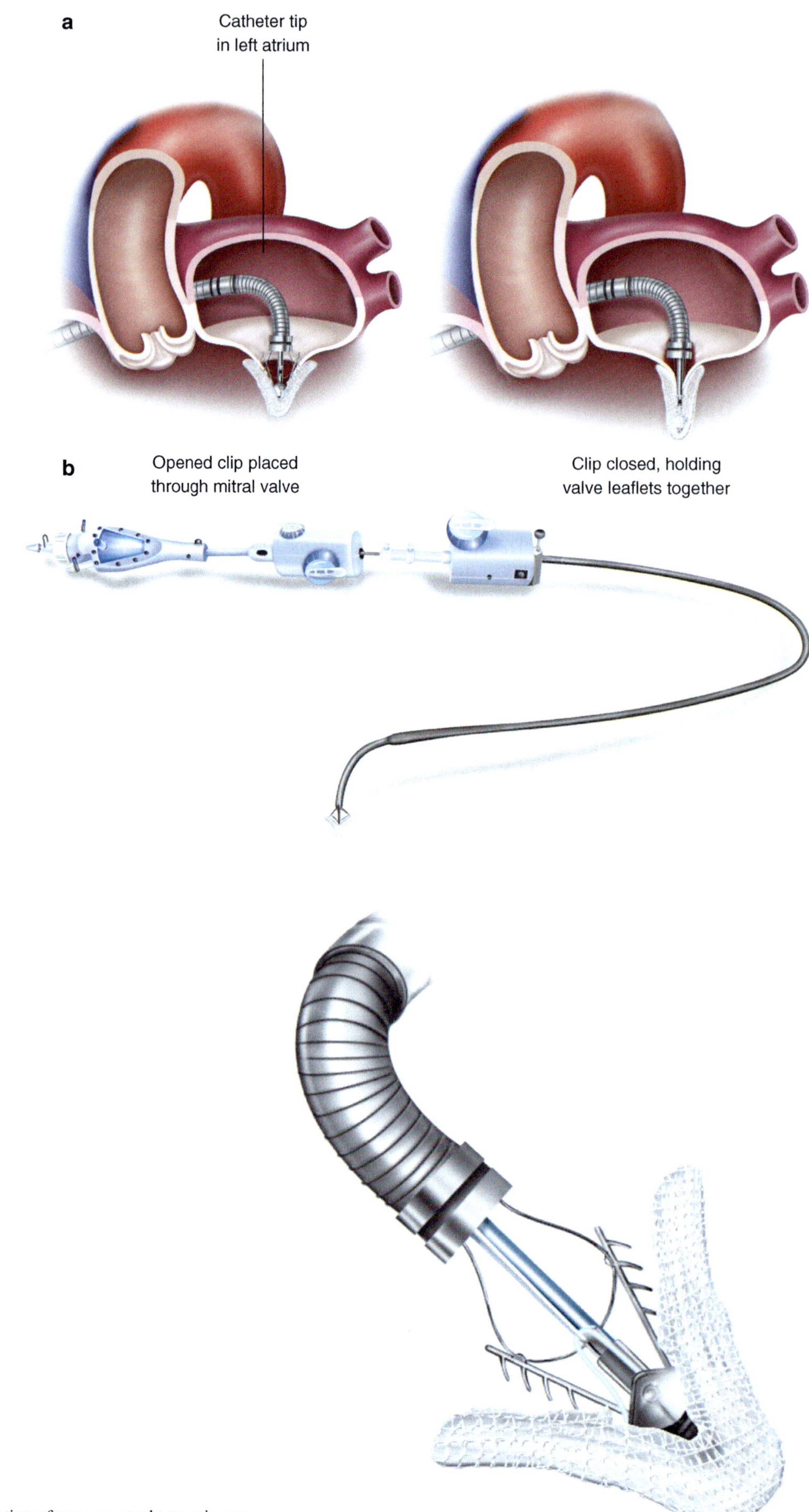

Fig. 6.3 MitraClip device, consisting of two arms and two grippers

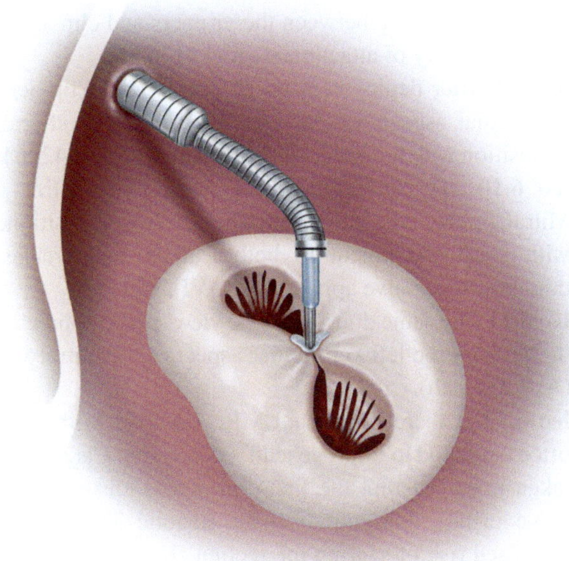

Fig. 6.4 The MitraClip is deployed perpendicular to the valve leaflets, with complete leaflet insertion bilaterally and stable leaflet tissue medial and lateral to the clip

6.1.2 Occluder Devices

The Amplatzer Vascular Plug II from St. Jude Medical is a representative example of the current generation of occluder devices (Fig. 6.5). These products are designed for precise, catheter-guided delivery and can be recaptured and repositioned to optimize orientation prior to final deployment. They typically have a Nitinol mesh design and come in a variety of different sizes. These features make them ideally suited for percutaneous closure of mitral paravalvular leaks, thereby allowing some patients to avoid redoing of open mitral valve surgery.

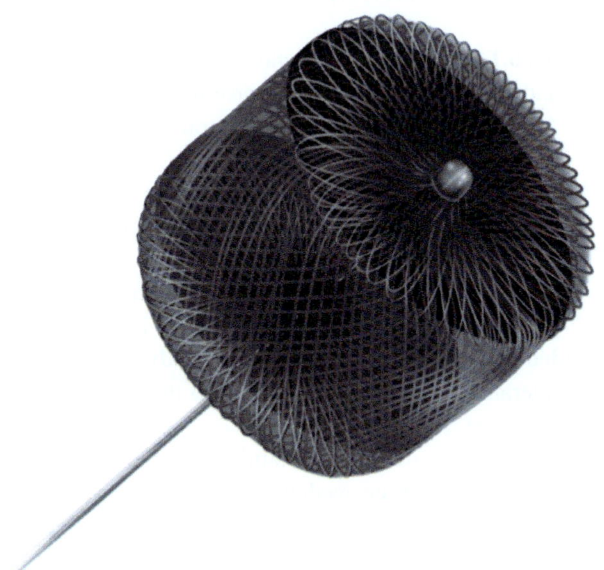

Fig. 6.5 The Amplatzer Vascular Plug II (St. Jude Medical) is a representative example of the current generation of occluder devices

6.2 Case 1. Procedural Steps for MitraClip Deployment

An 82-year-old man with a past history of coronary artery bypass graft surgery, chronic obstructive pulmonary disease (COPD) on home oxygen, an abdominal aortic aneurysm, and mitral valve prolapse presented for evaluation of worsening fatigue and shortness of breath at rest in the setting of severe mitral regurgitation. Because of his significant comorbidities, he had been previously managed medically for his mitral valve disease. He was referred for MitraClip, which was performed under transesophageal guidance (Figs. 6.6, 6.7, 6.8, 6.9, 6.10, 6.11, 6.12, 6.13, 6.14, 6.15, 6.16, 6.17, 6.18, 6.19, 6.20, 6.21, 6.22, 6.23, and 6.24).

Video 6.1 Transesophageal echo (TEE) biplane view at 125° and 11°, demonstrating excessive motion and flail of the A2 segment of the anterior mitral valve leaflet (AVI 3872 kb)

Video 6.2 TEE biplane view at 125° and 11°, demonstrating severe posterolaterally directed mitral regurgitation (AVI 1180 kb)

Video 6.3 Tenting of the interatrial septum to confirm the position prior to septostomy (AVI 7690 kb)

Video 6.4 The guide catheter is then advanced across the interatrial septum to gain access to the left atrium (AVI 4432 kb)

Video 6.5 The device is positioned in the left atrium to ensure appropriate medial-lateral and anterior-posterior alignment with the mitral valve (AVI 6117 kb)

Video 6.6 The device can be seen approaching the valve, using 3D imaging (AVI 2332 kb)

Video 6.7 3D imaging can be used to visualize the MitraClip crossing the mitral valve (AVI 1962 kb)

Video 6.8 When both clip arms are adequately aligned, the clip is positioned perpendicular to the line of leaflet coaptation Both leaflet tips must be fully inserted on both sides of the device between the grippers and clip arms to ensure stability of attachment (AVI 4108 kb)

Video 6.9 After deployment on an initial MitraClip across the medial aspects of A2 and P2, there is good leaflet opposition with moderate (2+) residual MR (AVI 4226 kb)

Video 6.10 3D zoom imaging is used to visualize the MitraClip from the left atrium The clip is well positioned, with good attachment to both leaflets, and creates a double-orifice valve appearance (AVI 2359 kb)

Video 6.11 The same double-orifice view can be appreciated in 3D from the left ventricular aspect of the mitral valve (AVI 2311 kb)

Video 6.12 If there is residual MR, a second MitraClip is often deployed to improve leaflet coaptation Care must be taken not to disrupt the first clip and to ensure that the valve orifice does not become stenotic There is also increased risk of snaring the second clip in the subvalvular apparatus, as the chordae are now more centrally positioned after deployment of the first clip In this example, deployment of a second clip is seen immediately adjacent to the first clip on the lateral aspect of the A2 and P2 scallops (biplane view) (AVI 4300 kb)

Video 6.13 An excellent final result is achieved, with only trivial MR seen on this bicommissural view with simultaneous gray-scale and color Doppler images (AVI 5098 kb)

Video 6.14 Trivial MR is confirmed on a long-axis view with simultaneous gray-scale and color Doppler images (AVI 5190 kb)

Video 6.15 The adjacent MitraClips create a double orifice mitral valve, which can be visualized in 3D from both the left ventricular (*left image*) and left atrial (*right image*) aspects (AVI 2534 kb)

Video 6.16 An expected trivial to mild residual left-to-right interatrial shunt was noted at the septostomy site on color Doppler imaging (AVI 5364 kb)

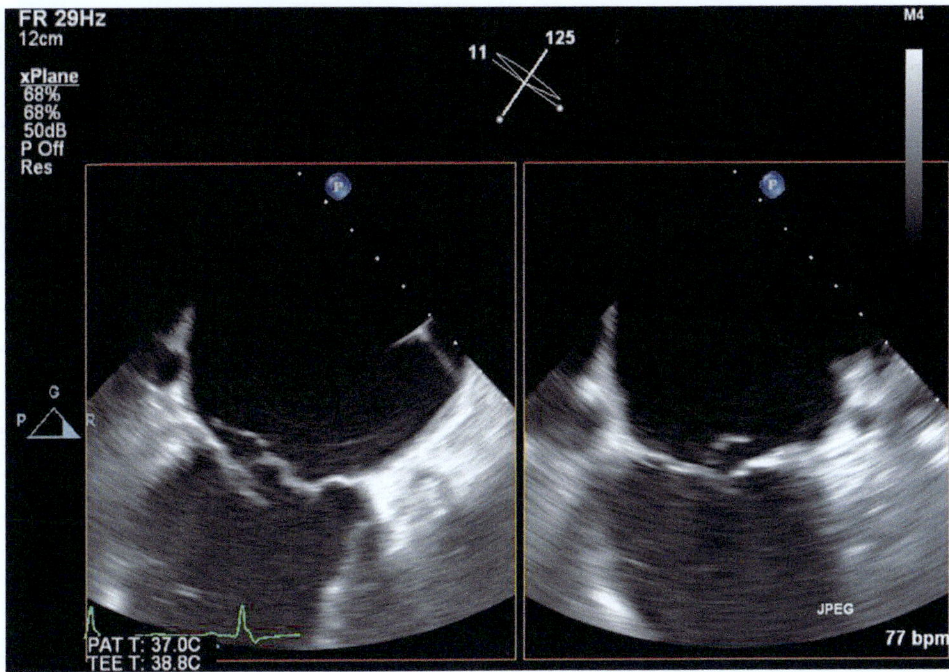

Fig. 6.6 Transesophageal echo (TEE) biplane view at 125° and 11°, demonstrating excessive motion and flail of the A2 segment of the anterior mitral valve leaflet

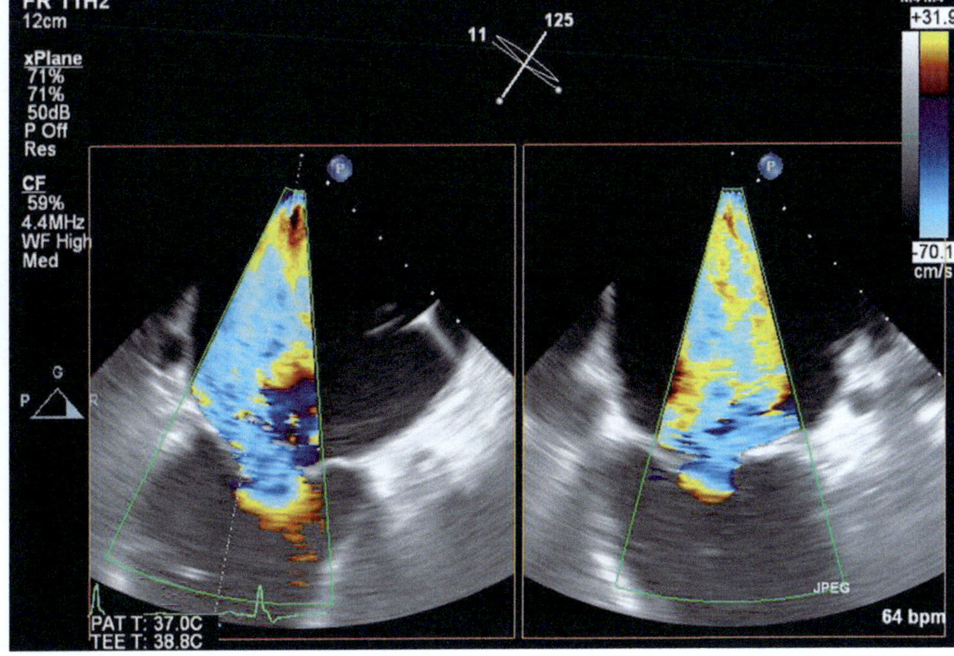

Fig. 6.7 TEE biplane view at 125° and 11°, demonstrating severe posterolaterally directed mitral regurgitation (MR)

Fig. 6.8 A proximal isovelocity surface area (PISA) of 1.7 cm^2 supports the diagnosis of severe MR

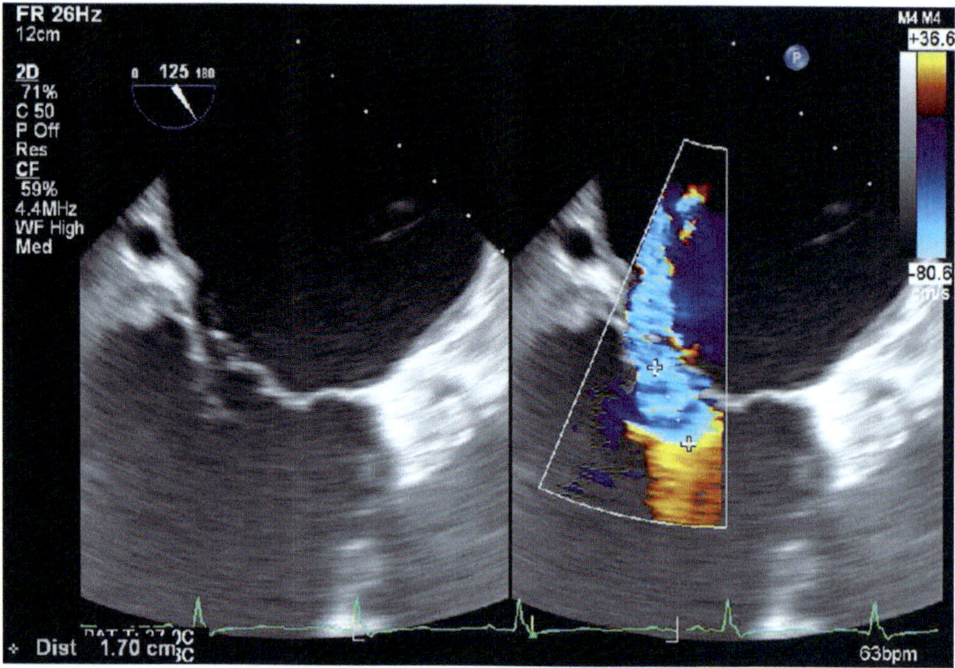

Fig. 6.9 Tenting of the interatrial septum to confirm the position prior to septostomy

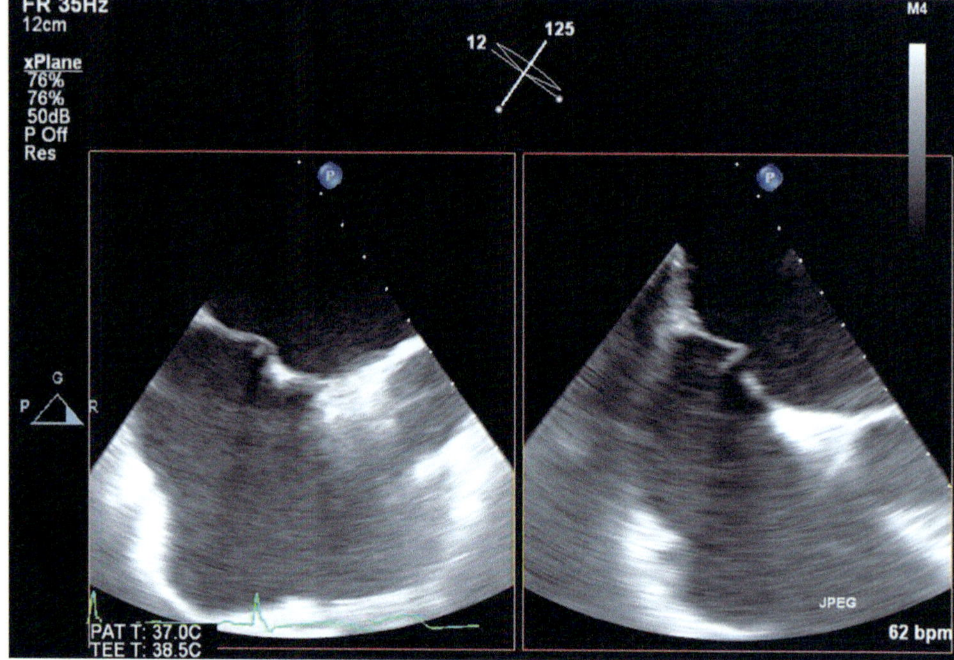

Fig. 6.10 The guide catheter is then advanced across the interatrial septum to gain access to the left atrium

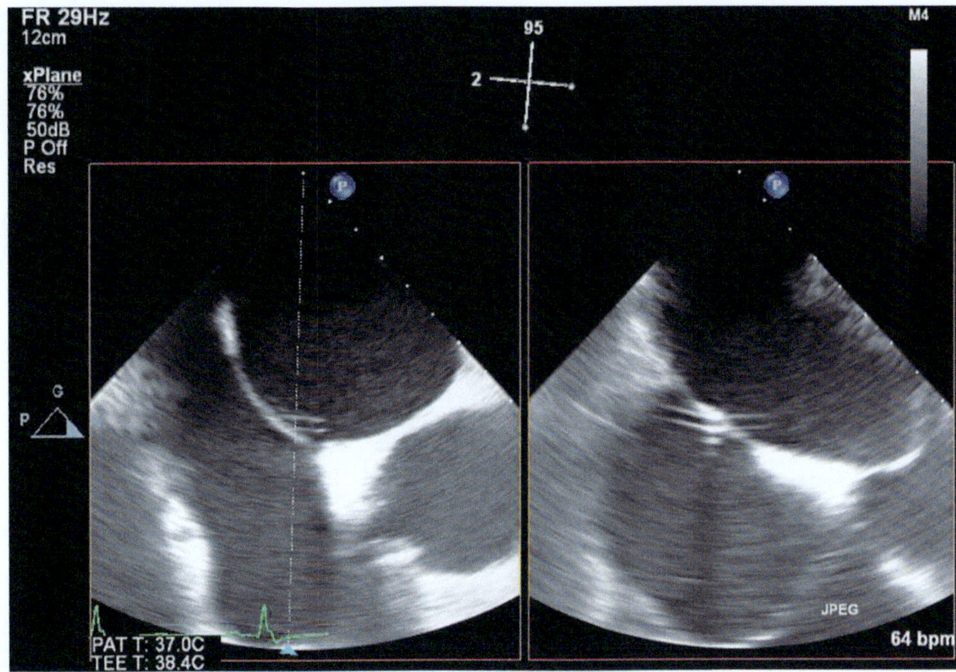

Fig. 6.11 The device is positioned in the left atrium to ensure appropriate medial-lateral and anterior-posterior alignment with the mitral valve

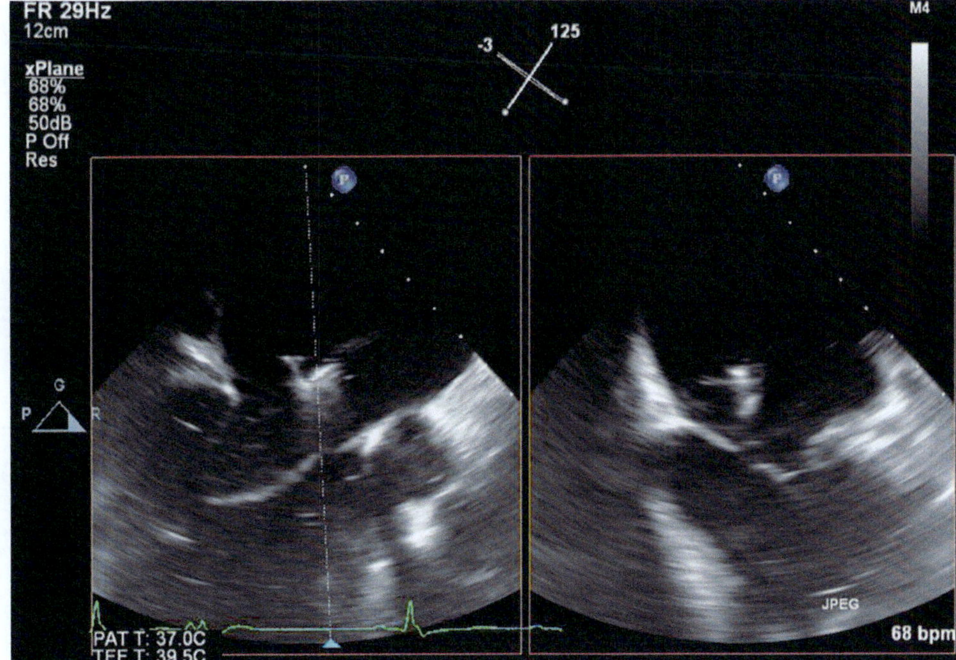

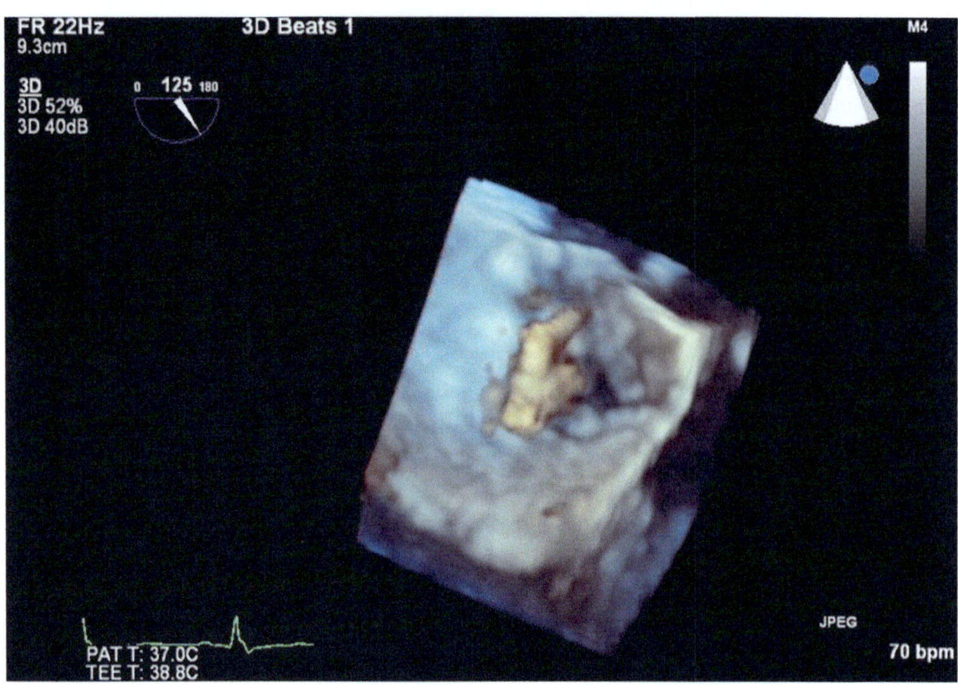

Fig. 6.12 The device can be seen approaching the valve, using 3D imaging

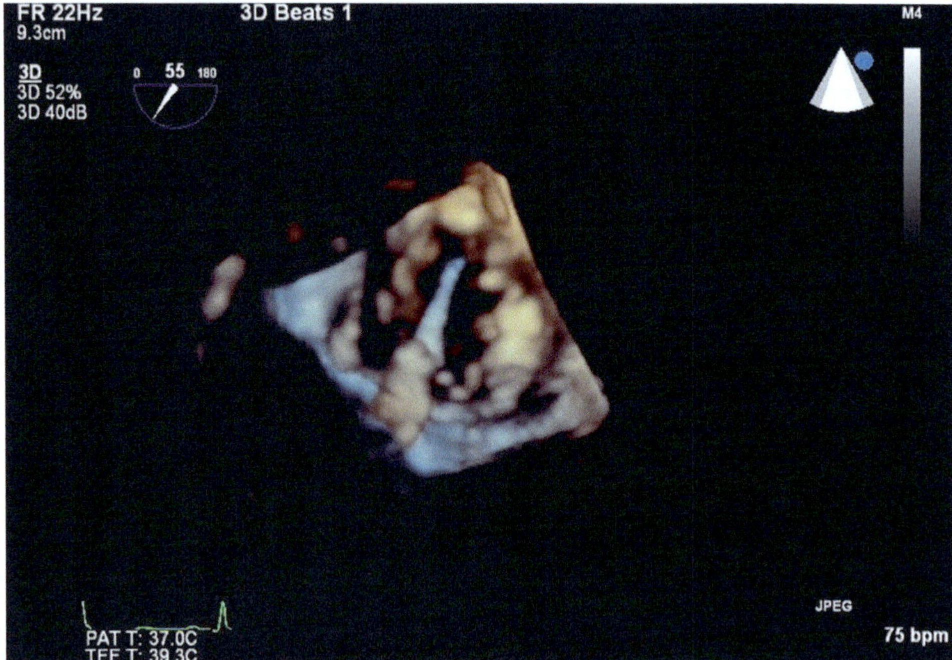

Fig. 6.13 3D imaging can be used to visualize the MitraClip crossing the mitral valve

Fig. 6.14 When both clip arms are adequately aligned, the clip is positioned perpendicular to the line of leaflet coaptation. Both leaflet tips must be fully inserted on both sides of the device between the grippers and clip arms to ensure stability of attachment

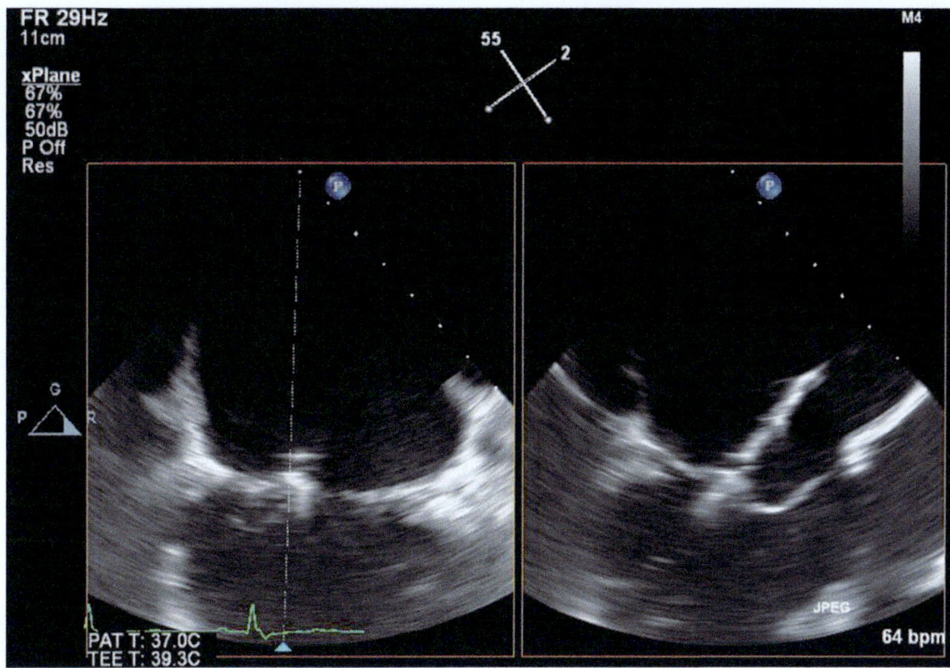

Fig. 6.15 After deployment on an initial MitraClip across the medial aspects of A2 and P2, there is good leaflet opposition with moderate (2+) residual MR

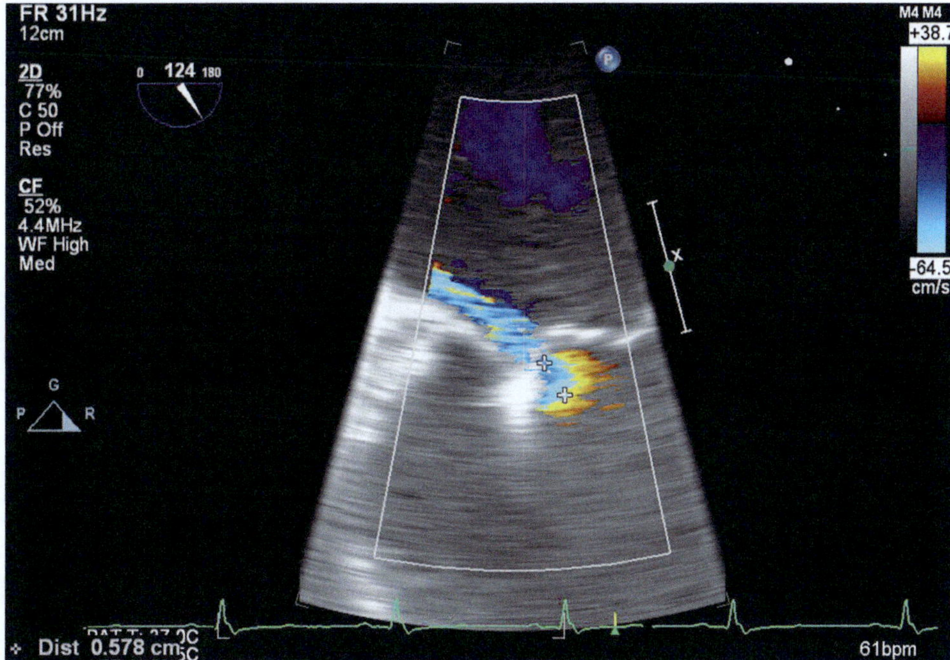

Fig. 6.16 3D zoom imaging is used to visualize the MitraClip from the left atrium. The clip is well positioned, with good attachment to both leaflets, and creates a double-orifice valve appearance

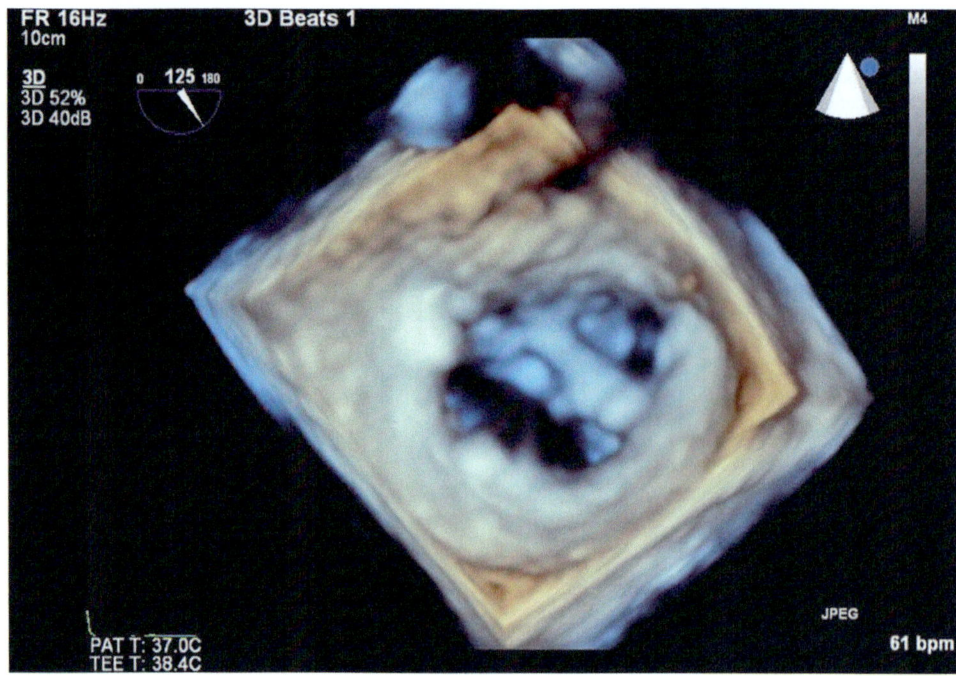

Fig. 6.17 The same double-orifice view can be appreciated in 3D from the left ventricular aspect of the mitral valve

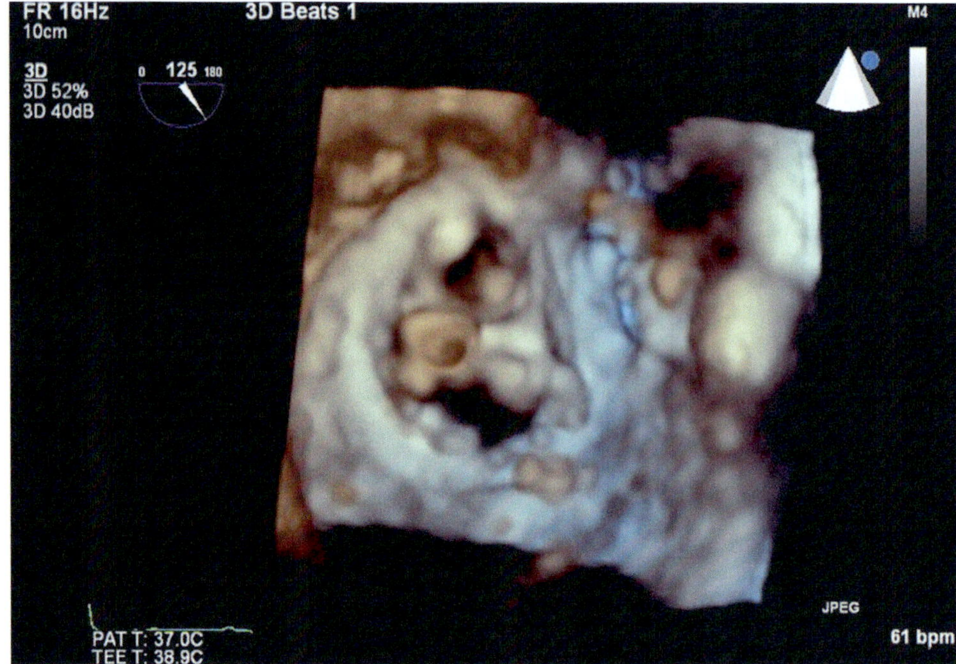

Fig. 6.18 If there is residual MR, a second MitraClip is often deployed to improve leaflet coaptation. Care must be taken not to disrupt the first clip and to ensure that the valve orifice does not become stenotic. There is also increased risk of snaring the second clip in the subvalvular apparatus, as the chordae are now more centrally positioned after deployment of the first clip. In this example, deployment of a second clip is seen immediately adjacent to the first clip on the lateral aspect of the A2 and P2 scallops (biplane view)

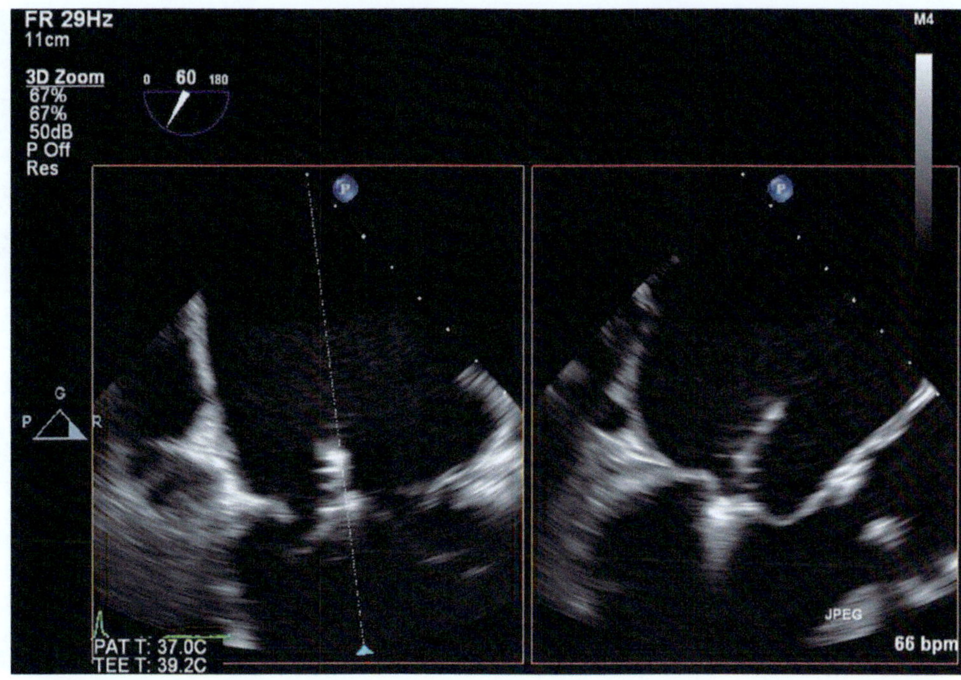

Fig. 6.19 An excellent final result is achieved, with only trivial MR seen on this bicommissural view with simultaneous gray-scale and color Doppler images

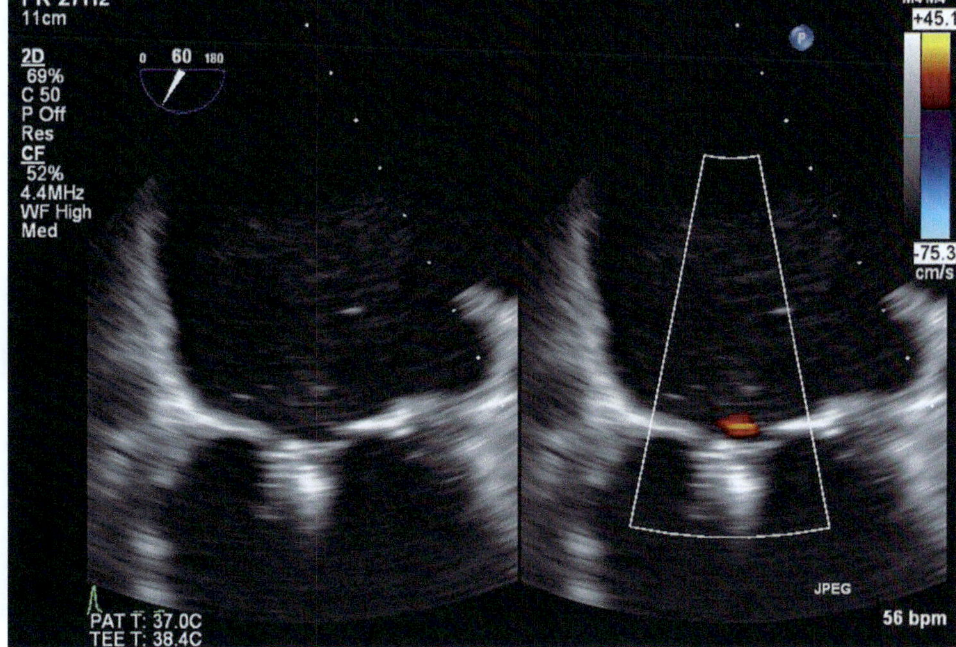

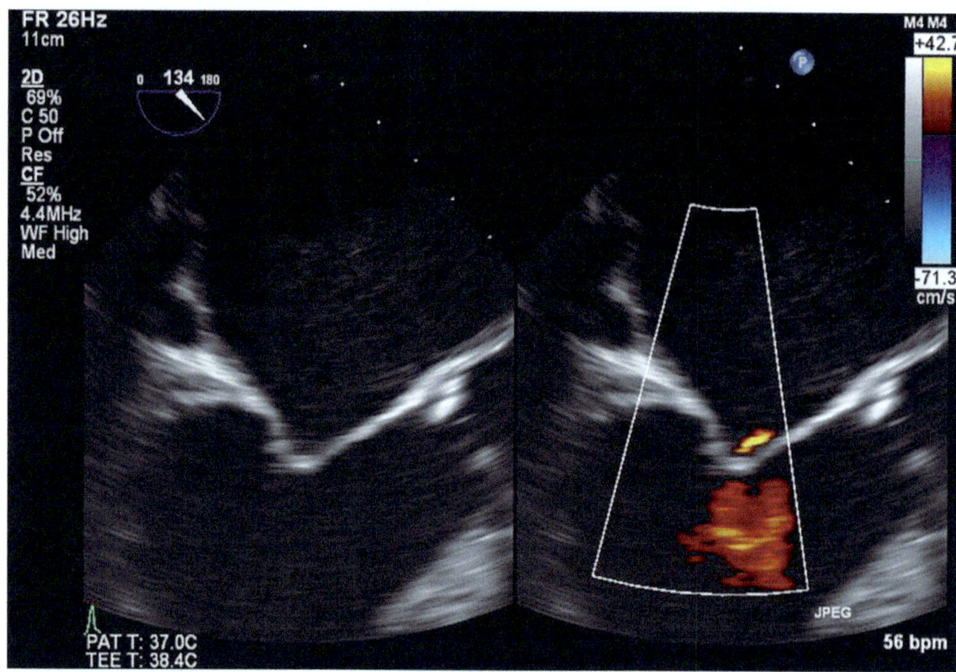

Fig. 6.20 Trivial MR is confirmed on a long-axis view with simultaneous gray-scale and color Doppler images

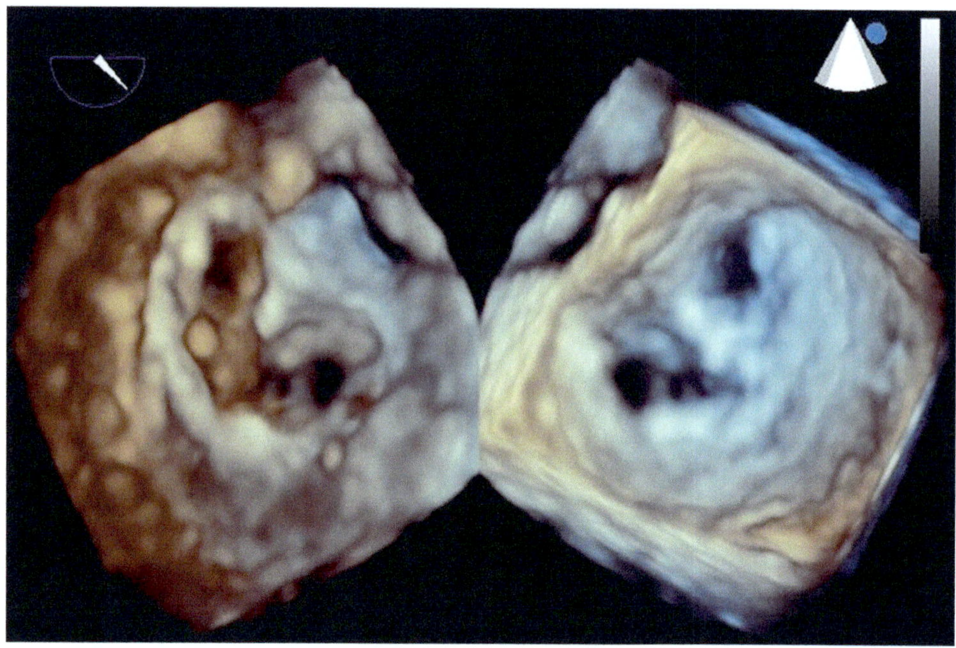

Fig. 6.21 The adjacent MitraClips create a double-orifice mitral valve, which can be visualized in 3D from both the left ventricular (*left image*) and left atrial (*right image*) aspects

Fig. 6.22 Continuous wave Doppler imaging across the mitral valve confirms that there is no hemodynamically significant stenosis related to deployment of the two MitraClips. Postprocedure transvalvular gradients were within normal limits (peak/mean 10/2 mmHg)

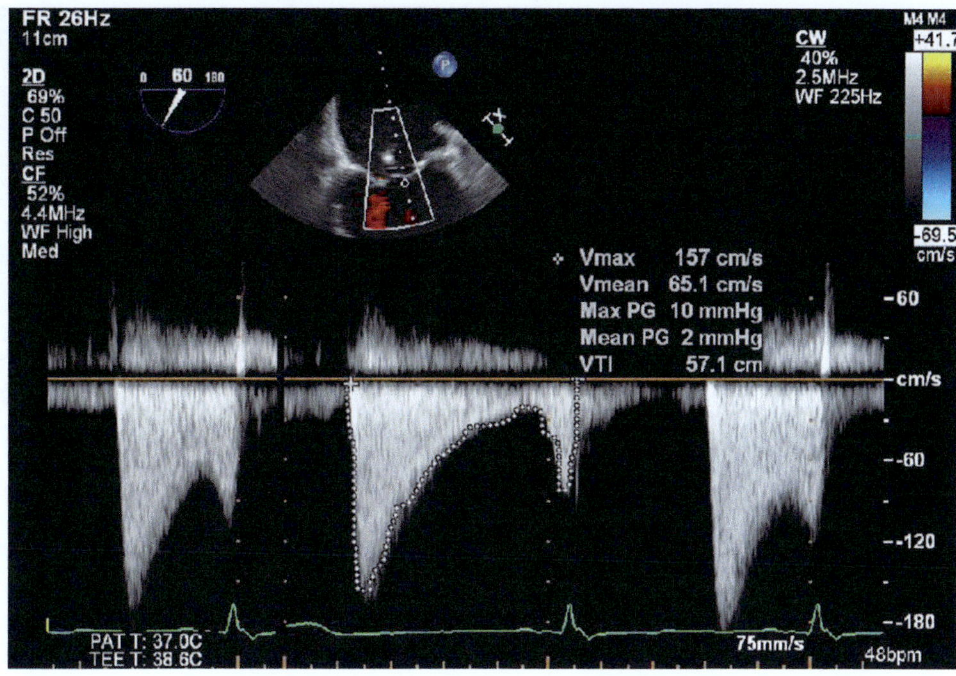

Fig. 6.23 Pulse wave Doppler imaging of the left upper pulmonary vein profile demonstrates normalization of the spectral trace, suggesting that left atrial pressures have already been reduced, related to the significant reduction in MR severity

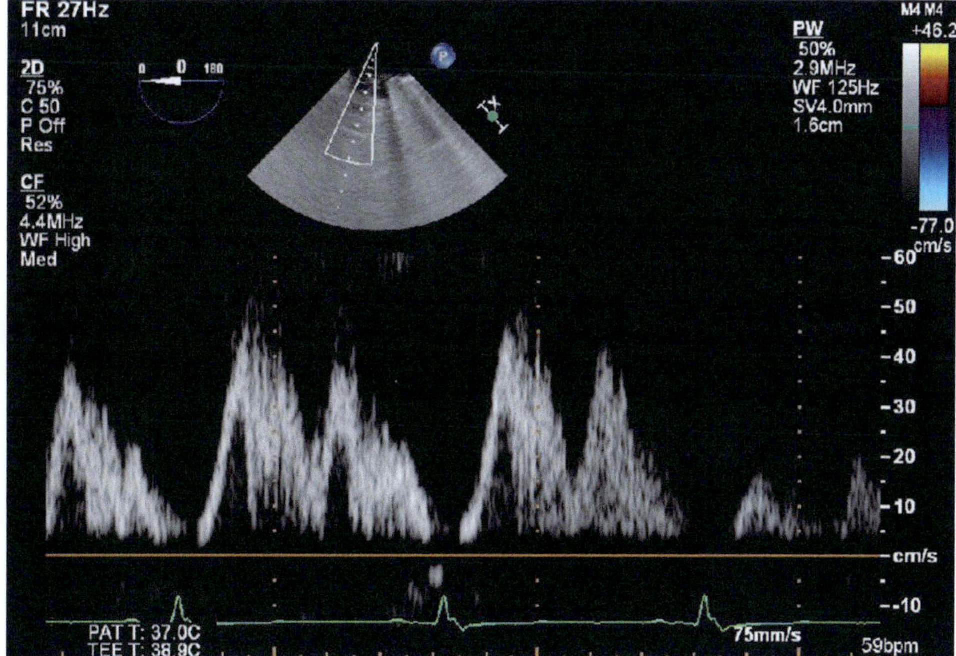

Fig. 6.24 An expected trivial to mild residual left-to-right interatrial shunt was noted at the septostomy site on color Doppler imaging

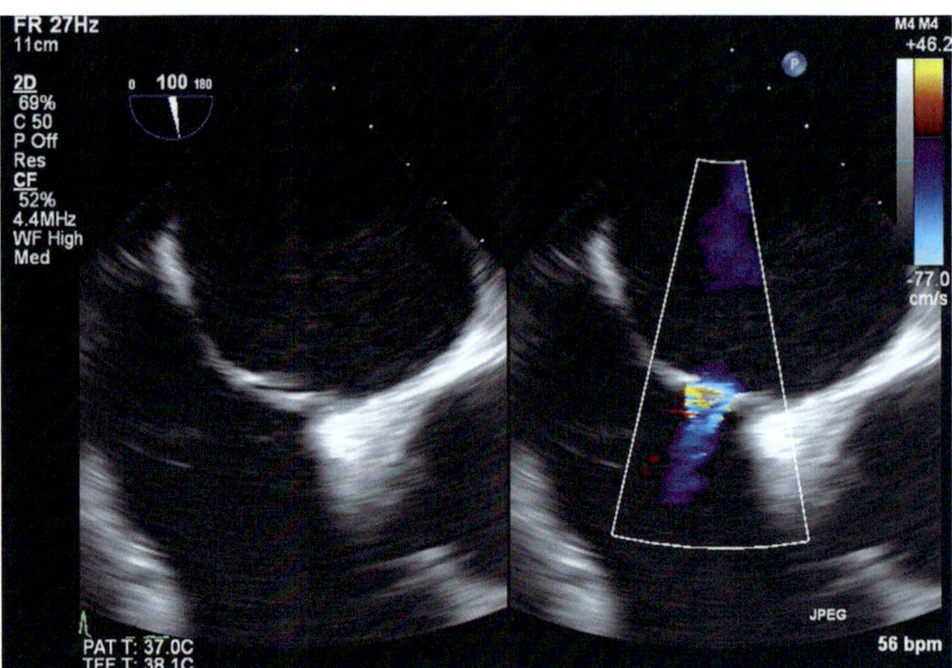

6.3   Case 2. MitraClip for Posterior Leaflet Prolapse

An 87-year-old man presented with progressive dyspnea on minimal exertion. He had known severe (4+) mitral regurgitation due to posterior leaflet prolapse with P2 flail and moderately severe pulmonary hypertension (right ventricular systolic pressure [RVSP] 73 mmHg). He declined surgery but was offered percutaneous mitral valve repair with a MitraClip. After the intervention, there was improvement in mitral regurgitation to 1+ and no associated stenosis (mean gradient of 2 mmHg) (Figs. 6.25, 6.26, 6.27, 6.28, 6.29, and 6.30).

Video 6.17 TEE 120° view shows the mitral valve with two MitraClips deployed side-by-side on the central and medial aspects of the valve, with good leaflet coaptation (AVI 10853 kb)

Video 6.18 TEE 120° view demonstrates mild (1+) residual central MR (AVI 2617 kb)

Video 6.19 Biplane view of the mitral valve in long-axis (125°) and off-axis (17°) four-chamber views, again showing the MitraClips (AVI 5001 kb)

Video 6.20 Biplane view of the mitral valve in long-axis (125°) and off-axis 4 chamber views (17°) with the MitraClips in situ and mild (1+) residual MR (AVI 1003 kb)

Video 6.21 3D zoom view of the mitral valve from the left atrial perspective The Mitraclips can be seen side-by-side, apposing the anterior and posterior leaflets (AVI 1076 kb)

Video 6.22 Use of Philips 3DQ reconstruction software demonstrates a multiplanar view of the mitral valve with the MitraClips in situ (AVI 1554 kb)

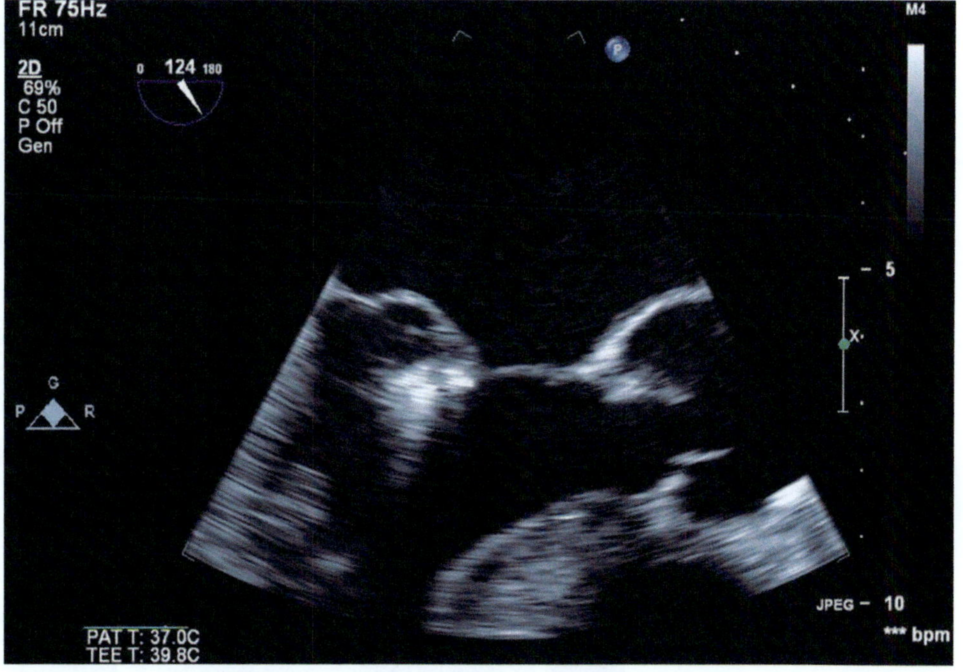

Fig. 6.25 TEE 120° view shows the mitral valve with two MitraClips deployed side-by-side on the central and medial aspects of the valve, with good leaflet coaptation

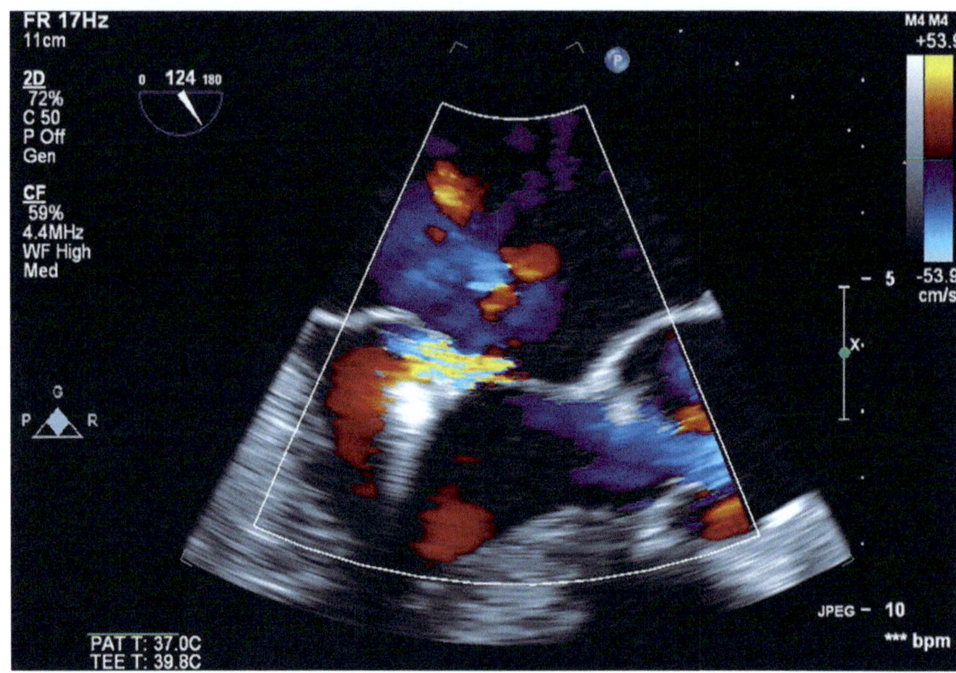

Fig. 6.26 TEE 120° view demonstrates mild (1+) residual central MR

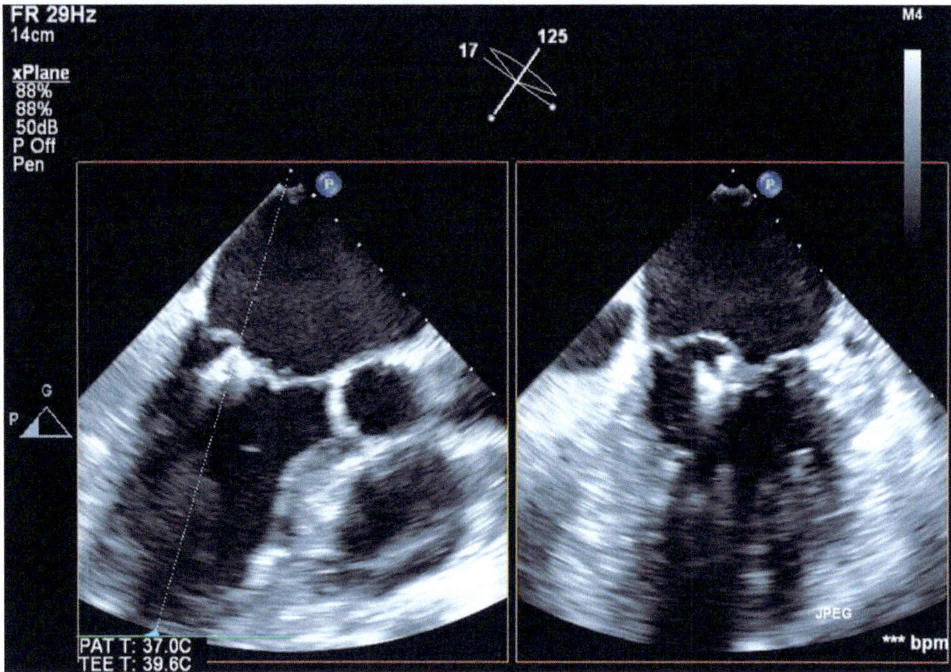

Fig. 6.27 Biplane view of the mitral valve in long-axis (125°) and off-axis four-chamber views (17°), again showing the MitraClips

Fig. 6.28 Biplane view of the mitral valve in long-axis (125°) and off-axis 4 chamber views (17°) with the MitraClips in situ and mild (1+) residual MR

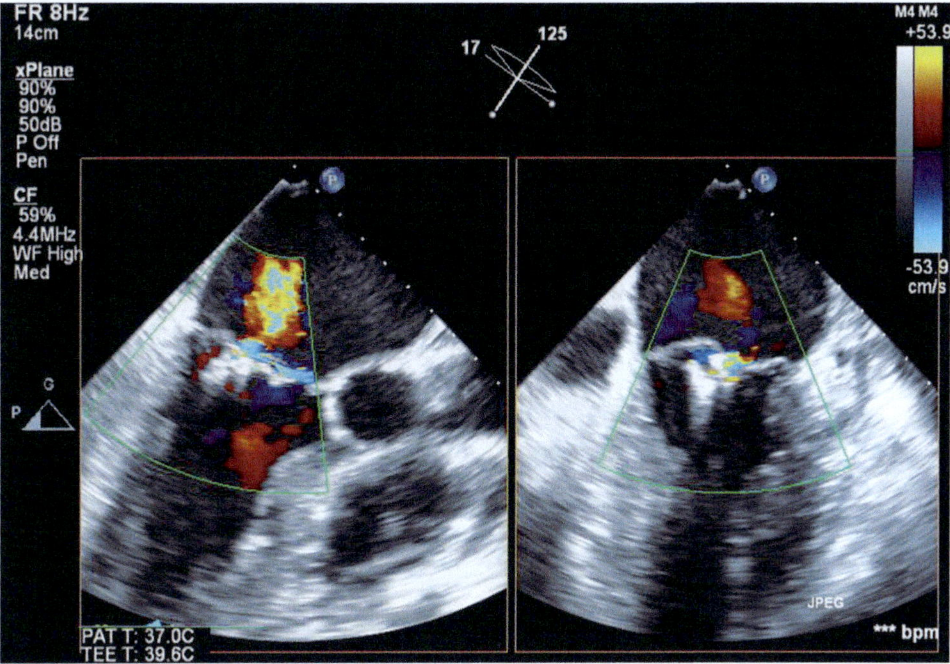

Fig. 6.29 3D zoom view of the mitral valve from the left atrial perspective. The Mitraclips can be seen side-by-side, apposing the anterior and posterior leaflets

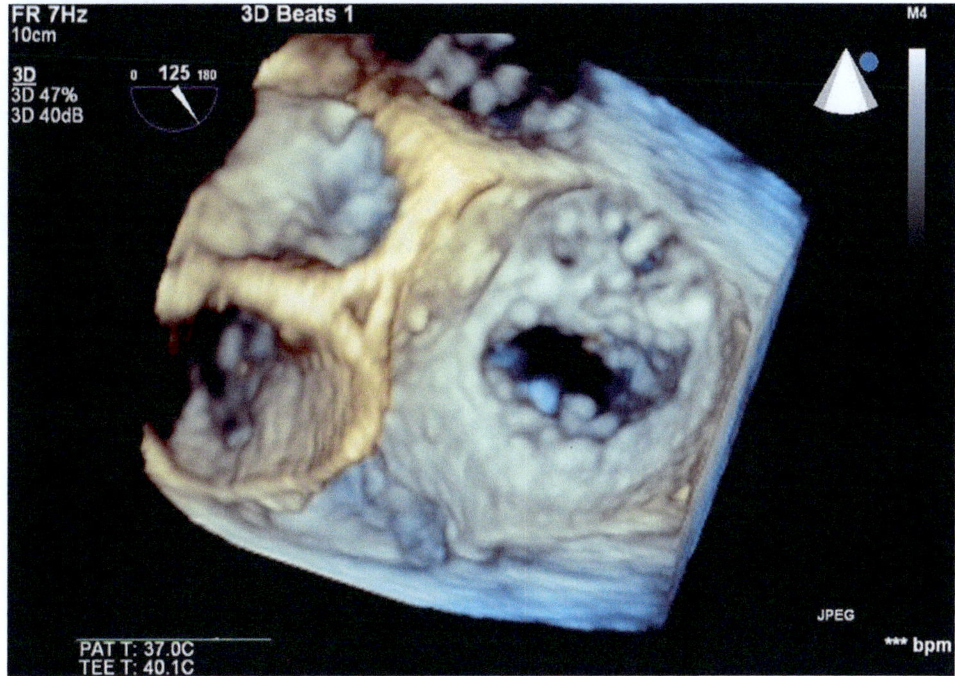

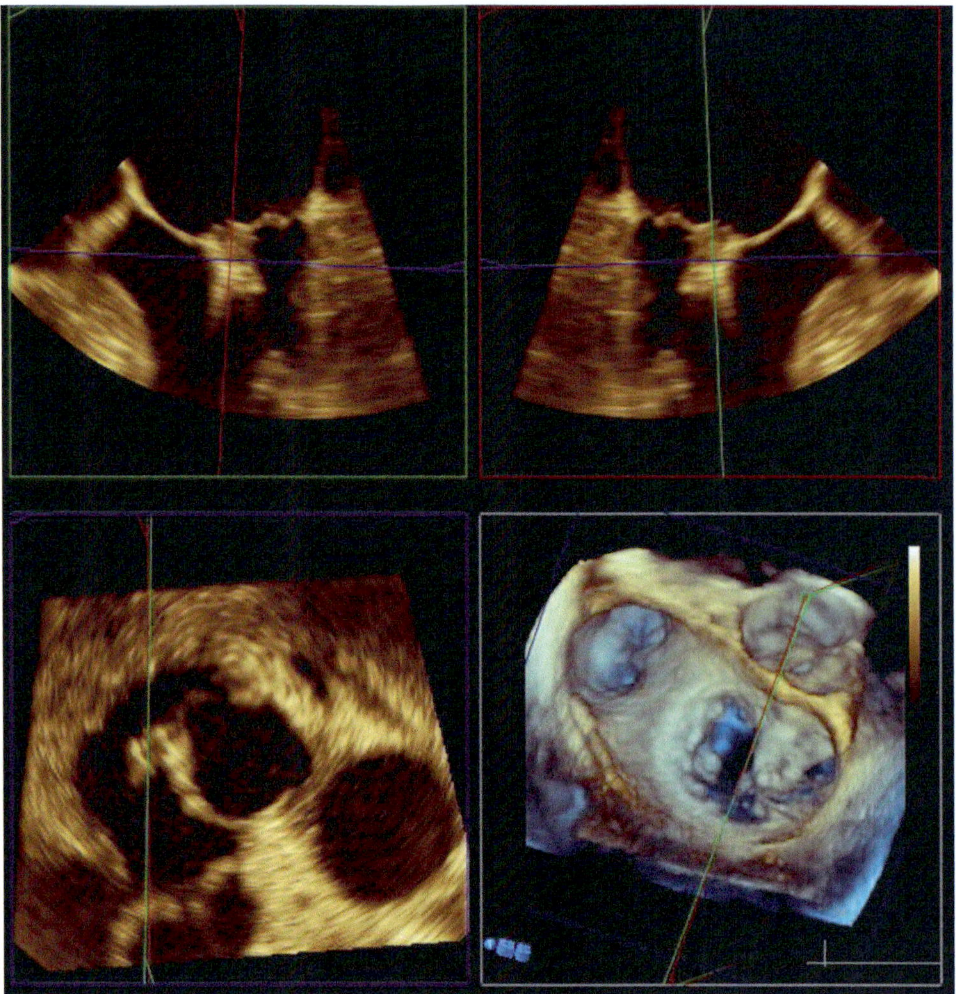

Fig. 6.30 Use of Philips 3DQ reconstruction software demonstrates a multiplanar view of the mitral valve with the MitraClips in situ

6.4 Case 3. MitraClip for Anterior Leaflet Prolapse

An 89-year-old man with a history of previous aortic valve replacement and known anterior mitral prolapse presents with increasing dyspnea (including paroxysmal nocturnal dyspnea), peripheral edema, and palpitations. He was noted to have an estimated RVSP of 95 mmHg, consistent with severe pulmonary hypertension. He was felt to be a very high-risk candidate for redoing open surgery, considering his age and problems with the previous surgery, so he was offered the option of MitraClip instead of open surgery (Figs. 6.31, 6.32, 6.33, 6.34, 6.35, 6.36, 6.37, 6.38, 6.39, 6.40, 6.41, and 6.42).

Video 6.23 Color Doppler imaging in a long-axis (120°) view confirmed severe (4+), posteriorly directed mitral regurgitation due to anterior leaflet prolapse and partial flail (AVI 1543 kb)

Video 6.24 3D imaging of the mitral valve from the left atrium confirmed predominant involvement of the A1/A2 scallops (AVI 621 kb)

Video 6.25 Atrial septostomy was performed (AVI 3546 kb)

Video 6.26 The device is aligned with the mitral valve using the steerable guide catheter, which bends at 90° in the left atrium after traversing the interatrial septum (AVI 7462 kb)

Video 6.27 The device is aligned perpendicular to the valve leaflets The long-axis (120°) view is helpful to visualize both device arms and both mitral valve leaflets simultaneously (AVI 7145 kb)

Video 6.28 Once the MitraClip is adequately positioned with optimal leaflet insertion between the grippers and arms, the clip is deployed (AVI 7453 kb)

Video 6.29 This transgastric TEE view shows a lateral view of the MitraClip with the clip arms perpendicular to the line of leaflet coaptation (AVI 7639 kb)

Video 6.30 Using 3D imaging of the mitral valve from a left atrial view, the clip can be seen apposing the lateral aspects of the leaflets (A1/P1 scallops) (AVI 1149 kb)

Video 6.31 To ensure optimal leaflet coaptation, a second MitraClip was deployed more medially Residual 1+ MR was noted on color Doppler imaging with TEE (AVI 1679 kb)

Video 6.32 Long-term follow-up with transthoracic echocardiography (TTE) demonstrates a good result, with only trivial residual MR noted on an apical four-chamber view (AVI 2897 kb)

Video 6.33 Color Doppler imaging in a parasternal long-axis view by TTE shows negligible regurgitation (AVI 2190 kb)

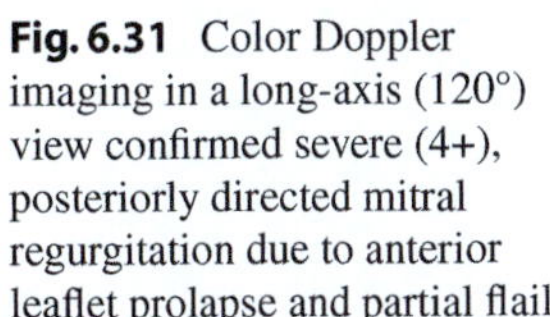

Fig. 6.31 Color Doppler imaging in a long-axis (120°) view confirmed severe (4+), posteriorly directed mitral regurgitation due to anterior leaflet prolapse and partial flail

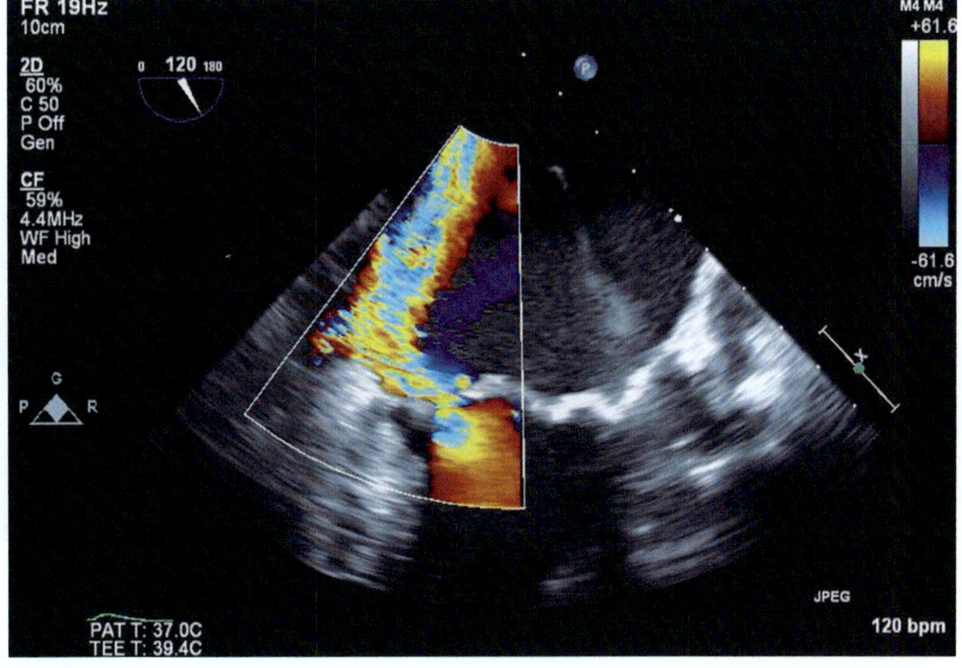

Fig. 6.32 3D imaging of the mitral valve from the left atrium confirmed predominant involvement of the A1/A2 scallops

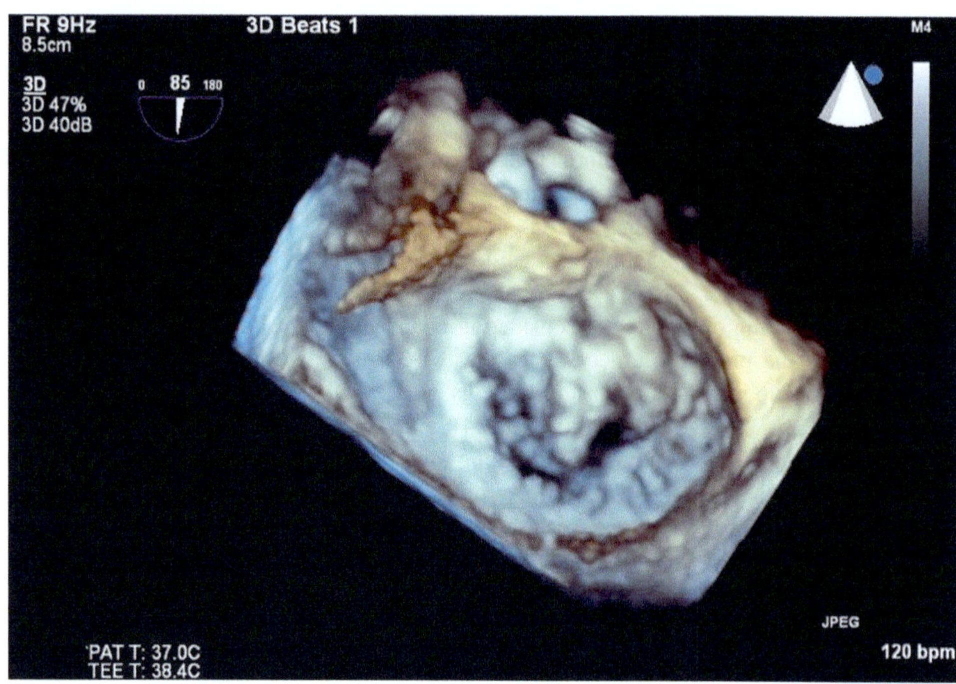

Fig. 6.33 Atrial septostomy was performed

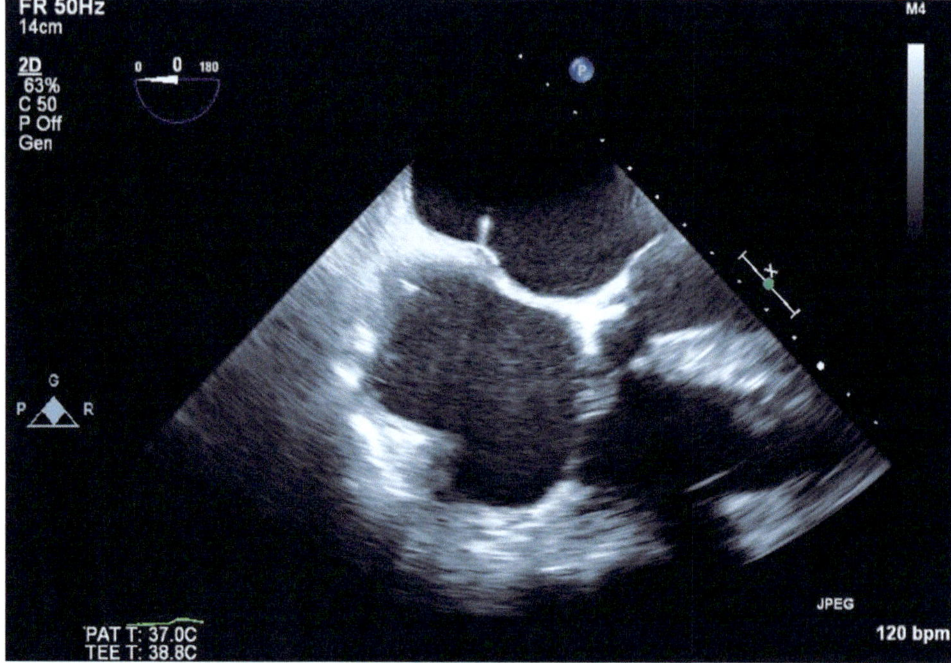

Fig. 6.34 The device is aligned with the mitral valve using the steerable guide catheter, which bends at 90° in the left atrium after traversing the interatrial septum

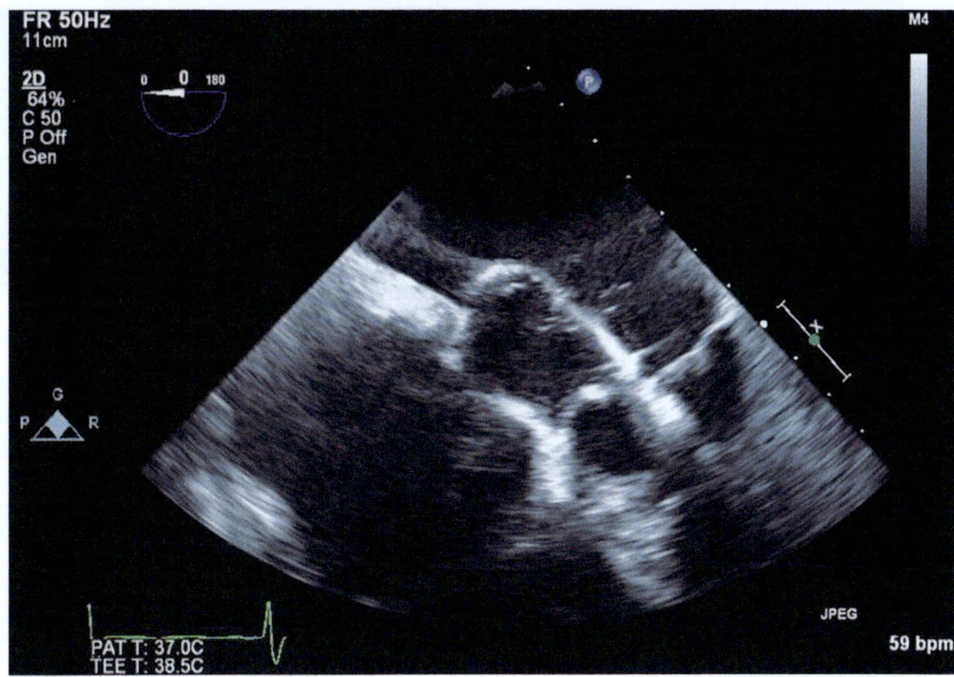

Fig. 6.35 The device is aligned perpendicular to the valve leaflets. The long-axis (120°) view is helpful to visualize both device arms and both mitral valve leaflets simultaneously

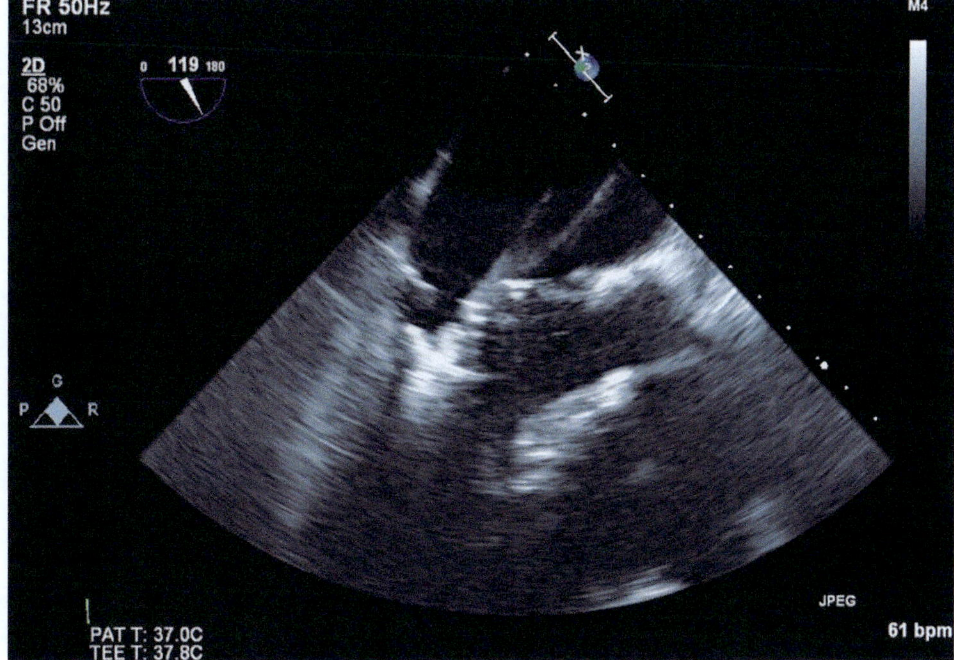

Fig. 6.36 Once the MitraClip is adequately positioned with optimal leaflet insertion between the grippers and arms, the clip is deployed

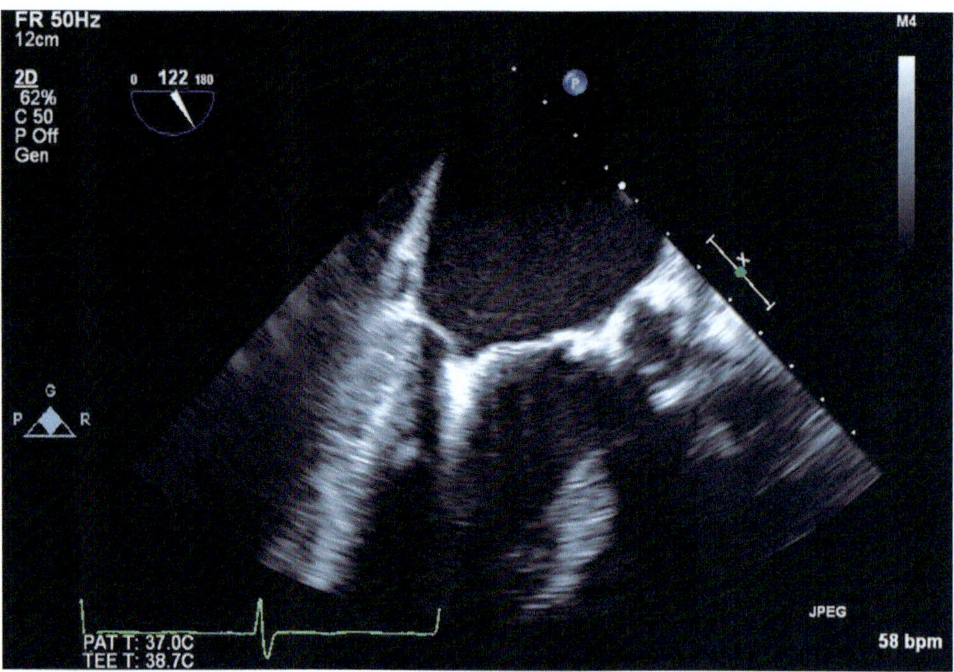

Fig. 6.37 This transgastric TEE view shows a lateral view of the MitraClip with the clip arms perpendicular to the line of leaflet coaptation

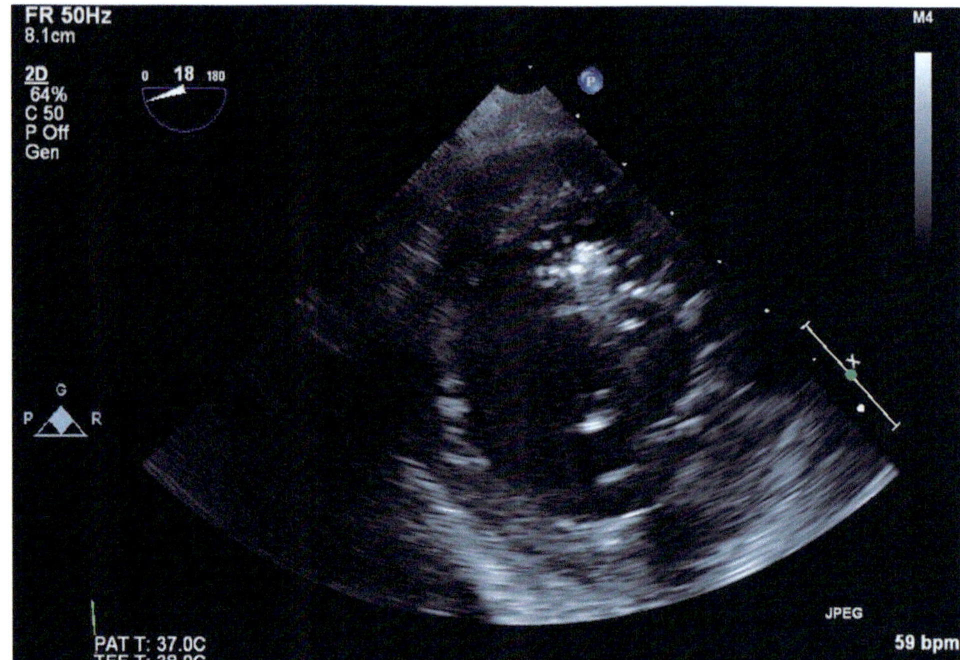

Fig. 6.38 Using 3D imaging of the mitral valve from a left atrial view, the clip can be seen apposing the lateral aspects of the leaflets (A1/P1 scallops)

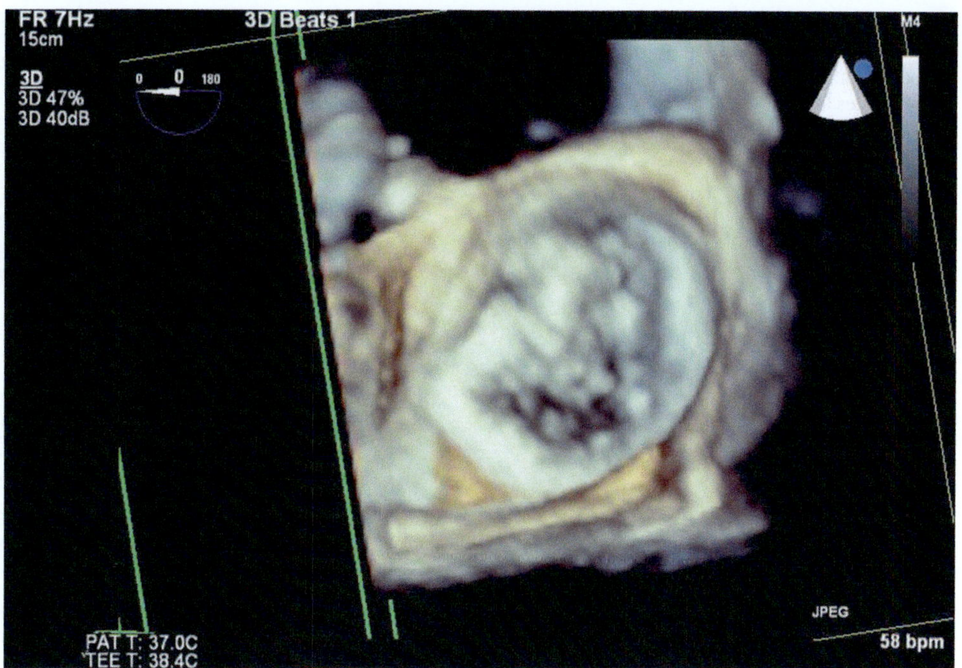

Fig. 6.39 To ensure optimal leaflet coaptation, a second MitraClip was deployed more medially. Residual 1+ MR was noted on color Doppler imaging with TEE

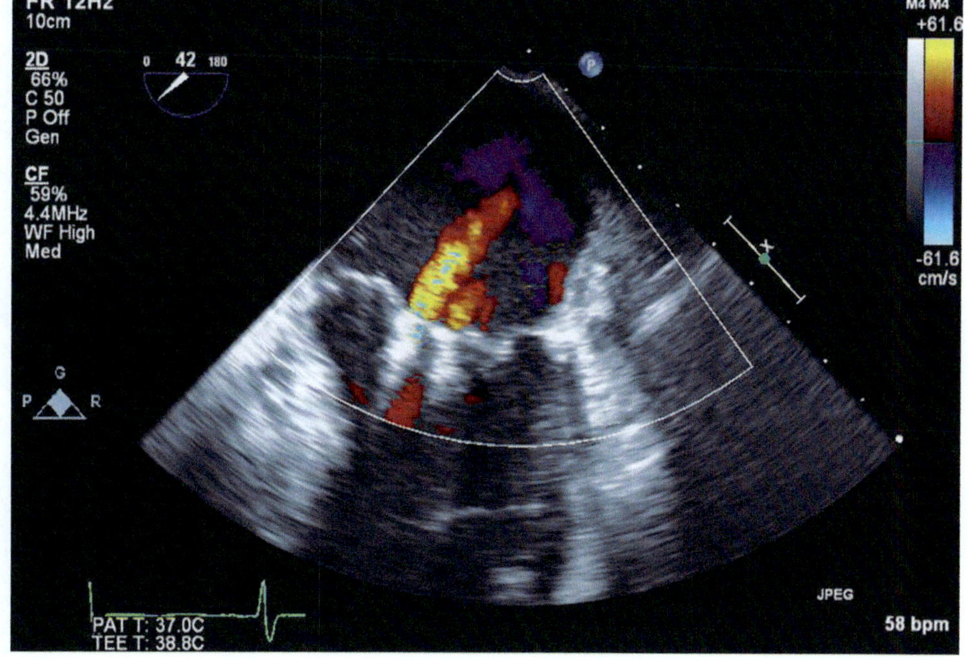

Fig. 6.40 Long-term follow-up with transthoracic echocardiography (TTE) demonstrates a good result, with only trivial residual MR noted on an apical four-chamber view

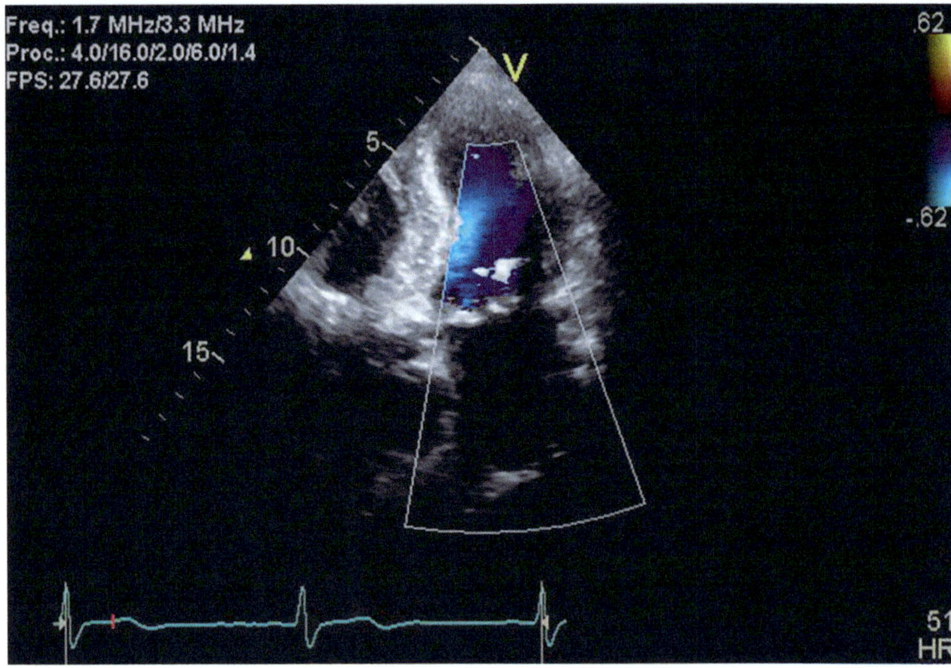

Fig. 6.41 Color Doppler imaging in a parasternal long-axis view by TTE shows negligible regurgitation

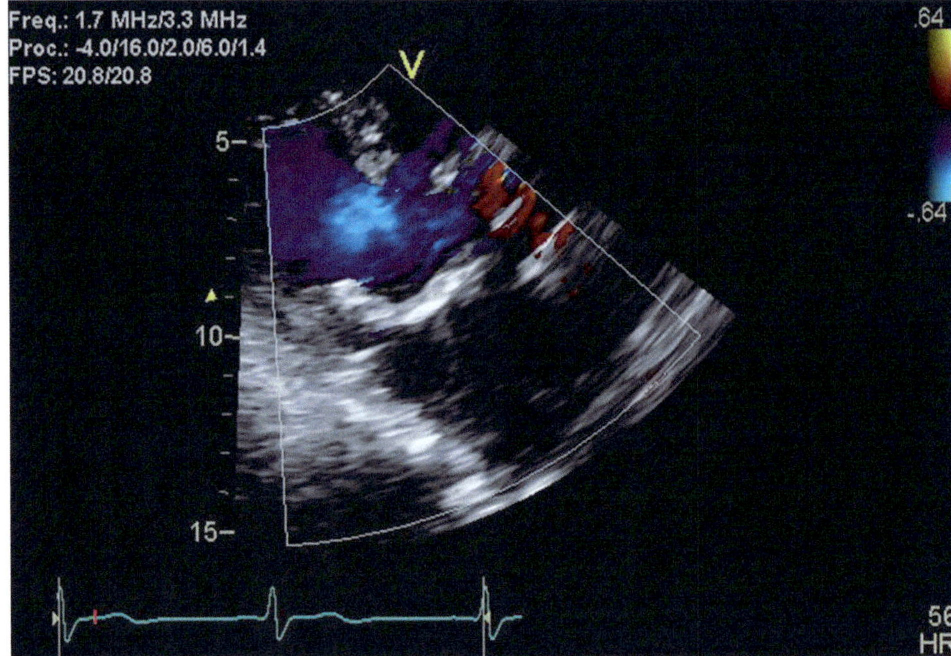

Fig. 6.42 Continuous wave Doppler imaging through the mitral valve confirms that there is no evidence of valvular stenosis (peak/mean gradients of 11/3 mmHg)

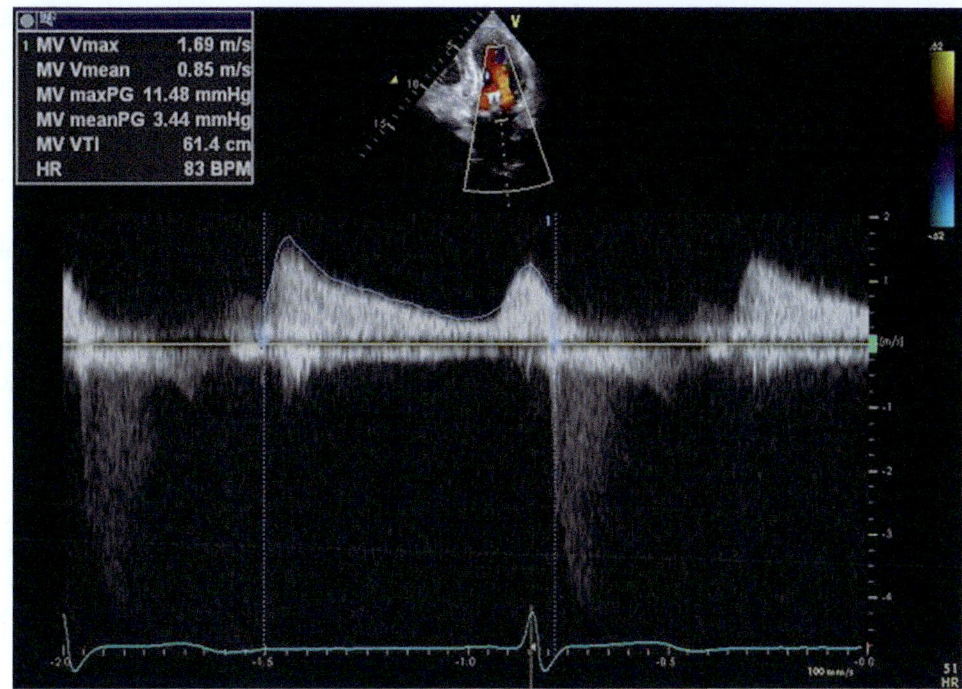

6.5 Case 4. 3D Guidance of MitraClip

An 87-year-old male ex-smoker with a past history of coronary artery disease (coronary artery bypass graft surgery), atrial fibrillation, pulmonary hypertension, hypertension, and hyperlipidemia presented with multifactorial dyspnea. On echocardiography, he was noted to have mild right ventricular systolic dysfunction with moderately severe (3+) posteriorly directed mitral valve regurgitation secondary to anterior (A2 scallop) leaflet prolapse, moderately severe (3+) tricuspid valve regurgitation, and moderately severe pulmonary hypertension (RVSP 70 mmHg). Because of his significant comorbidities, he was not felt to be a surgical candidate, so he was referred for MitraClip (Figs. 6.43, 6.44, 6.45, 6.46, 6.47, 6.48, 6.49, and 6.50).

Video 6.34 TEE view of the mitral valve at 112°, demonstrating anterior leaflet prolapse (A2 scallop) (AVI 6904 kb)

Video 6.35 Color Doppler imaging demonstrates resultant moderately severe (3+) MR due to failure of leaflet coaptation (AVI 2187 kb)

Video 6.36 Baseline 3D image of the mitral valve viewed from the left atrium (AVI 1482 kb)

Video 6.37 3D image showing the guide catheter in the left atrium approaching the mitral valve The position and trajectory are adjusted to optimize perpendicular alignment of the MitraClip with the valve leaflets (AVI 979 kb)

Video 6.38 A TEE two dimensional (2D) long-axis view of the mitral valve demonstrates that the MitraClip is well positioned, with stable attachment to both leaflets, and is ready for deployment (AVI 6948 kb)

Video 6.39 (**a**) After MitraClip deployment, 3D imaging shows the guide catheter retracted into the left atrium (AVI 2360 kb)

Video 6.39 (**b**) The MitraClip can be seen apposing the valve leaflets centrally across the A2 and P2 scallops to create a double-orifice mitral valve (AVI 1634 kb)

Video 6.40 2D imaging of the mitral valve in long-axis view demonstrates 1+ residual MR (AVI 3942 kb)

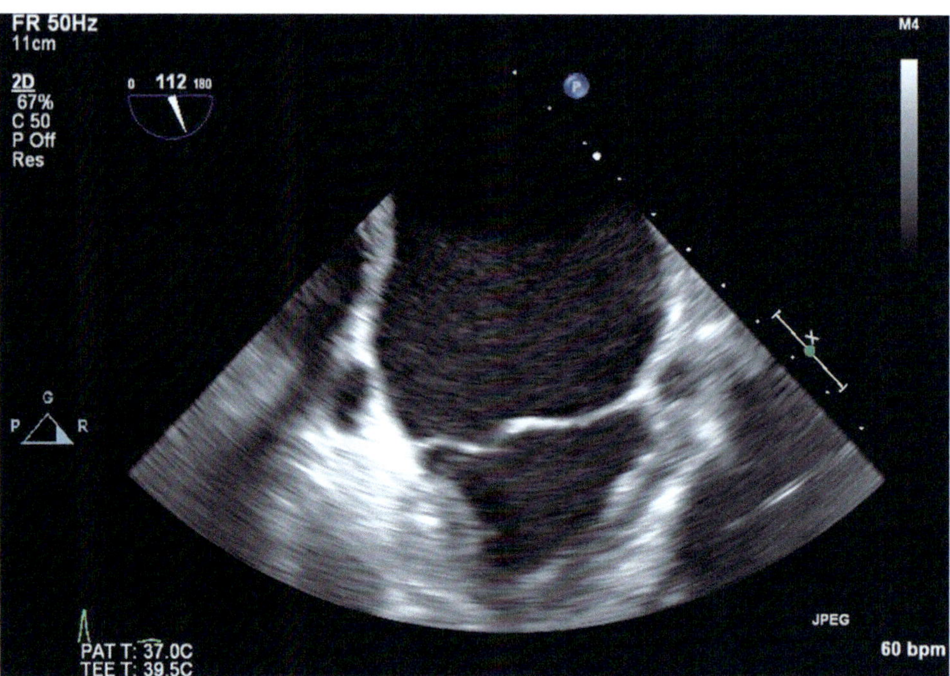

Fig. 6.43 TEE view of the mitral valve at 112°, demonstrating anterior leaflet prolapse (A2 scallop)

Fig. 6.44 Color Doppler imaging demonstrates resultant moderately severe (3+) MR due to failure of leaflet coaptation

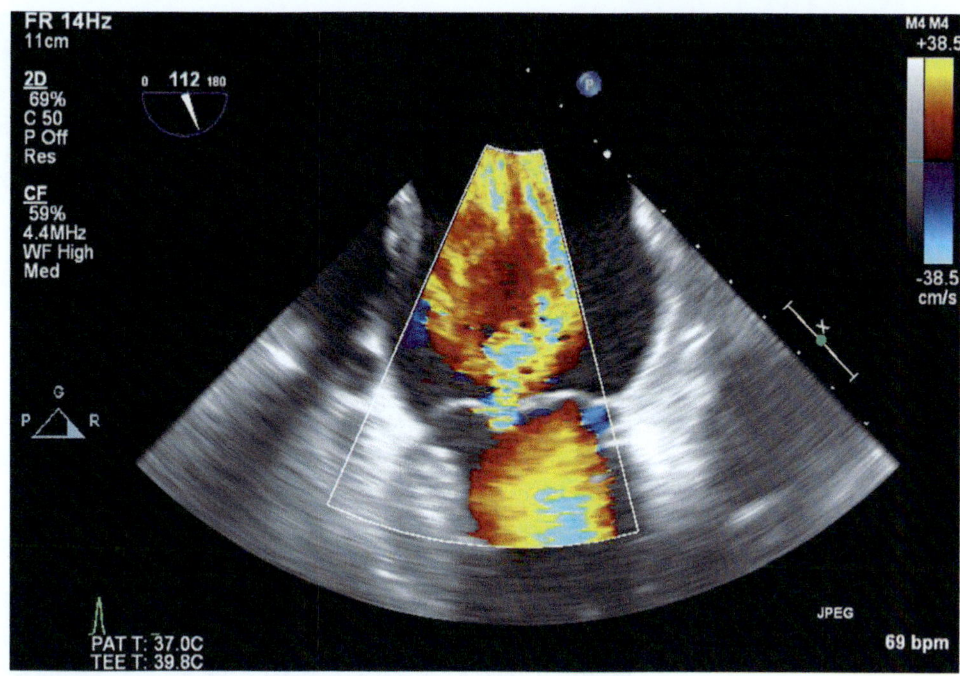

Fig. 6.45 Baseline 3D image of the mitral valve viewed from the left atrium

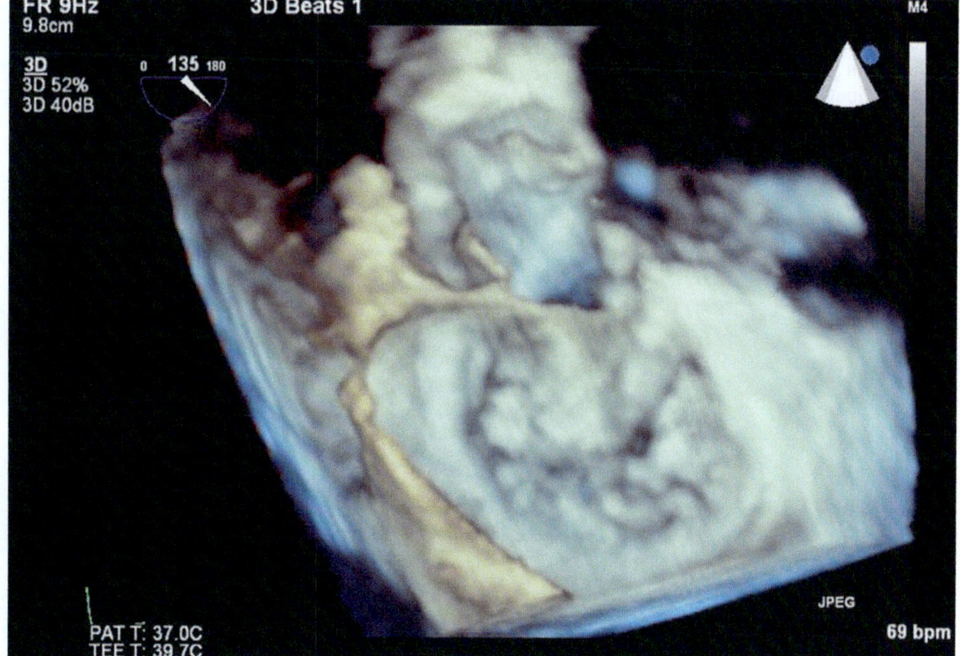

Fig. 6.46 3D image showing the guide catheter in the left atrium approaching the mitral valve. The position and trajectory are adjusted to optimize perpendicular alignment of the MitraClip with the valve leaflets

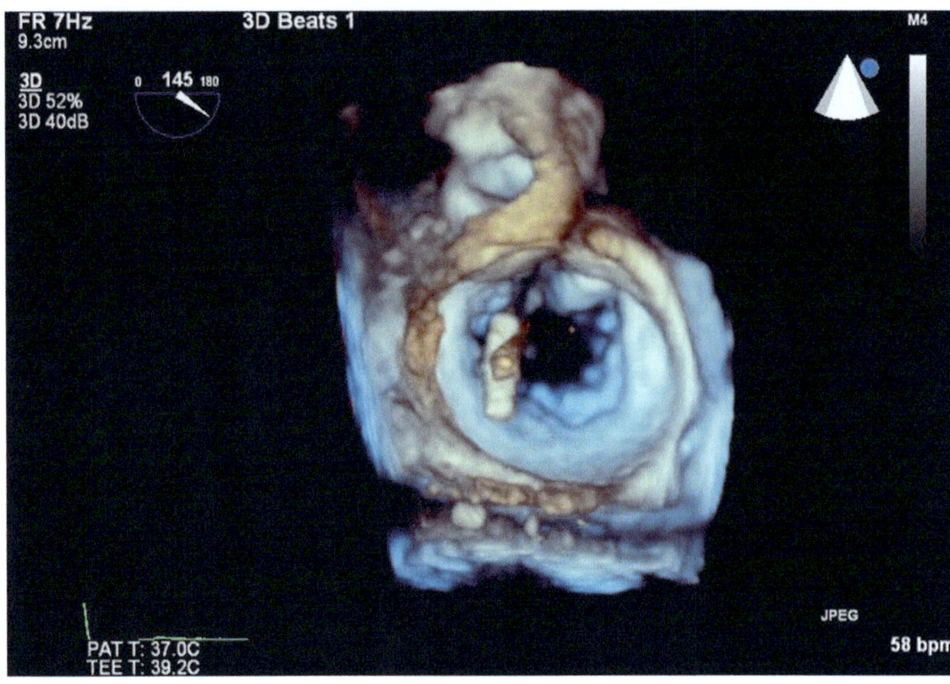

Fig. 6.47 A TEE two dimensional (2D) long-axis view of the mitral valve demonstrates that the MitraClip is well positioned, with stable attachment to both leaflets, and is ready for deployment

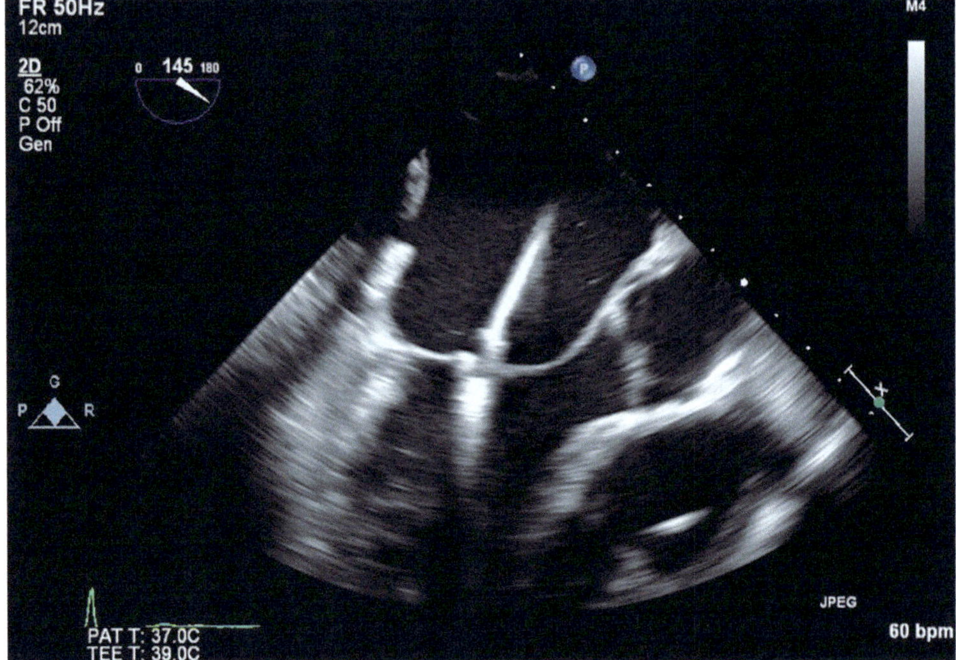

Fig. 6.48 (**a**) After MitraClip deployment, 3D imaging shows the guide catheter retracted into the left atrium. (**b**) The MitraClip can be seen apposing the valve leaflets centrally across the A2 and P2 scallops to create a double-orifice mitral valve

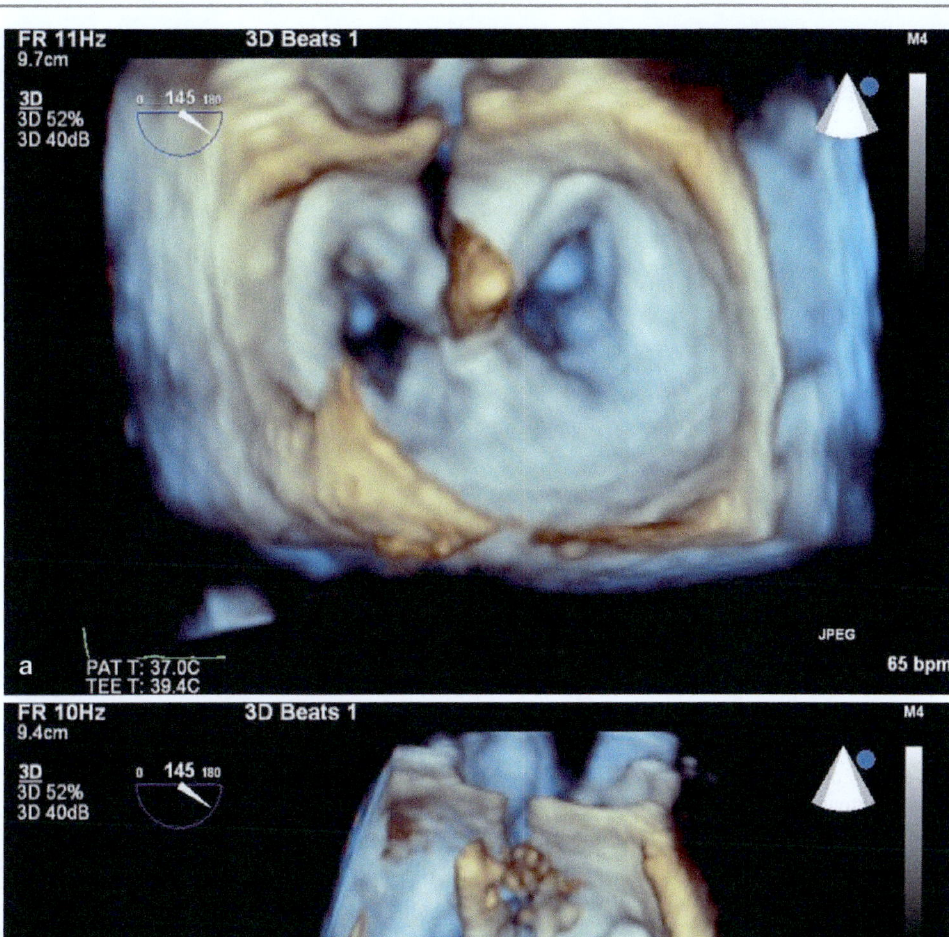

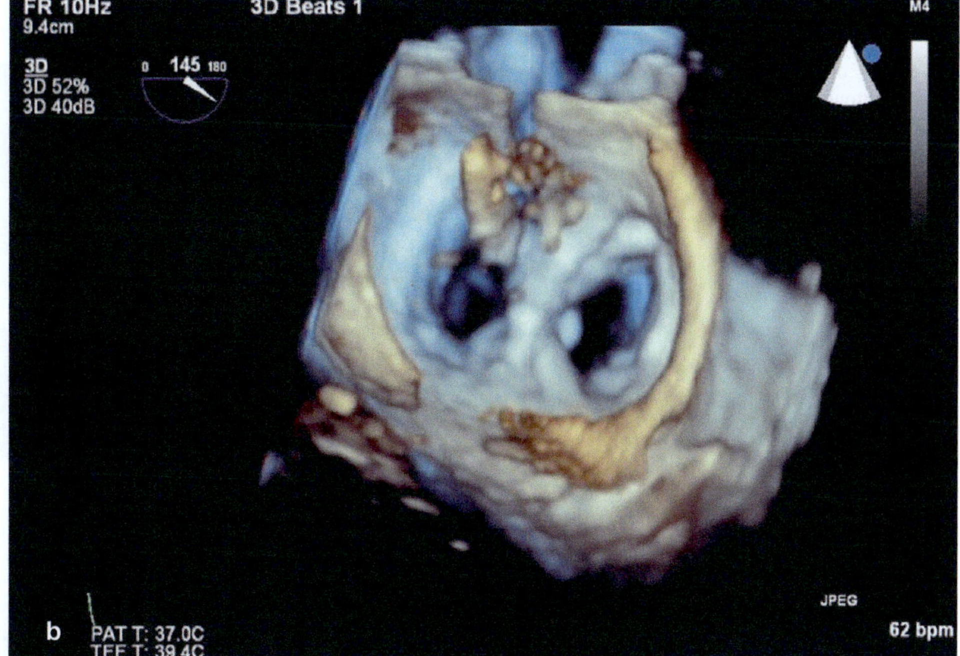

Fig. 6.49 2D imaging of the mitral valve in long-axis view demonstrates 1+ residual MR

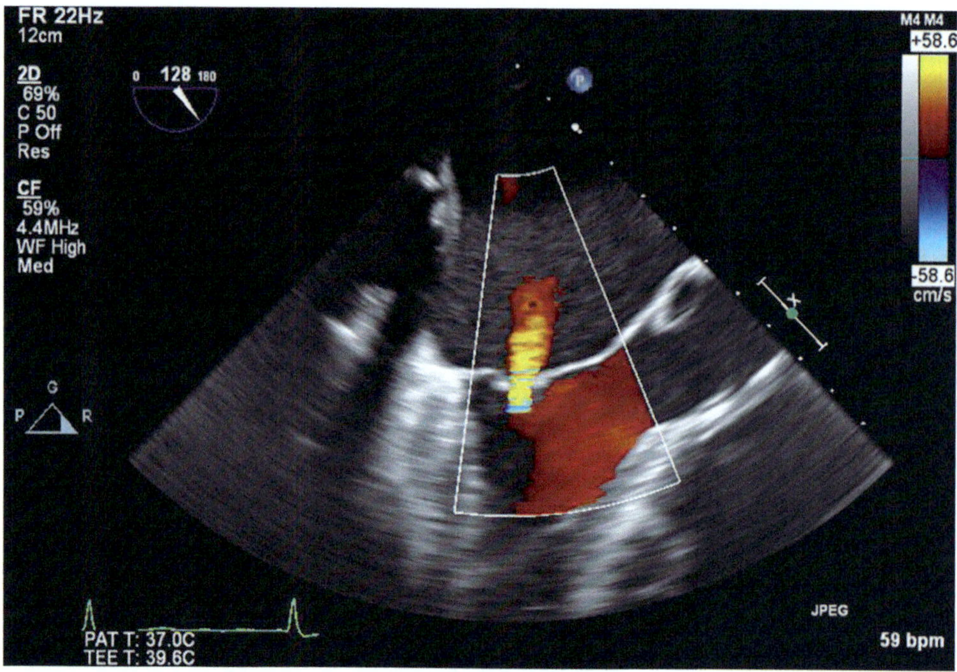

Fig. 6.50 Continuous wave Doppler through the mitral valve confirms that the MitraClip is not causing hemodynamically significant stenosis (peak/mean gradients of 12/3 mmHg)

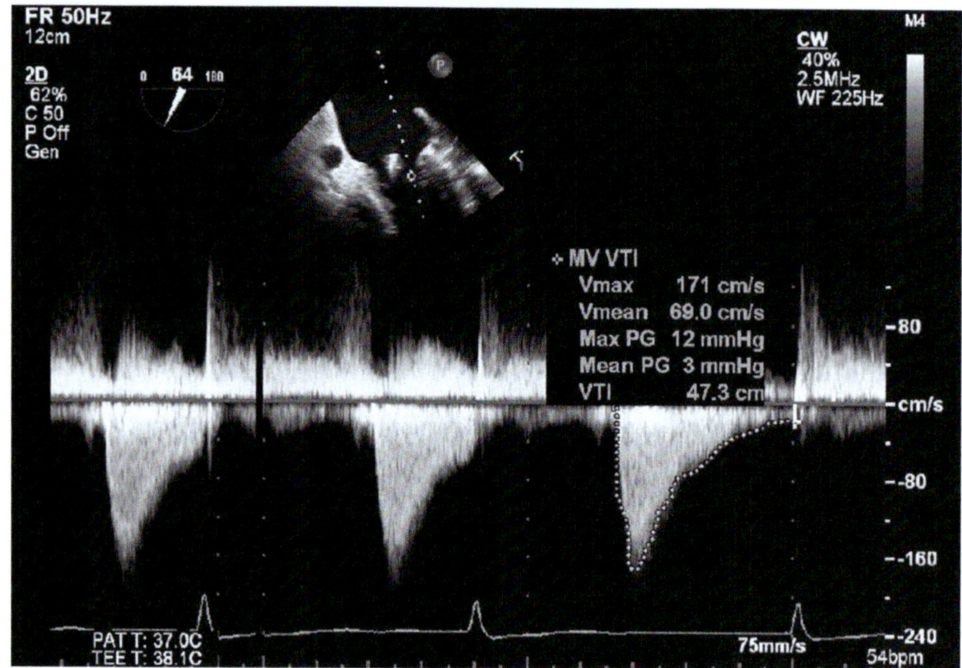

6.6   Case 5. Paravalvular Leak After Mechanical Mitral Valve Replacement

A 54-year-old man with a past history of coronary artery bypass graft surgery, St. Jude mechanical aortic and mitral valve replacements, and pacemaker insertion for heart block was transferred for evaluation regarding possible redo mitral valve replacement. He had presented to another hospital with pulmonary edema and respiratory acidosis and had been found to have a severe paravalvular leak at the antero-lateral aspect of the mitral valve annulus. He underwent Amplatzer closure of the paravalvular leak using guidance by real-time 3D imaging (Figs. 6.51, 6.52, 6.53, 6.54, 6.55, and 6.56).

Video 6.41 2D TEE image at 90° of the St Jude bileaflet mitral valve replacement (AVI 6519 kb)

Video 6.42 Color Doppler imaging demonstrates a severe, eccentric, paravalvular leak at the anterolateral aspect of the prosthetic valve annulus (AVI 1893 kb)

Video 6.43 3D imaging of the left atrial aspect of the mitral valve prosthesis The *arrow* points to a region of dehiscence from which the paravalvular leak originates (AVI 3399 kb)

Video 6.44 Color 3D imaging demonstrates color flow through the region of dehiscence, representative of the paravalvular leak (AVI 529 kb)

Video 6.45 A 3D view of the mitral valve from the anterolateral aspect demonstrates the region of dehiscence (AVI 466 kb)

Video 6.46 3D image of the bileaflet mitral valve prosthesis with the occluder device in situ, adjacent to the anterolateral aspect of the valve (AVI 438 kb)

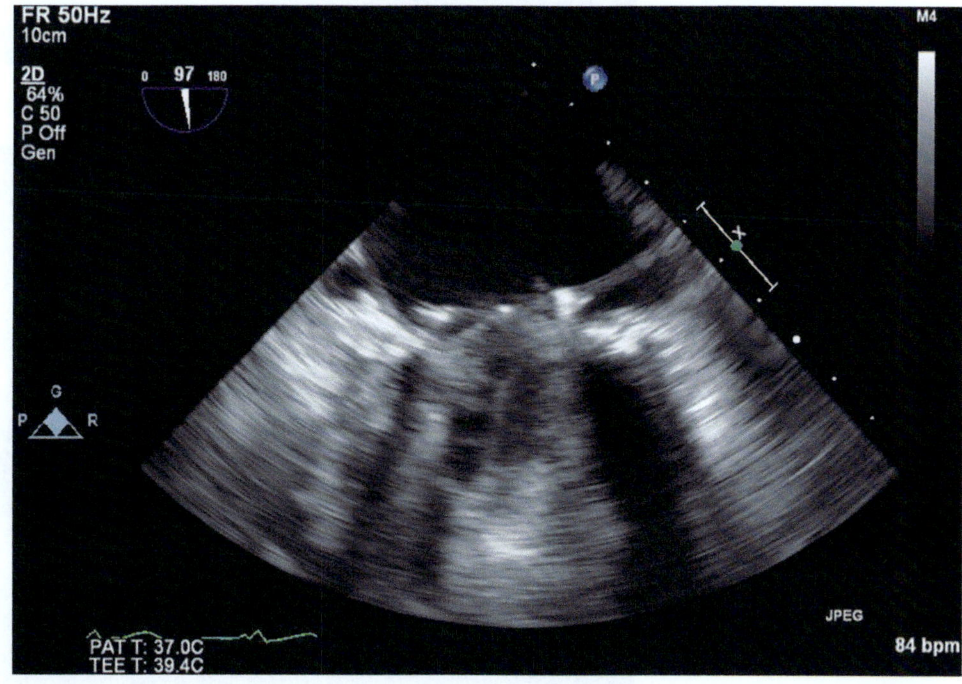

Fig. 6.51 2D TEE image at 90° of the St. Jude bileaflet mitral valve replacement

Fig. 6.52 Color Doppler imaging demonstrates a severe, eccentric, paravalvular leak at the anterolateral aspect of the prosthetic valve annulus

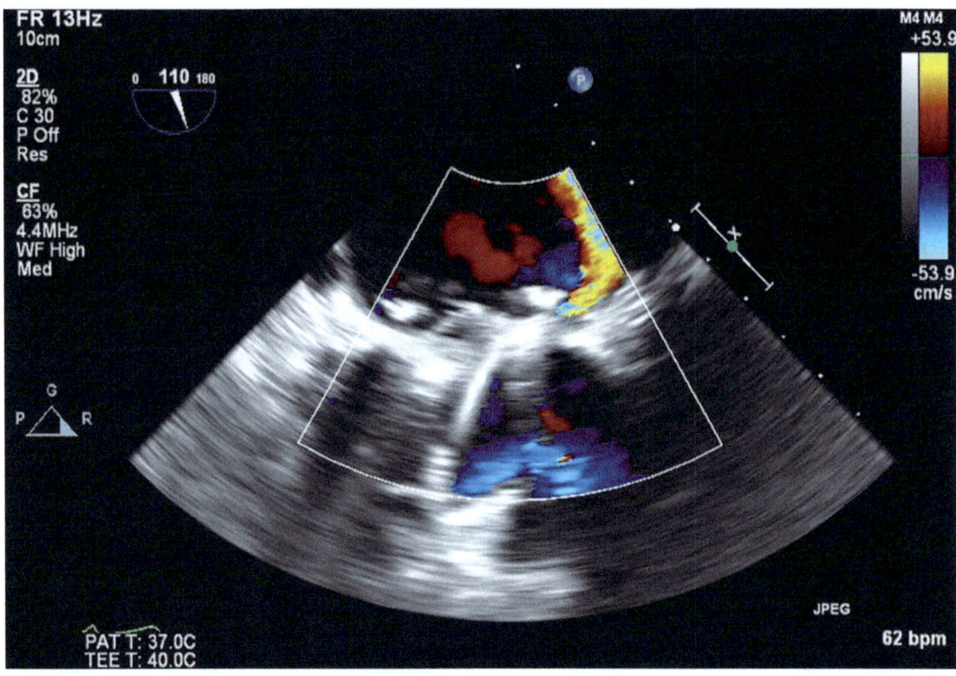

Fig. 6.53 3D imaging of the left atrial aspect of the mitral valve prosthesis. The arrow points to a region of dehiscence from which the paravalvular leak originates

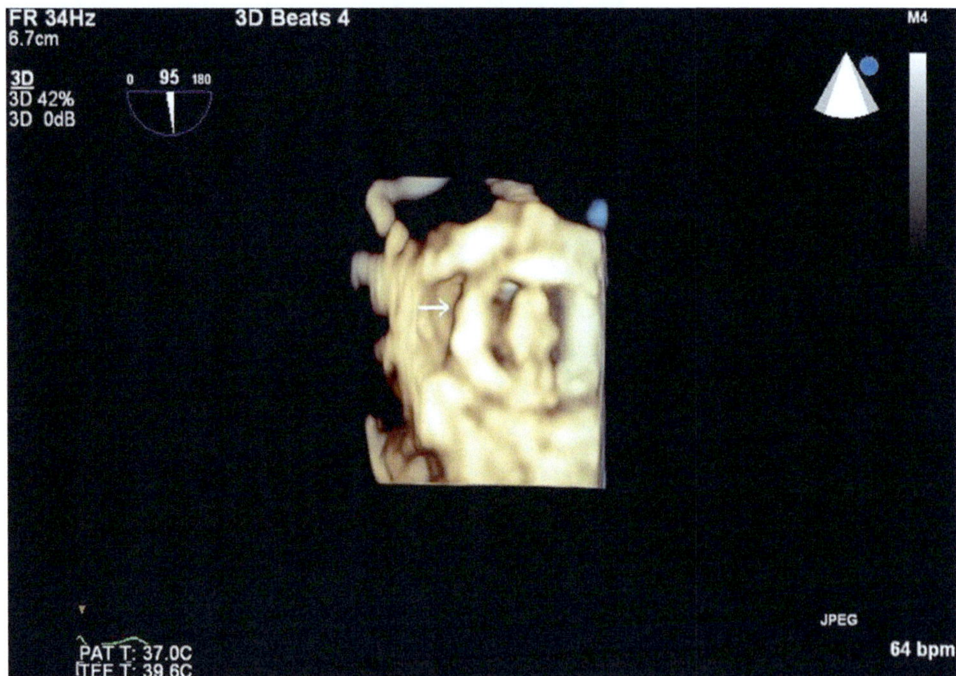

Fig. 6.54 Color 3D imaging demonstrates color flow through the region of dehiscence, representative of the paravalvular leak

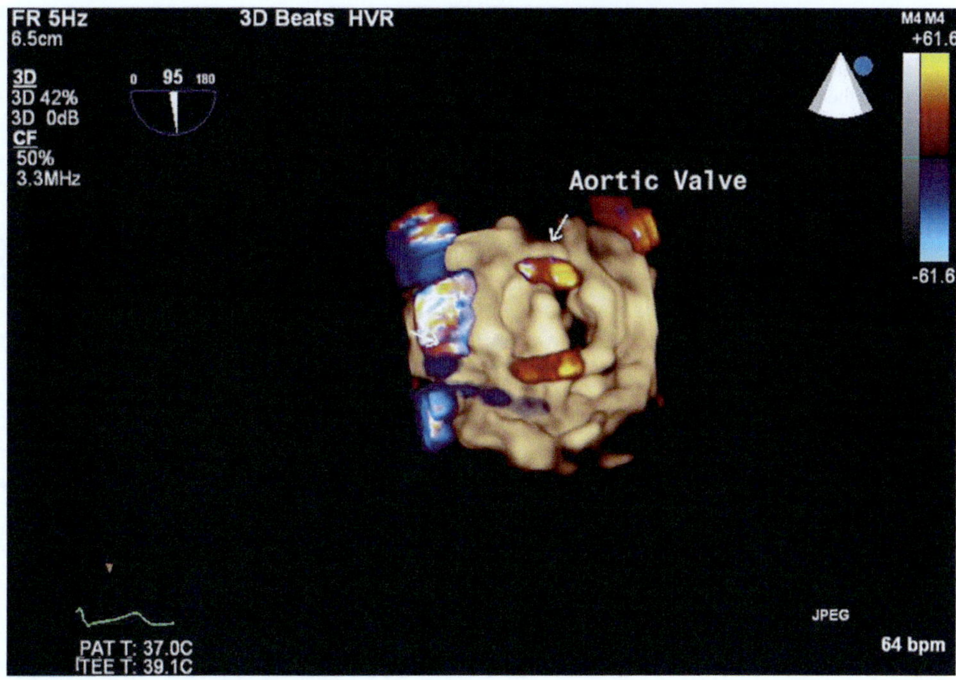

Fig. 6.55 A 3D view of the mitral valve from the anterolateral aspect. The arrow demonstrates a small region of dehiscence

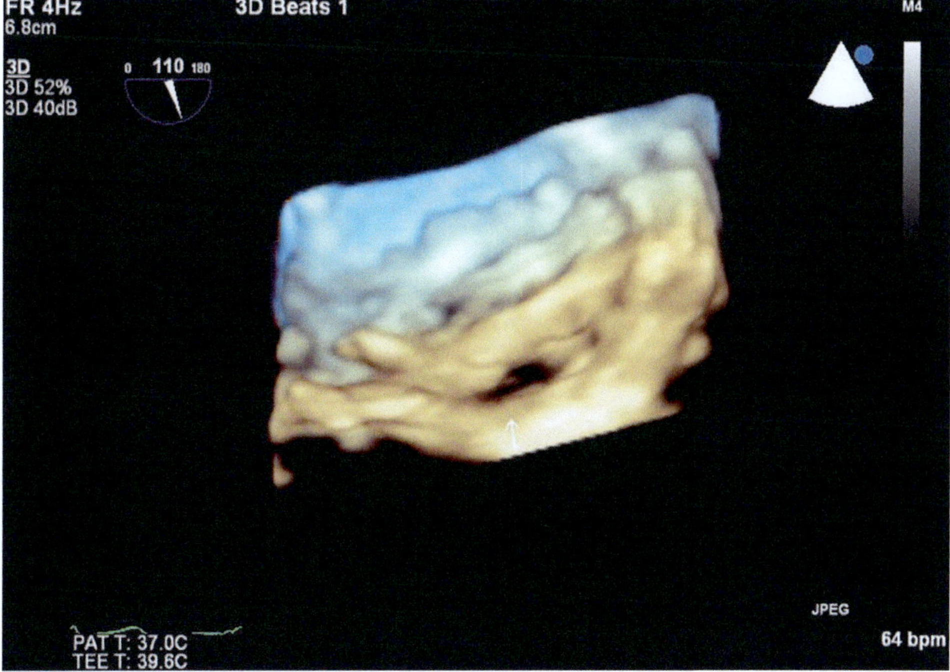

Fig. 6.56 3D image of the bileaflet mitral valve prosthesis with the occluder device in situ, adjacent to the anterolateral aspect of the valve

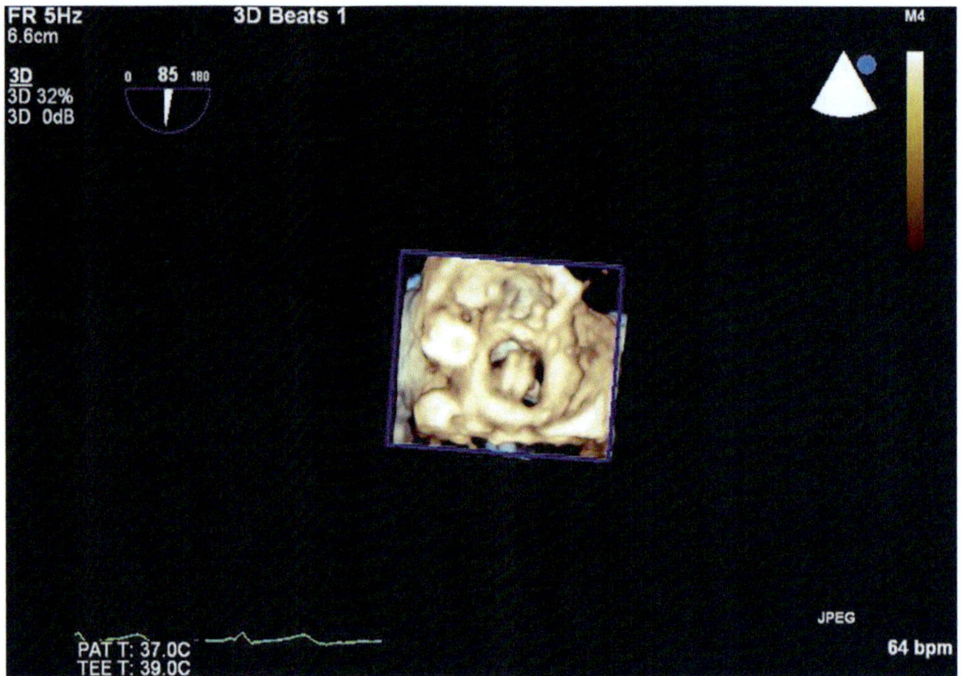

6.7 Case 6. Paravalvular Leak Closure: Bioprosthetic Mitral Valve Replacement

64-year-old man presented for percutaneous closure of a mitral paravalvular leak. His past history included bioprosthetic mitral valve replacement and coronary artery bypass graft surgery 3 years earlier, hyperlipidemia, hypertension, pulmonary embolism, history of smoking, and family history of coronary artery disease. His prior sternotomy had been complicated by infection, which had required extensive débridement and muscle flap repair. He had reported recent increasing dyspnea with exertion, and echocardiography had demonstrated a moderate (2–3+) paraprosthetic leak in the anterolateral region at the base of the prosthetic valve annulus. Otherwise the stented bioprosthetic valve (Carpentier-Edwards prosthetic valve size #29) was functioning normally (Figs. 6.57, 6.58, 6.59, 6.60, and 6.61).

Video 6.47 Biplane color Doppler TEE image at 130° and 11°, showing a bileaflet prosthetic mitral valve with moderate (2–3+) anterolateral paravalvular leak (AVI 1150 kb)

Video 6.48 Color 3D reconstruction image of the paravalvular jet of mitral regurgitation (AVI 134 kb)

Video 6.49 3D image of the mitral valve from a left atrial view, showing a guide catheter through the anterolateral region of valve dehiscence (2 o'clock position) (AVI 567 kb)

Video 6.50 3D reconstruction of the mitral valve from the left atrial view The paravalvular leak was successfully closed using 10-mm and 12-mm Amplatzer Vascular Plug II devices at the 2 and 3 o'clock positions (AVI 754 kb)

Video 6.51 Biplane color Doppler TEE image at 125° and 14° after deployment of the occluder in the anterolateral region of valve dehiscence The Amplatzer occluder devices can be seen adjacent to the valve replacement, with only a trivial residual paravalvular leak (AVI 501 kb)

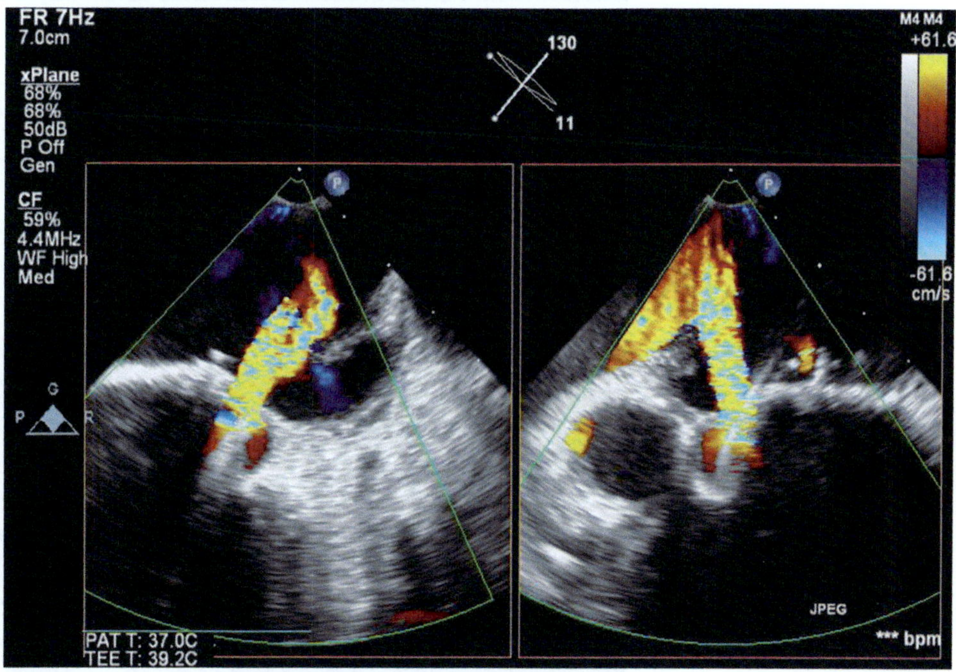

Fig. 6.57 Biplane color Doppler TEE image at 130° and 11°, showing a bileaflet prosthetic mitral valve with moderate (2–3+) anterolateral paravalvular leak

Fig. 6.58 Color 3D reconstruction image of the paravalvular jet of mitral regurgitation

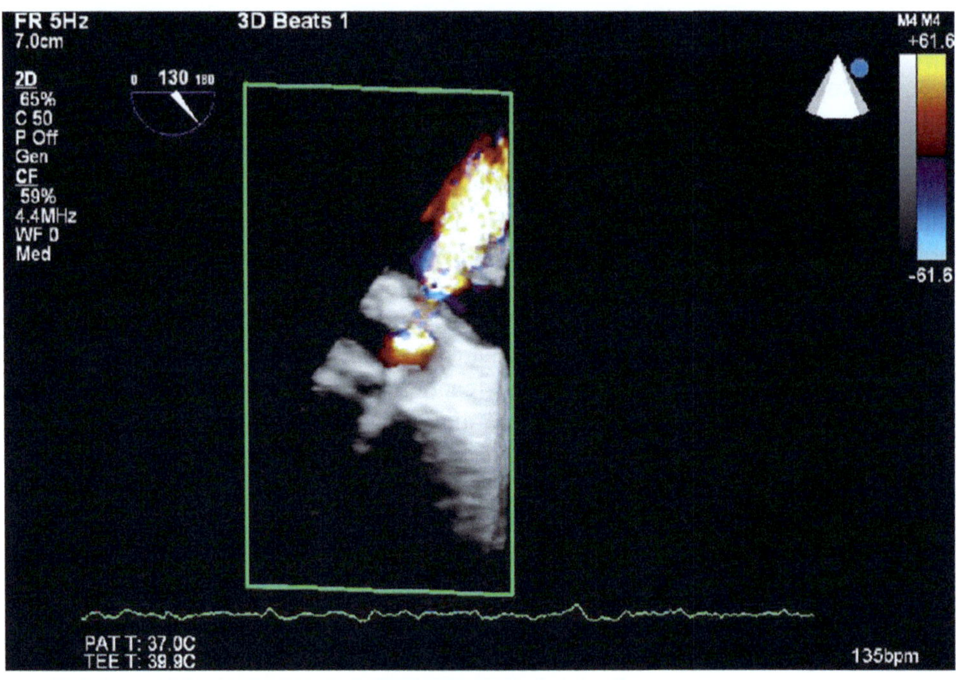

Fig. 6.59 3D image of the mitral valve from a left atrial view, showing a guide catheter through the anterolateral region of valve dehiscence (2 o'clock position)

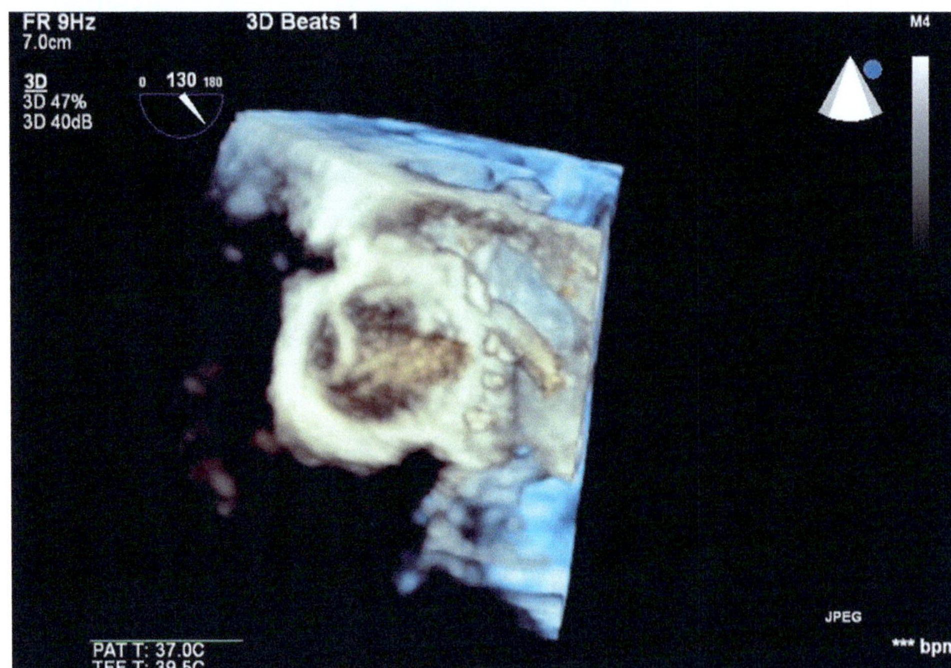

Fig. 6.60 3D reconstruction of the mitral valve from the left atrial view. The paravalvular leak was successfully closed using 10 and 12-mm Amplatzer Vascular Plug II devices at the 2 and 3 o'clock positions

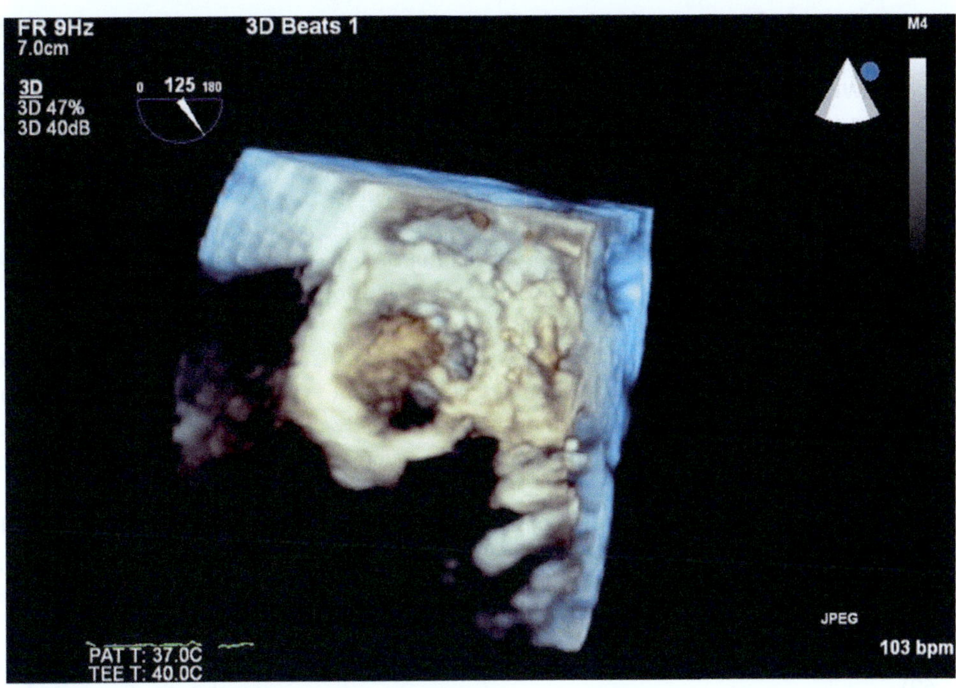

Fig. 6.61 Biplane color Doppler TEE image at 125° and 14° after deployment of the occluder in the anterolateral region of valve dehiscence. The Amplatzer occluder devices can be seen adjacent to the valve replacement, with only a trivial residual paravalvular leak

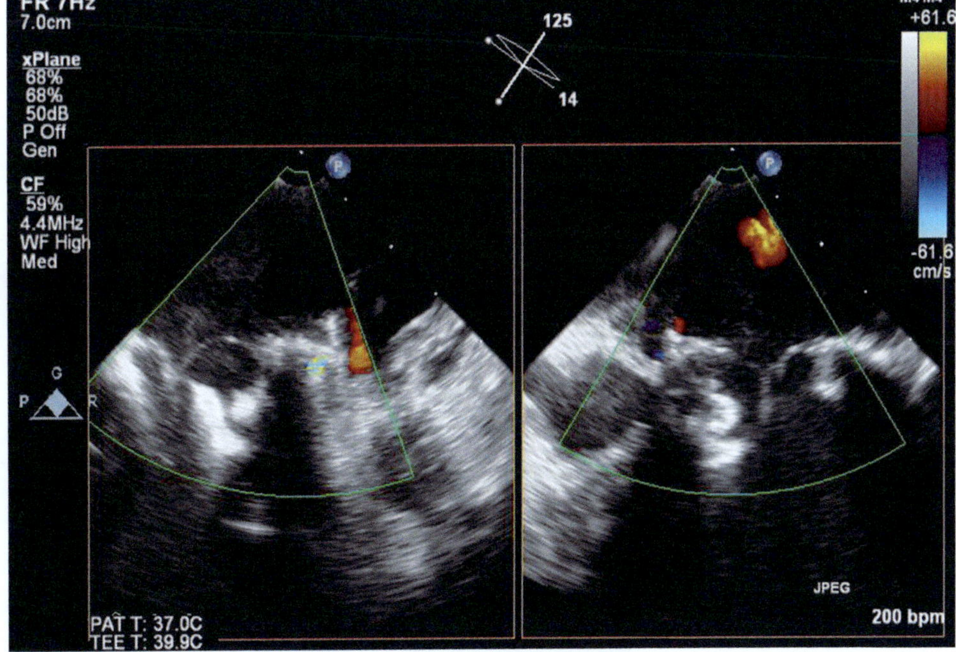

6.8 Case 7. Paravalvular Leak Closure: Mechanical Mitral Valve Replacement with Hemolysis

A 60-year-old woman with a past cardiac history of atrial fibrillation and previous valve surgery (mechanical aortic and mitral valve replacements and a tricuspid valve repair) for rheumatic heart disease presented for evaluation of significant nausea, vomiting, and jaundice. She was noted to have a normocytic anemia with no obvious source of bleeding, new acute renal insufficiency, and elevated liver function tests. Colonoscopy, esophagogastroduodenoscopy, and ERCP were unremarkable. TEE demonstrated normally functioning mechanical valves, but a mild to moderate (1–2+) paravalvular leak was noted adjacent to the inferoposterior aspect of the mitral valve sewing ring. Prosthetic valve–related hemolysis was diagnosed. She was determined to be too high-risk for additional open heart surgery and was offered percutaneous device closure of the paravalvular leak (Figs. 6.62, 6.63, 6.64, 6.65, 6.66, 6.67, 6.68, and 6.69).

Video 6.52 TEE image at 61° demonstrating a normally functioning bileaflet St Jude prosthetic mitral valve (AVI 4737 kb)

Video 6.53 TEE image at 61° demonstrating the mild to moderate paravalvular leak (AVI 1882 kb)

Video 6.54 Valve dehiscence is not evident on 3D reconstruction (Philips 3DQ) of the mitral valve replacement from a left atrial view, owing to the small size of the orifice of the leak (AVI 1249 kb)

Video 6.55 Magnified view of the 3D mitral valve reconstruction from Fig. 6.64 (AVI 929 kb)

Video 6.56 Transesophageal 72° view demonstrating a trivial residual paravalvular leak after deployment of the occluder device (AVI 1646 kb)

Video 6.57 3D zoom view of the mitral valve, showing the 12-mm Amplatzer Vascular Plug II device deployed inferoposteriorly (AVI 3809 kb)

Video 6.58 TTE parasternal long-axis view with simultaneous 2D and color Doppler imaging demonstrating the occluder device in situ adjacent to the posterior aspect of the valve ring No significant residual mitral regurgitation is visible (AVI 4244 kb)

Video 6.59 Transthoracic parasternal short-axis view just apical to the true mitral valve annulus with simultaneous 2D and color Doppler imaging The ventricular aspect of the occluder device can be seen inferoposteriorly (AVI 6442 kb)

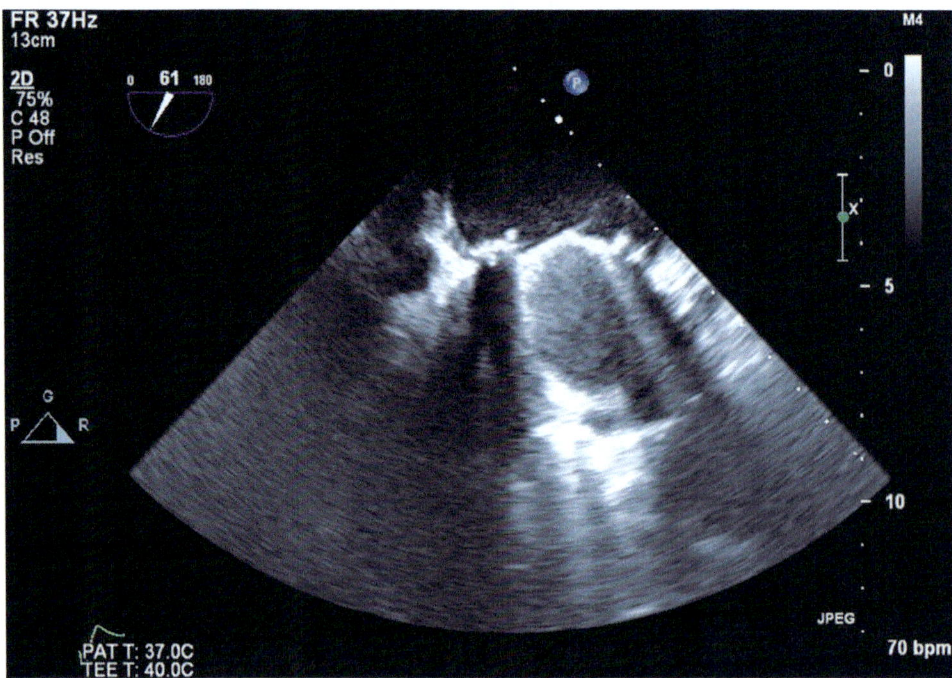

Fig. 6.62 TEE image at 61° demonstrating a normally functioning bileaflet St. Jude prosthetic mitral valve

Fig. 6.63 TEE image at 61° demonstrating the mild to moderate paravalvular leak

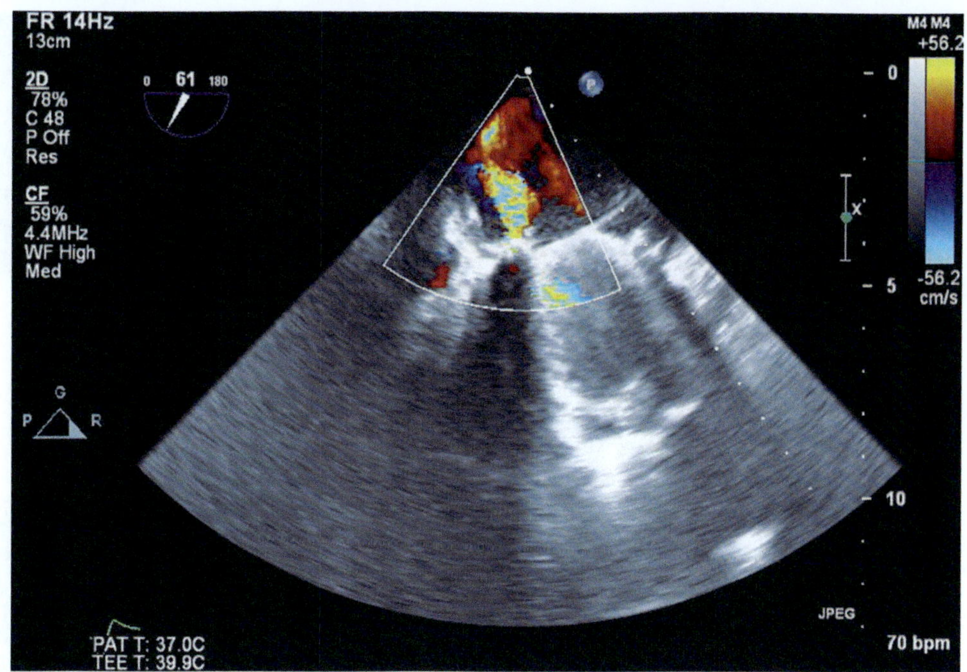

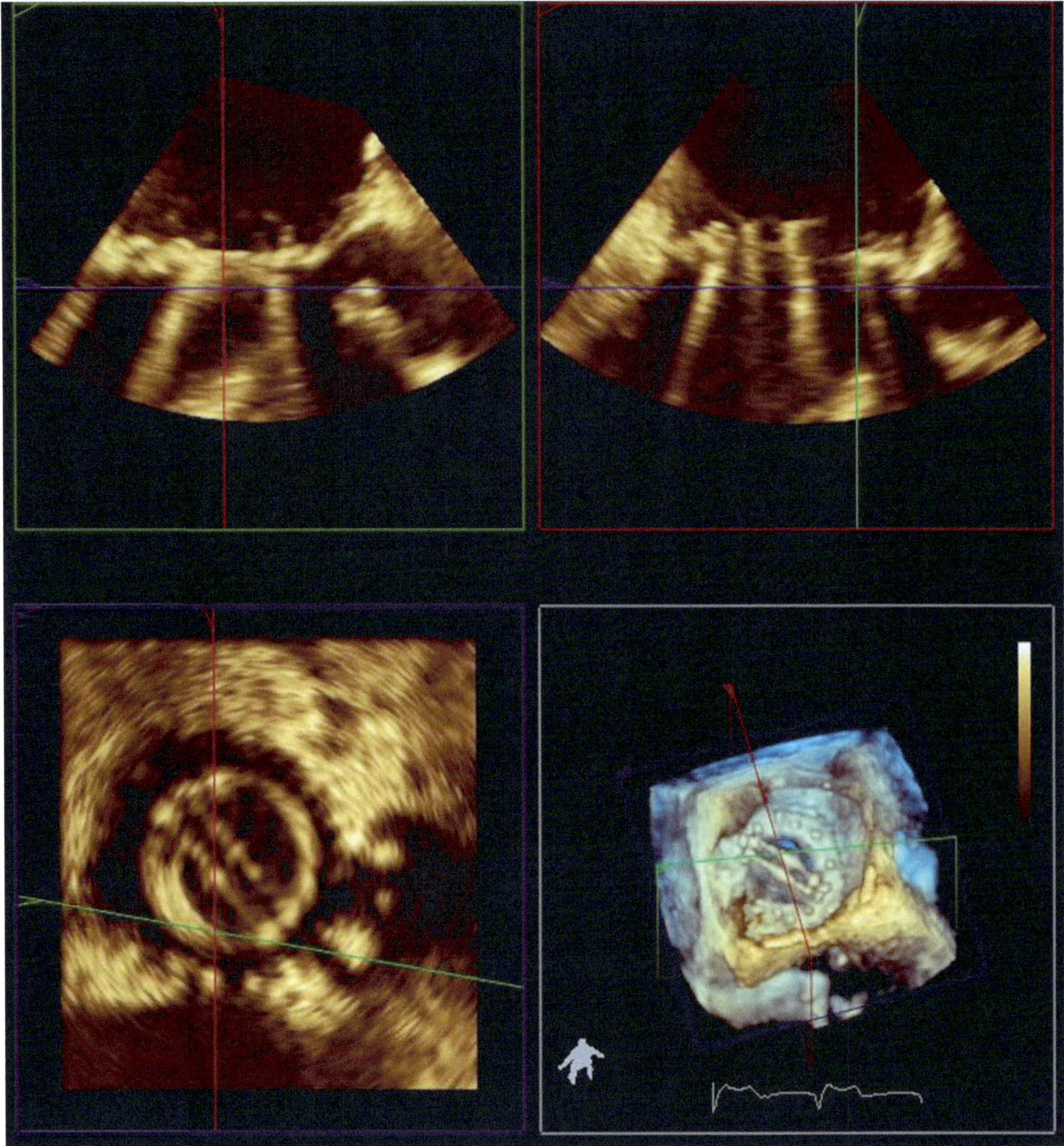

Fig. 6.64 Valve dehiscence is not evident on 3D reconstruction (Philips 3DQ) of the mitral valve replacement from a left atrial view, owing to the small size of the orifice of the leak

Fig. 6.65 Magnified view of the 3D mitral valve reconstruction from Fig. 6.64

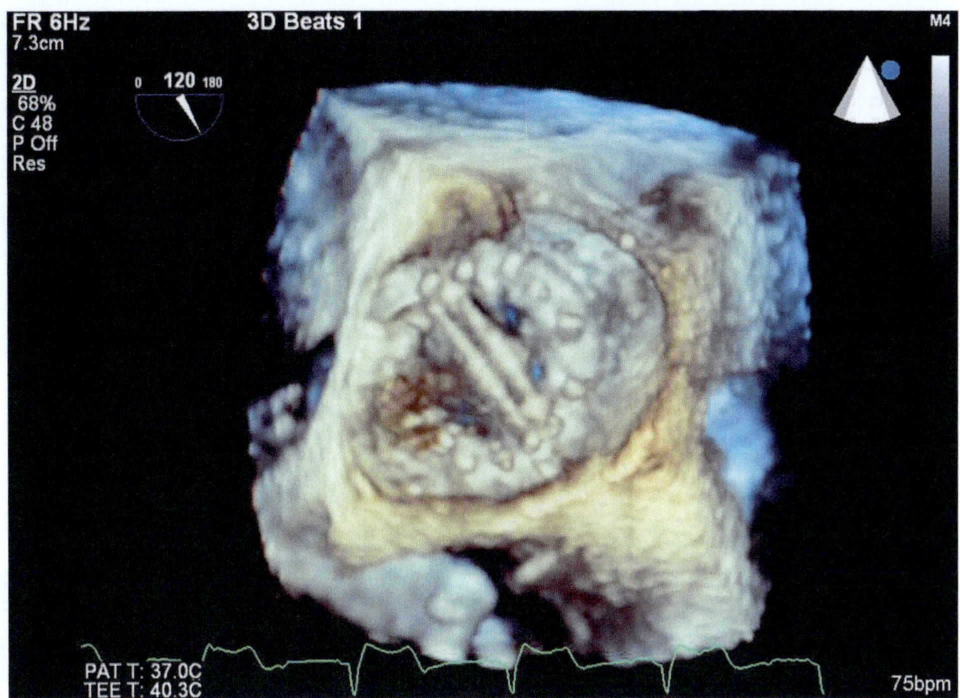

Fig. 6.66 Transesophageal 72° view demonstrating no significant residual paravalvular leak after deployment of the occluder device

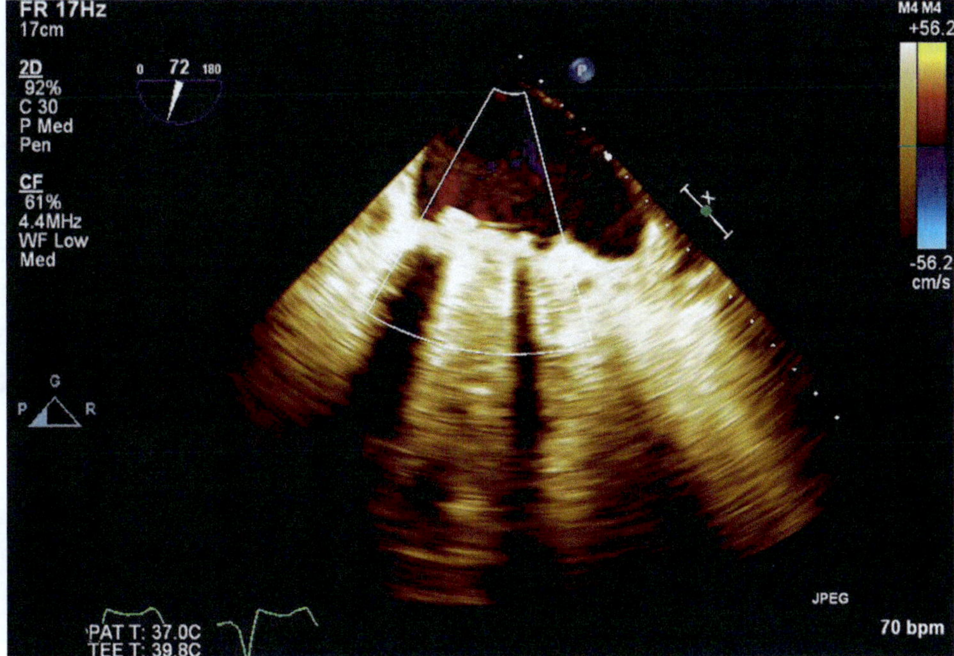

Fig. 6.67 3D zoom view of the mitral valve, showing the 12-mm Amplatzer Vascular Plug II device deployed inferoposteriorly

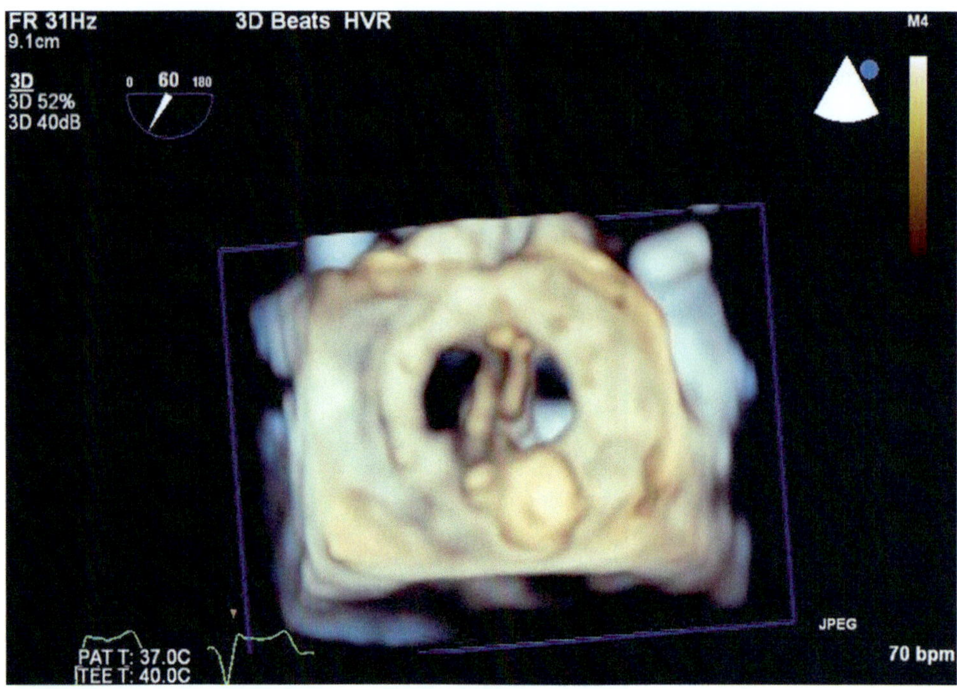

Fig. 6.68 TTE parasternal long-axis view with simultaneous 2D and color Doppler imaging demonstrating the occluder device in situ adjacent to the posterior aspect of the valve ring. No significant residual mitral regurgitation is visible

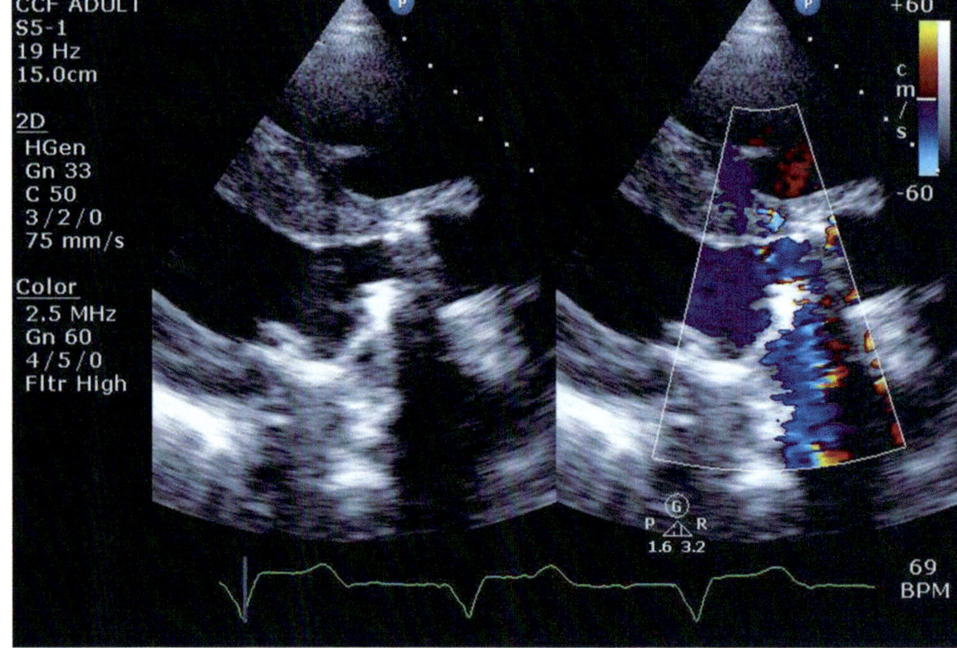

Fig. 6.69 Transthoracic parasternal short-axis view just apical to the true mitral valve annulus with simultaneous 2D and color Doppler imaging. The ventricular aspect of the occluder device can be seen inferoposteriorly

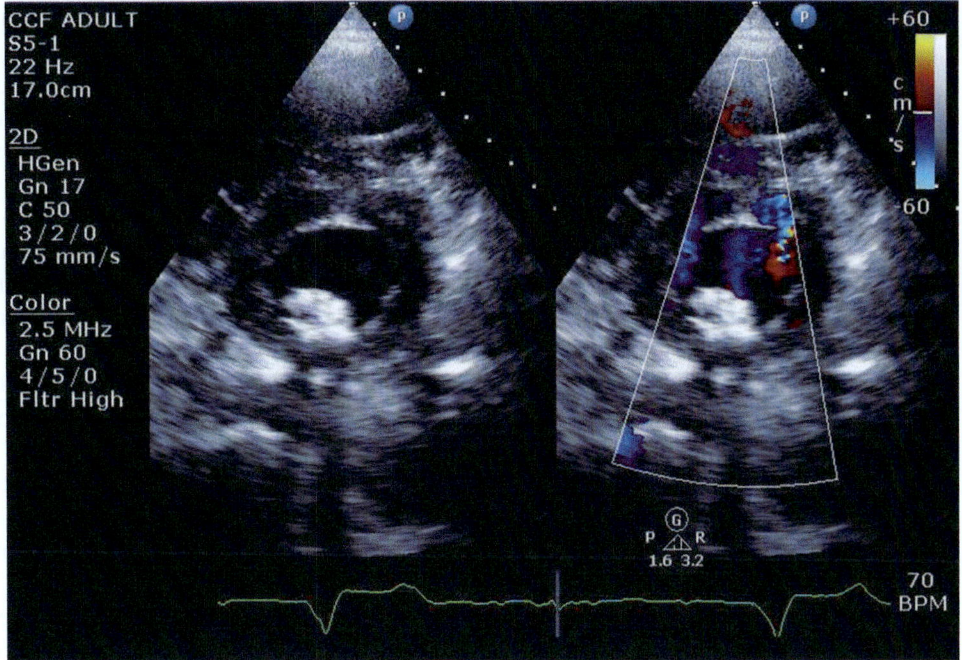

6.9   Case 8. Transcutaneous Mitral Valve Replacement: "Valve in Valve"

An 80-year-old woman with a past history of rheumatic heart disease presented with congestive cardiac failure due to prosthetic mitral and native aortic valve stenosis. She had a past history of previous open heart surgery, including open mitral commissurotomy 42 years ago, pericardiectomy for constrictive pericarditis 22 years ago, and bioprosthetic mitral valve replacement (Carpentier-Edwards 27 mm) 11 years ago. She was deemed to be high risk for redo of open surgery and underwent transcutaneous aortic and mitral valve replacements via a transapical approach (Figs. 6.70, 6.71, 6.72, 6.73, 6.74, 6.75, 6.76, 6.77, and 6.78).

Video 6.60 Transesophageal 0° view demonstrating the Carpentier-Edwards prosthetic mitral valve in situ, with calcification and immobility of the posteromedial leaflet (AVI 5076 kb)

Video 6.61 3D zoom of the bioprosthetic mitral valve from the left atrium, demonstrating thickening and immobility of the posteromedial prosthetic leaflet (AVI 996 kb)

Video 6.62 3D imaging of the guidewire across the mitral valve (AVI 1835 kb)

Video 6.63 3D imaging of the mitral valve prosthesis being fed along the guide wire into position (AVI 862 kb)

Video 6.64 3D imaging during balloon inflation and deployment of the new 26-mm Edwards Sapien bioprosthetic valve prosthesis (AVI 505 kb)

Video 6.65 3D imaging after deployment of the fully expanded and normally functioning mitral valve prosthesis; the guidewire is still in situ (AVI 1006 kb)

Video 6.66 3D imaging after removal of the guidewire demonstrates unrestricted opening of the new transcutaneous "valve in valve" mitral valve replacement (AVI 1933 kb)

Video 6.67 Transesophageal 2D biplane view (0° and 90°) demonstrating the new transcutaneous mitral valve replacement opening normally (AVI 4148 kb)

Video 6.68 Transesophageal biplane view (0° and 90°) with color Doppler imaging demonstrating mild residual valvular mitral regurgitation and a trace anterior paravalvular leak (AVI 912 kb)

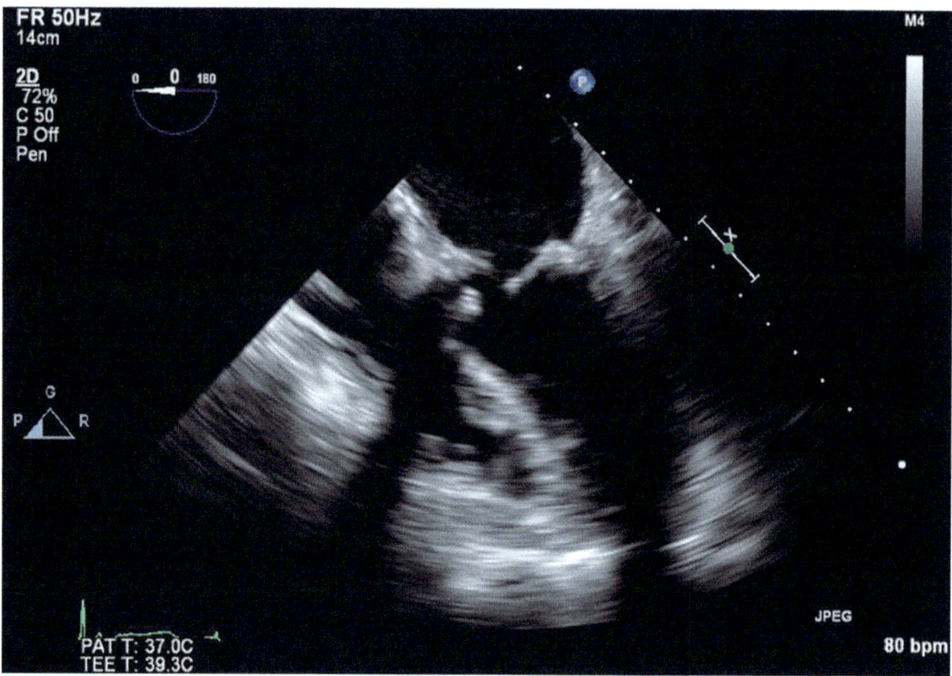

Fig. 6.70 Transesophageal 0° view demonstrating the Carpentier-Edwards prosthetic mitral valve in situ, with calcification and immobility of the posteromedial leaflet

Fig. 6.71 3D zoom of the bioprosthetic mitral valve from the left atrium, demonstrating thickening and immobility of the posteromedial prosthetic leaflet

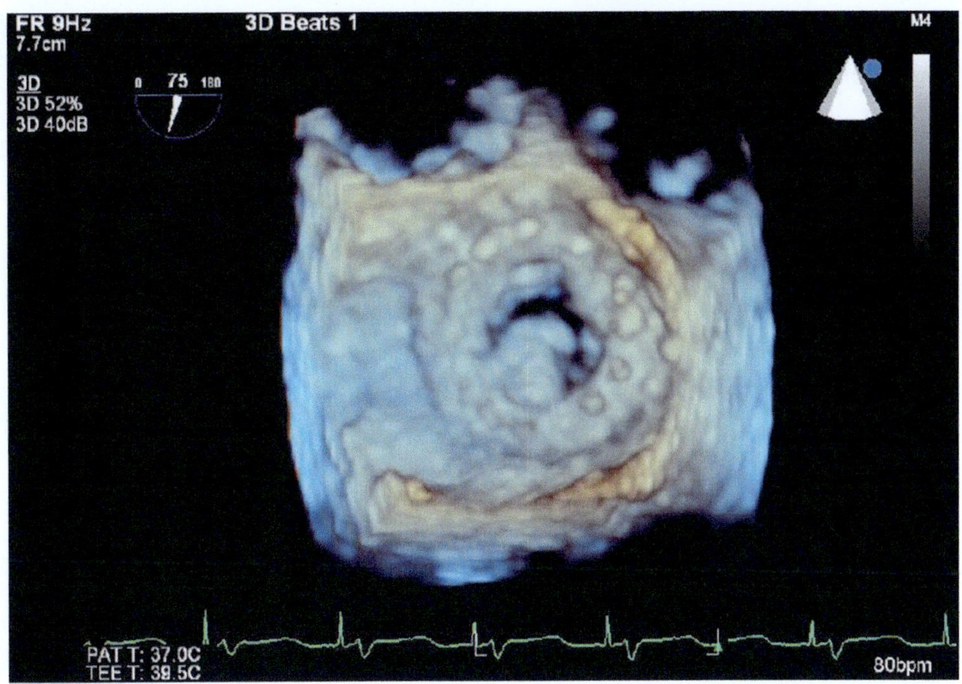

Fig. 6.72 3D imaging of the guidewire across the mitral valve

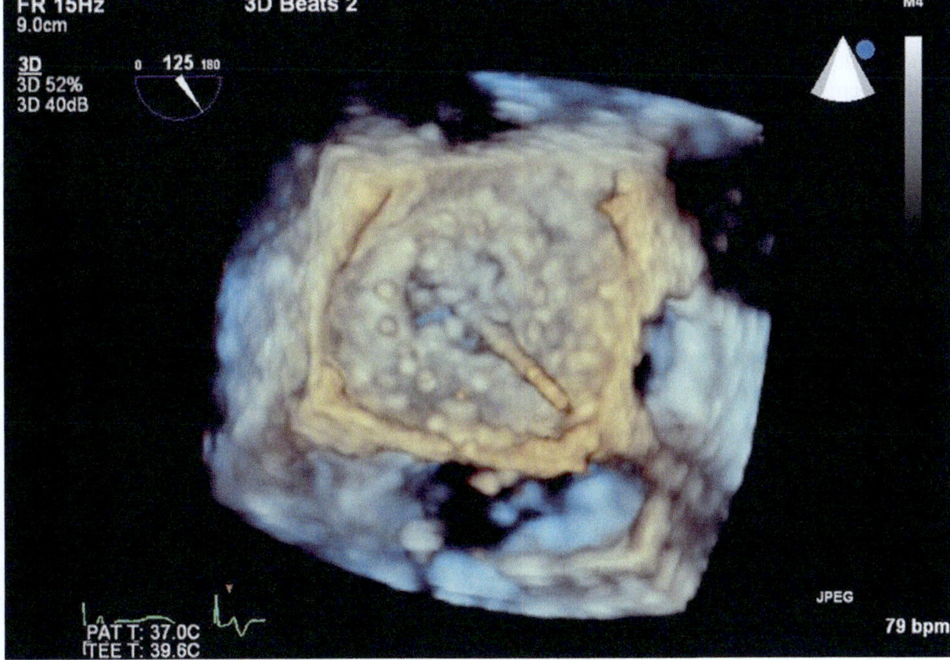

Fig. 6.73 3D imaging of the mitral valve prosthesis being fed along the guide wire into position

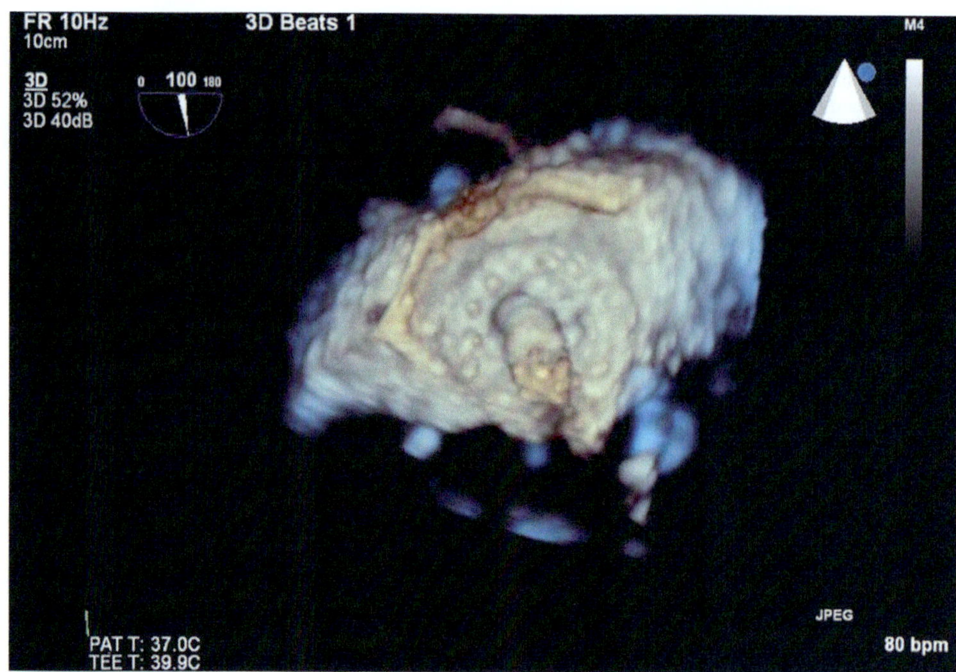

Fig. 6.74 3D imaging during balloon inflation and deployment of the new 26-mm Edwards Sapien bioprosthetic valve prosthesis

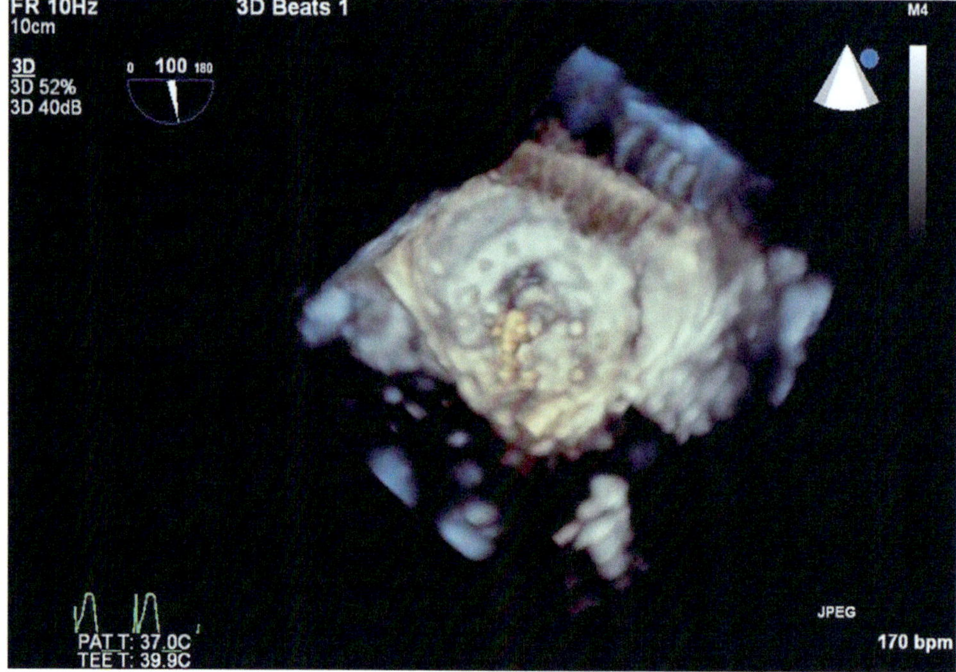

Fig. 6.75 3D imaging after deployment of the fully expanded and normally functioning mitral valve prosthesis; the guidewire is still in situ

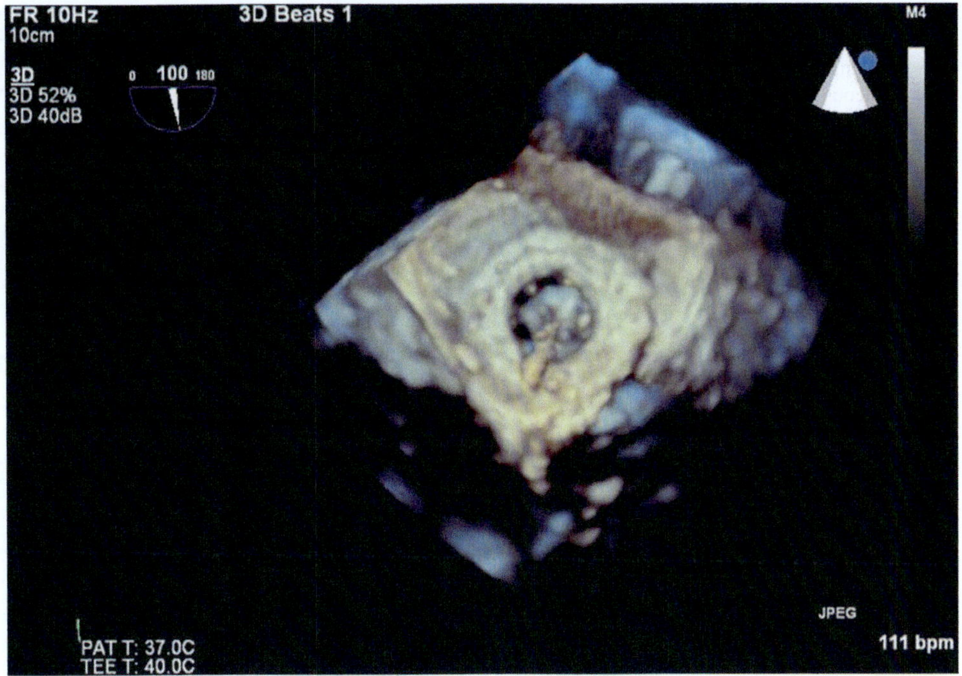

Fig. 6.76 3D imaging after removal of the guidewire demonstrates unrestricted opening of the new transcutaneous "valve in valve" mitral valve replacement

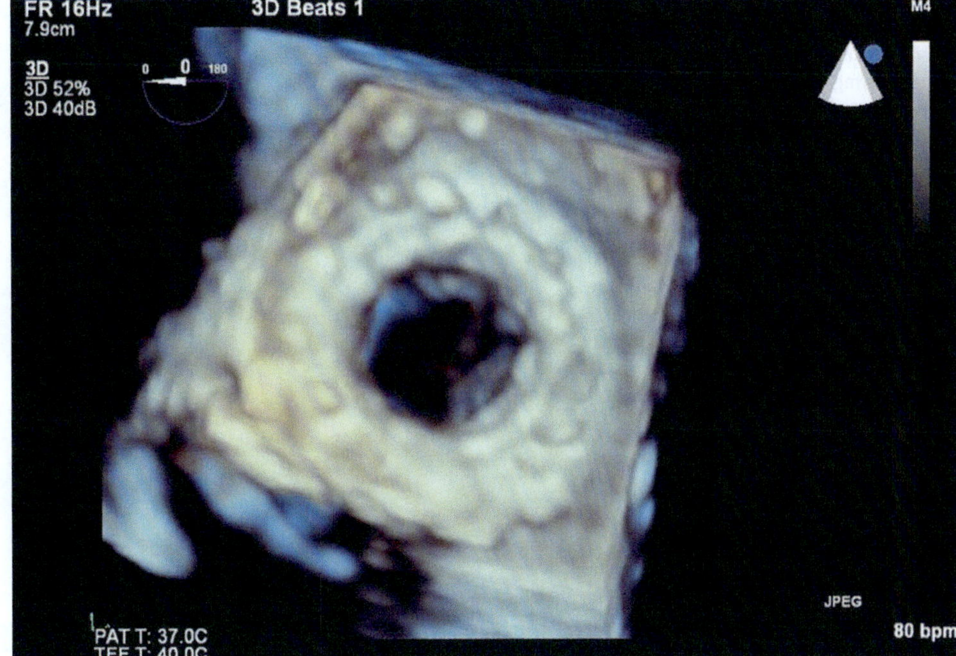

Fig. 6.77 Transesophageal 2D biplane view (0° and 90°) demonstrating the new transcutaneous mitral valve replacement opening normally

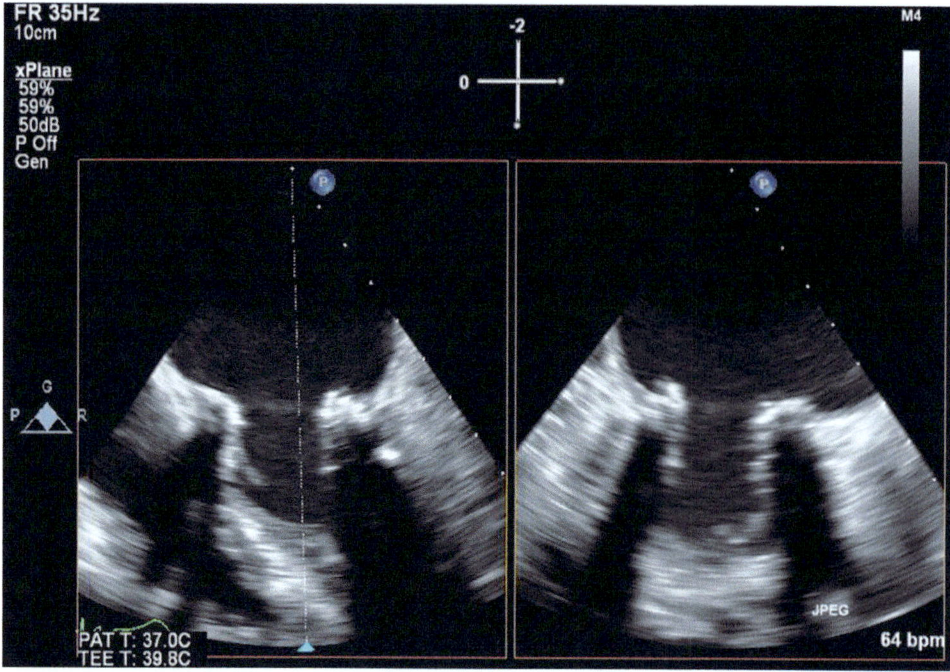

Fig. 6.78 Transesophageal biplane view (0° and 90°) with color Doppler imaging demonstrating mild residual valvular mitral regurgitation and a trace anterior paravalvular leak

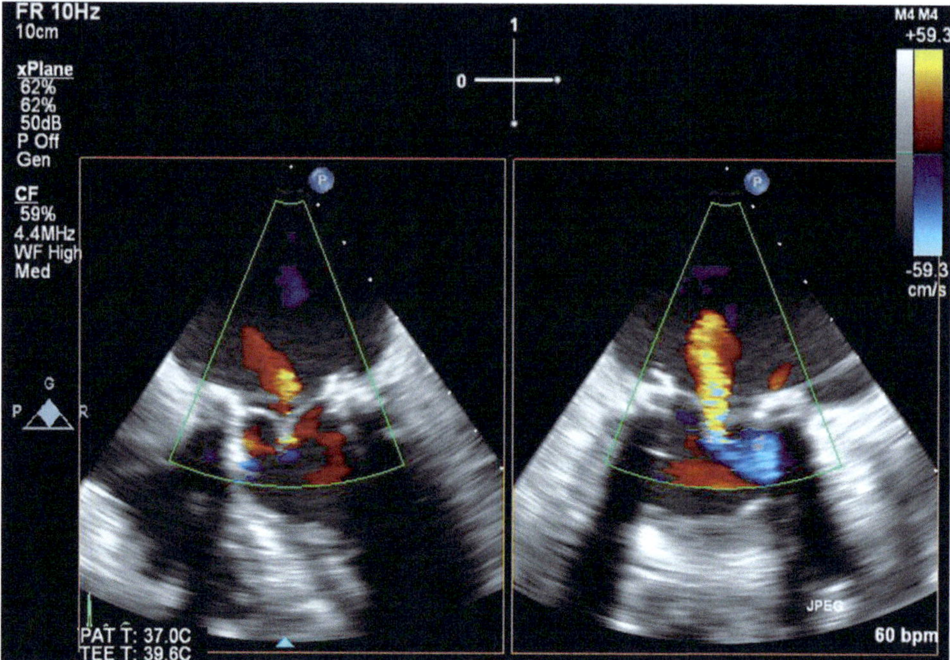

6.10   Case 9. Mitral Balloon Valvuloplasty

63-year-old woman with a history of rheumatic fever as a child presented with worsening dyspnea after only mild exertion. She was noted to have severe mitral stenosis (mean gradient 10 mmHg) with moderate to severe thickening and restriction of the anterior leaflet tip and posterior leaflet tip and body. A degree of valve mobility was preserved (anterior > posterior), there was negligible calcification, and the subvalvular apparatus was minimally involved. Given this constellation of findings, she was felt to be a good candidate for balloon valvuloplasty (Figs. 6.79, 6.80, 6.81, 6.82, 6.83, 6.84, 6.85, and 6.86).

Video 6.69 Transesophageal four-chamber (0°) view demonstrating moderate to severe thickening of both leaflet tips and restriction of leaflet mobility (posterior > anterior) (MPG 503 kb)

Video 6.70 Transesophageal view of the mitral valve at 60°, demonstrating moderate bileaflet thickening with restriction of posterior leaflet movement (P1) but relative preservation of anterior leaflet excursion (A1 and A2 scallops) (MPG 504 kb)

Video 6.71 Transesophageal view of the mitral valve at 60° with color Doppler imaging, demonstrating turbulent diastolic forward flow associated with the stenosis but minimal regurgitation (MPG 498 kb)

Video 6.72 Transesophageal imaging of the mitral valve at 108° during balloon valvuloplasty (MPG 539 kb)

Video 6.73 Transesophageal four-chamber (−5°) view of the mitral valve after balloon valvuloplasty demonstrates improved anterior leaflet excursion (MPG 1080 kb)

Video 6.74 After valvuloplasty, a transesophageal view of the mitral valve at 20° with color Doppler imaging demonstrates reduced turbulence of the diastolic forward flow and only trivial to mild regurgitation (MPG 414 kb)

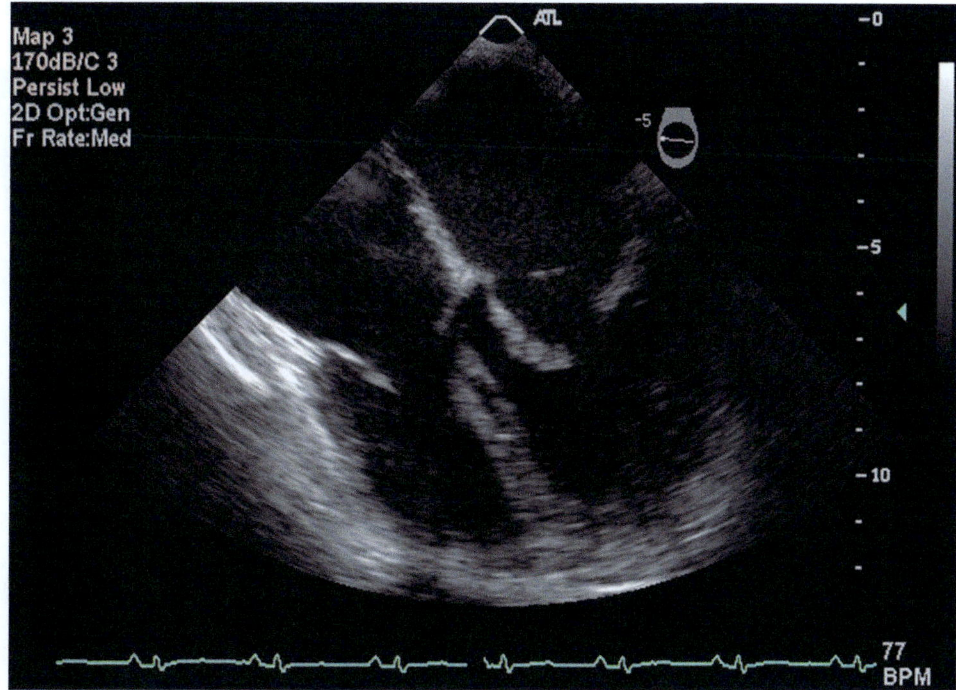

Fig. 6.79 Transesophageal four-chamber (0°) view demonstrating moderate to severe thickening of both leaflet tips and restriction of leaflet mobility (posterior > anterior)

Fig. 6.80 Transesophageal view of the mitral valve at 60°, demonstrating moderate bileaflet thickening with restriction of posterior leaflet movement (P1) but relative preservation of anterior leaflet excursion (A1 and A2 scallops)

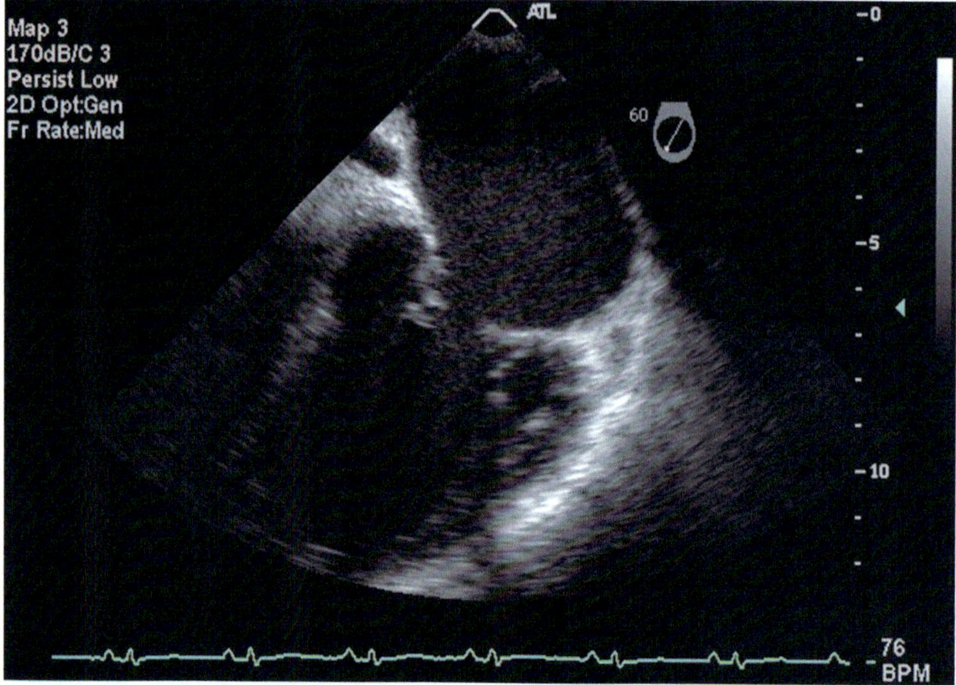

Fig. 6.81 Transesophageal view of the mitral valve at 60° with color Doppler imaging, demonstrating turbulent diastolic forward flow associated with the stenosis but minimal regurgitation

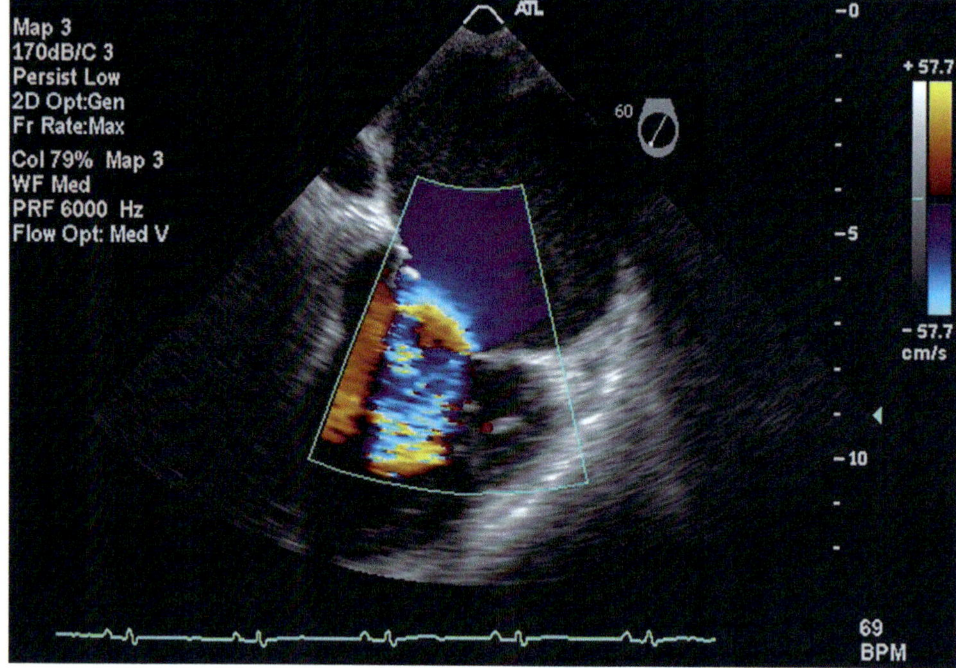

Fig. 6.82 Continuous wave Doppler trace across the mitral valve demonstrates severe stenosis (peak transvalvular gradient, 19 mmHg; mean gradient, 10 mmHg)

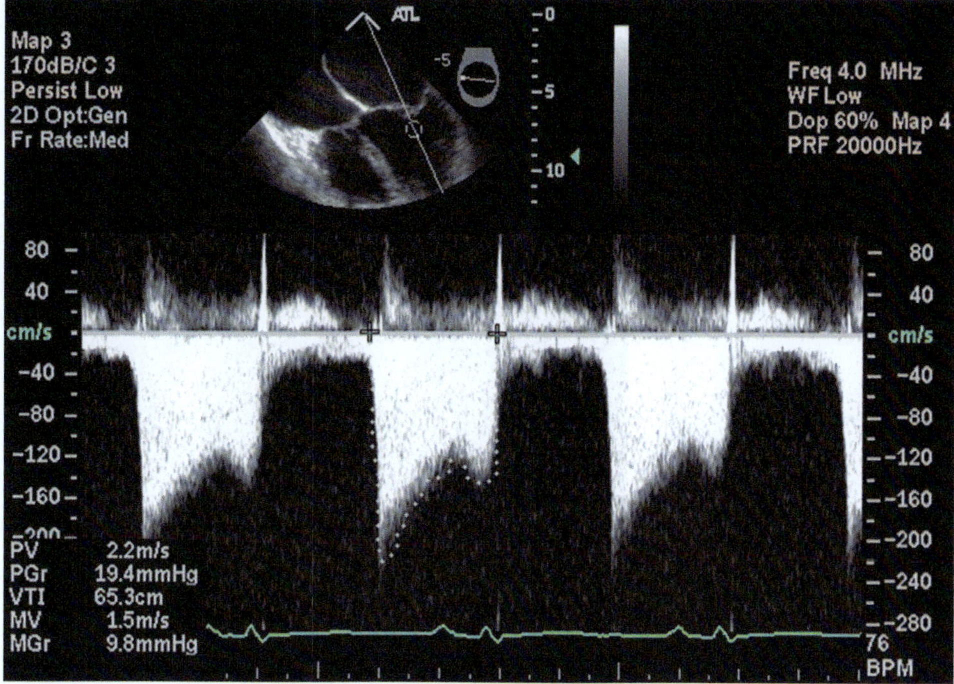

Fig. 6.83 Transesophageal imaging of the mitral valve at 108° during balloon valvuloplasty

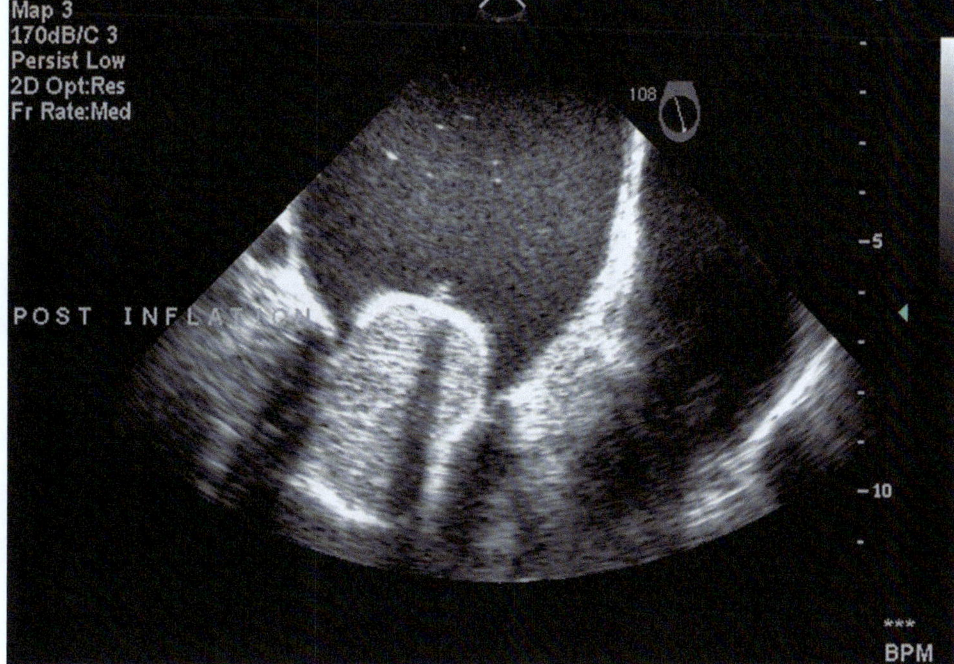

Fig. 6.84 Transesophageal four-chamber (−5°) view of the mitral valve after balloon valvuloplasty demonstrates improved anterior leaflet excursion

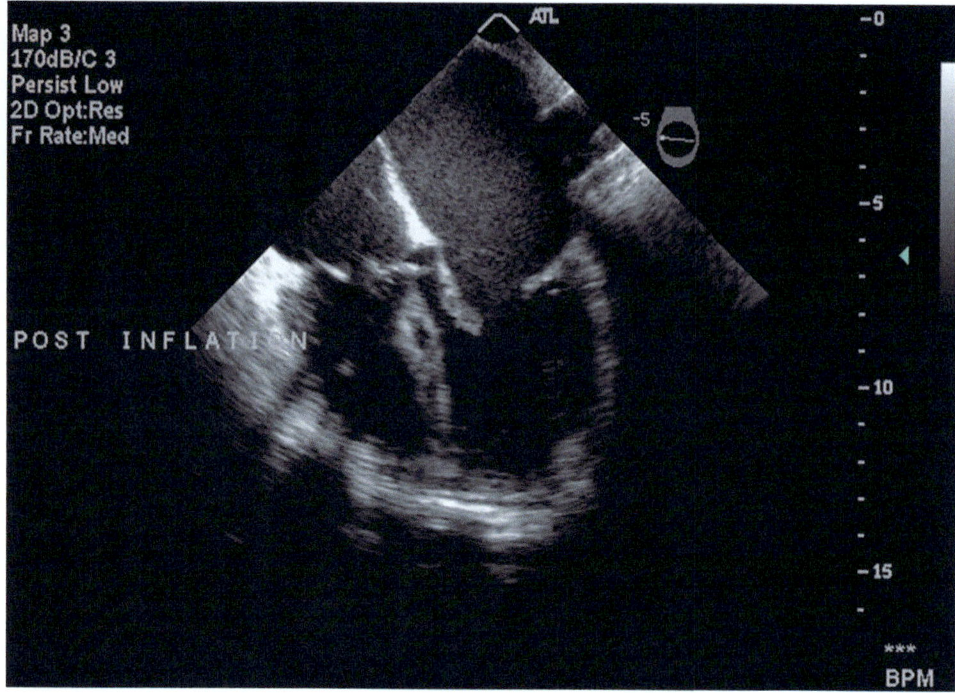

Fig. 6.85 After valvuloplasty, a transesophageal view of the mitral valve at 20° with color Doppler imaging demonstrates reduced turbulence of the diastolic forward flow and only trivial to mild regurgitation

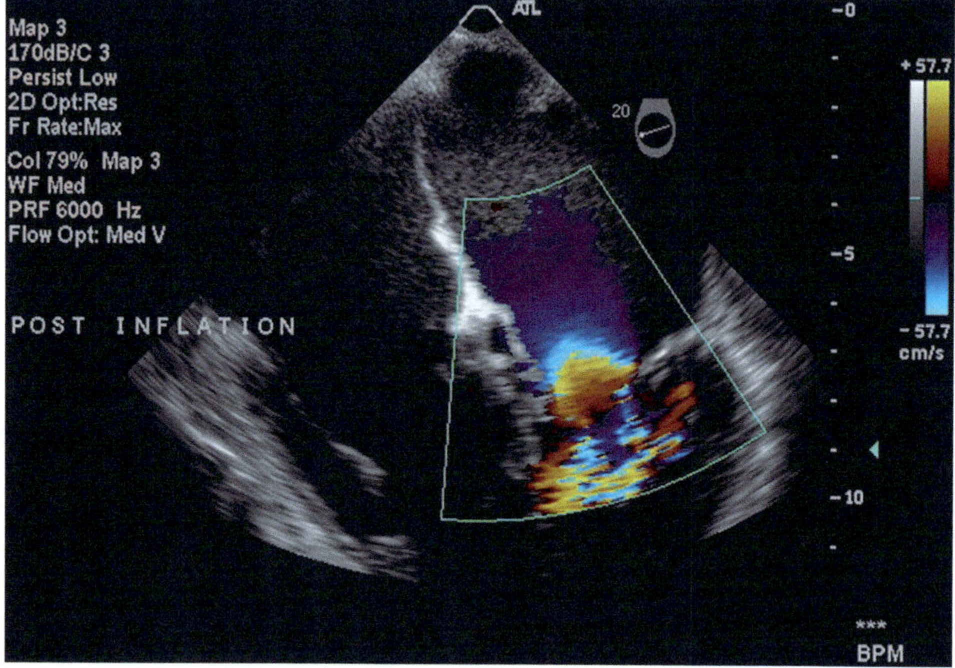

Fig. 6.86 After valvuloplasty, a continuous wave Doppler trace across the mitral valve demonstrates a reduction in peak and mean transvalvular gradients to 14 and 7 mmHg respectively

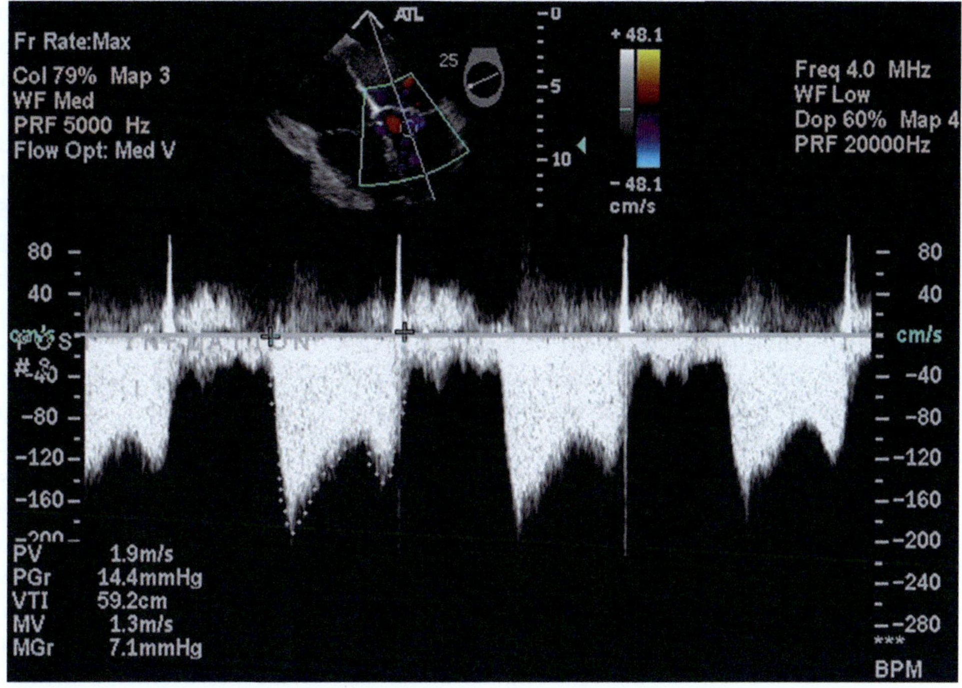

6.11 Case 10. Device Therapy: Cardiac Resynchronization Therapy

A 67-year-old man with a known ischemic cardiomyopathy, an ejection fraction of 20 %, and a QRS duration of 130 msec presented for consideration of biventricular pacemaker/implantable defibrillator (CRT-D) implantation. He reported New York Heart Association (NYHA) Class III symptoms and had a past history of remote coronary artery bypass graft surgery without further options for revascularization. At baseline, he was noted to have extensive regional wall motion abnormalities, including an aneurysmal basal inferior wall. Associated severe left ventricular enlargement lead to apical tethering of the mitral valve and posterior leaflet restriction. In combination, this resulted in severe (3–4+) mitral regurgitation. He underwent CRT-D implantation. After 6 months of cardiac resynchronization therapy, he underwent repeat echocardiographic assessment, which showed evidence of left ventricular remodeling with a reduction in left ventricular size and improvement in left ventricular function (ejection fraction 25–30 %). His mitral regurgitation had also significantly improved and was now graded as mild to moderate (1–2+) in severity. Clinically, these echocardiographic changes were mirrored by improvement in symptoms to NYHA Class I (Figs. 6.87 and 6.88).

Video 6.75 Apical long-axis image with color Doppler imaging demonstrates a severely dilated left ventricle with extensive regional wall motion abnormalities consistent with multivessel coronary artery disease An aneurysmal basal inferior wall is noted There is severe (3–4+) central mitral regurgitation secondary to apical tethering and leaflet restriction (AVI 10546 kb)

Video 6.76 Apical long-axis 2 chamber (B) image with color Doppler imaging demonstrate a severely dilated left ventricle with extensive regional wall motion abnormalities consistent with multivessel coronary artery disease An aneurysmal basal inferior wall is noted There is severe (3–4+) central mitral regurgitation secondary to apical tethering and leaflet restriction (AVI 5689 kb)

Video 6.77 Apical long-axis 3 chamber image with color Doppler imaging demonstrate a severely dilated left ventricle with extensive regional wall motion abnormalities consistent with multivessel coronary artery disease There is severe (3–4+) central mitral regurgitation secondary to apical tethering and leaflet restriction (AVI 7420 kb)

Video 6.78 After 6 months of cardiac resynchronization therapy, a marked decrease in left ventricular size, improvement in left ventricular function, and reduction in mitral regurgitation severity to mild to moderate (1–2+) were observed (AVI 3127 kb)

Fig. 6.87 Apical long-axis 4 chamber (**a**), 2 chamber (**b**), and 3 chamber (**c**) images with color Doppler imaging demonstrate a severely dilated left ventricle with extensive regional wall motion abnormalities consistent with multivessel coronary artery disease. An aneurysmal basal inferior wall is noted. There is severe (3–4+) central mitral regurgitation secondary to apical tethering and leaflet restriction

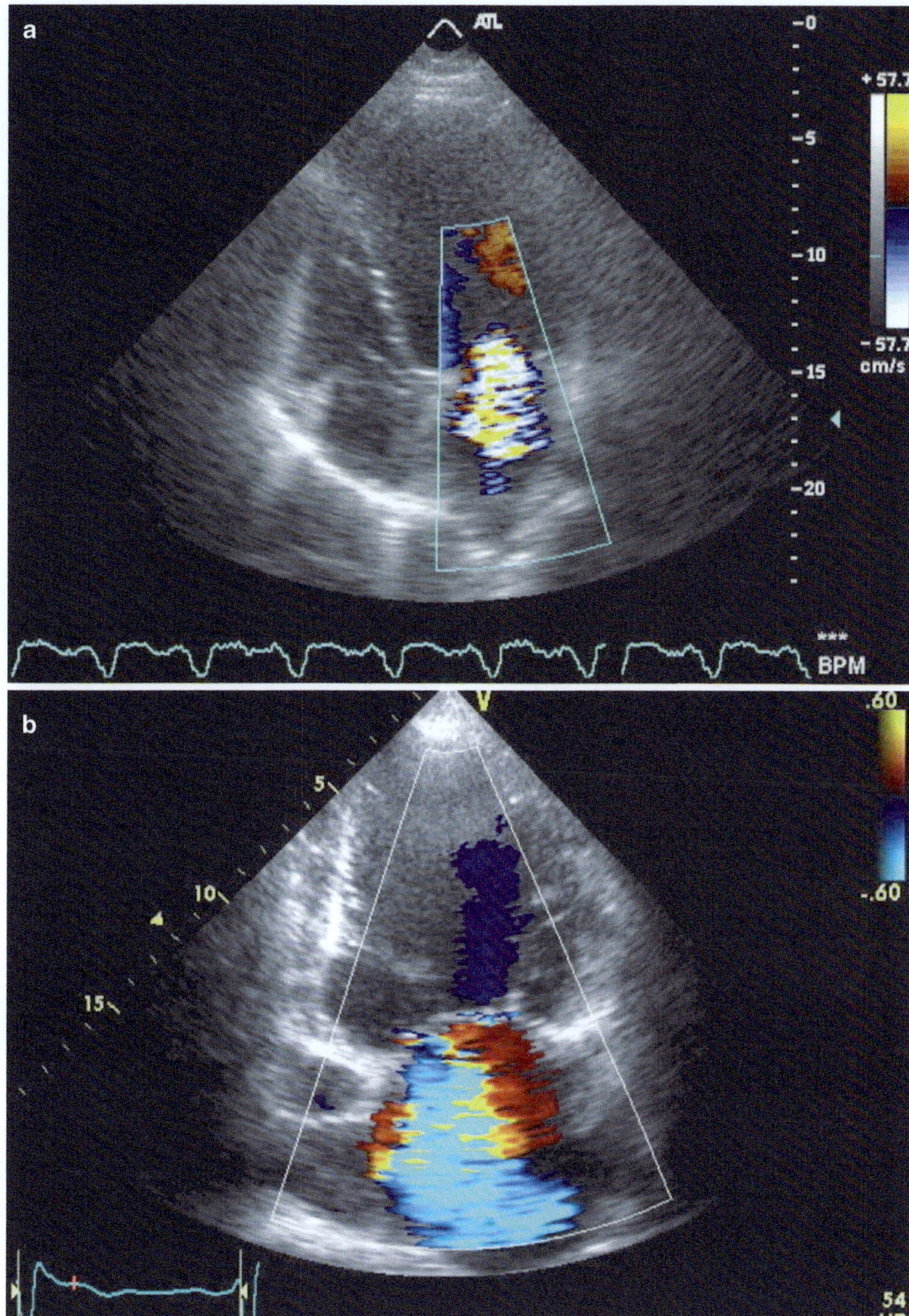

Fig. 6.87 (continued)

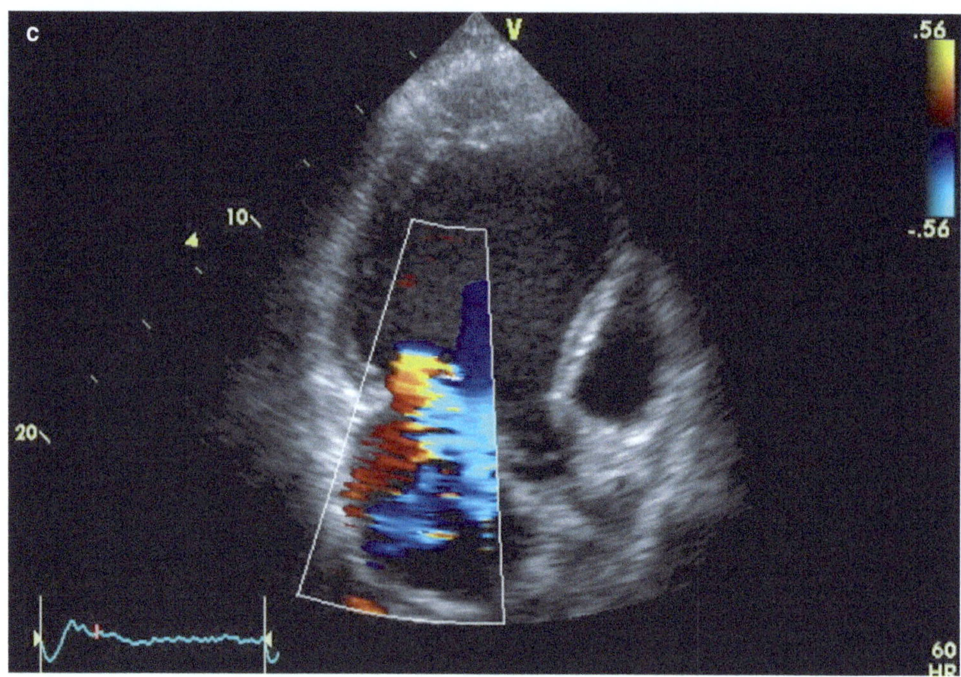

Fig. 6.88 After 6 months of cardiac resynchronization therapy, a marked decrease in left ventricular size, improvement in left ventricular function, and reduction in mitral regurgitation severity to mild to moderate (1–2+) were observed and can be seen on the 4-chamber (**a**) and 2-chamber (**b**) apical long-axis views

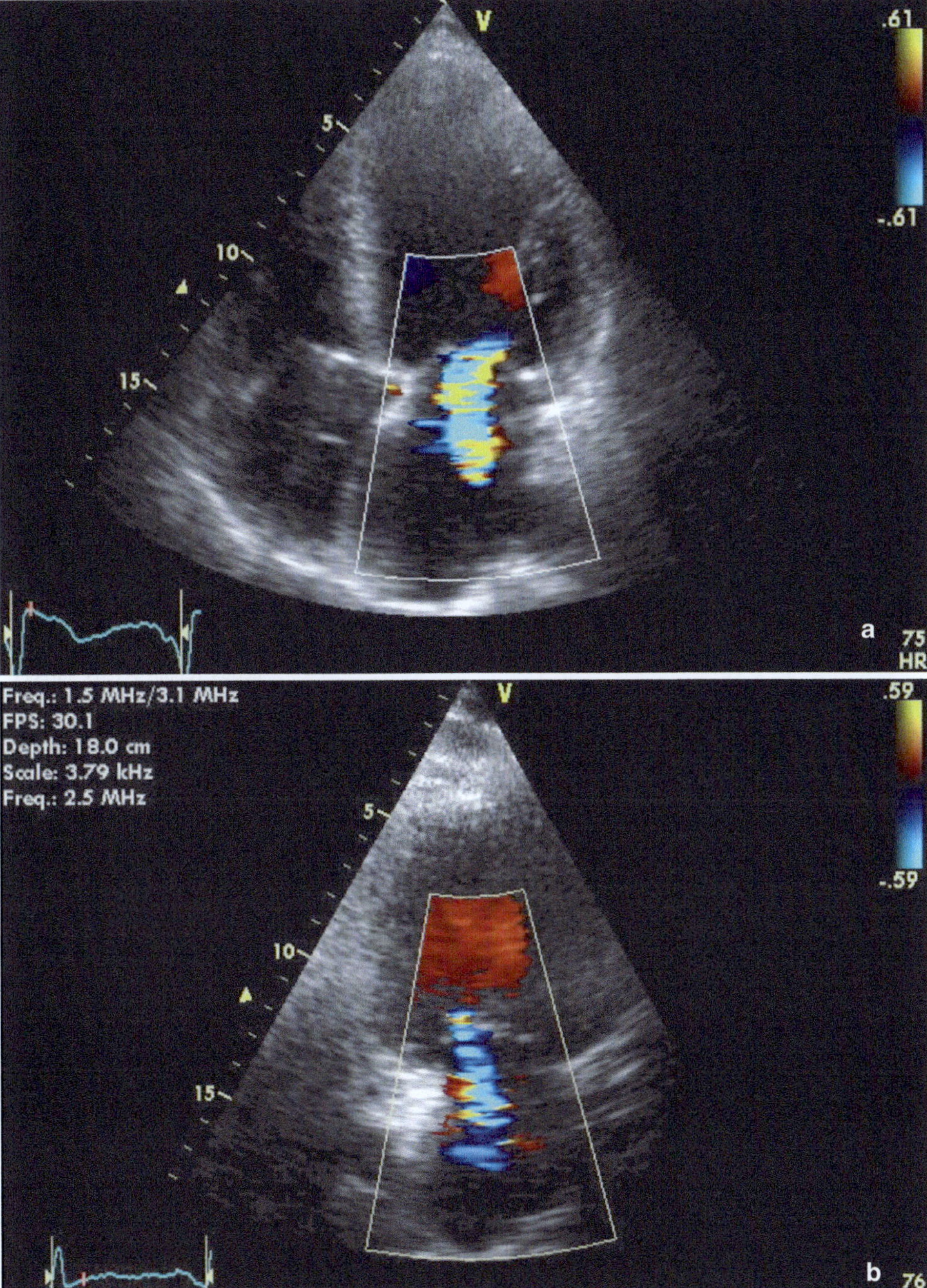

6.12 Teaching Points

- Percutaneous devices such as the MitraClip offer alternative, nonsurgical treatment strategies for patients with valvular mitral regurgitation. Occluder plugs offer a similar alternative strategy for patients with paravalvular regurgitation. These devices must be reserved for appropriate individuals based upon surgical risk, long-term goals, and informed patient preference [1, 2].
- Adequate training in the deployment of these percutaneous devices is mandatory for all practitioners. Outcomes are typically associated with initial operator-specific and site-specific learning phases, so procedural experience and case volume are important considerations when referring patients.
- Echocardiography is essential for intraprocedural guidance. New echo platform features, including biplane and 3D capabilities with real-time imaging, continue to improve our spatial awareness and enable ongoing implementation of more complex device therapies.
- Hybrid interventional suites are becoming more common and will facilitate a new era of cooperation between interventionalists and surgeons, thereby allowing more complex procedures to be safely undertaken.
- Multiple clips or occluder devices may be required in the same patient to achieve an acceptable final result, with obvious cost and technical implications.
- Small paravalvular leaks may cause increased jet turbulence and therefore greater associated hemolysis than larger, more laminar jets.
- Mitral balloon valvuloplasty is a well validated procedure, which can significantly improve patient symptoms. It can be employed as destination therapy or as a bridge to surgical or transcutaneous valve replacement. When determining suitability for valvuloplasty, it is important to consider valve characteristics, which are summarized by the "Splitability Score" which rates (from 0 to 4) parameters of leaflet thickness, leaflet calcification, leaflet mobility, and subvalvular apparatus [3].
- Transcutaneous mitral valve replacement, including "valve in valve" procedures, remain off-label and require long-term outcome studies.

References

1. Mauri L, Foster E, Glower DD, Apruzzese P, Massaro JM, Herrmann HC, et al. 4-year results of a randomized controlled trial of percutaneous repair versus surgery for mitral regurgitation. J Am Coll Cardiol. 2013;62:317–28.
2. Krishnaswamy A, Kapadia SR, Tuzcu EM. Percutaneous paravalvular leak closure– imaging, techniques and outcomes. Circ J. 2013;77:19–27.
3. Wilkins GT, Weyman AE, Abascal VM, Block PT, Palacios IF. Percutaneous balloon dilatation of the mitral valve: an analysis of echocardiographic variables related to the outcome and mechanism of dilatation. Br Heart J. 1988;60:299–308.

Teerapat Yingchoncharoen

7.1 Case 1. Native Valve Infective Endocarditis

A 62-year-old man with a history of degenerative mitral valve disease for several years presented to his local primary care physician due to fever, night sweats, chills, shortness of breath, and lethargy for 1 week. He was diagnosed with viral illness and treated with azithromycin twice a day for 1 week. His fever persisted despite good compliance with antibiotics therapy. He went to see a cardiologist, where blood cultures were drawn and echocardiography was performed. His blood culture grew group B *Streptococcus* and transthoracic echocardiography (TTE) showed severe mitral regurgitation with possible torn chordae tendinae. He was treated with intravenous ceftriaxone and gentamicin for 1 month and referred to our institute for mitral valve surgery. Intraoperatively, degenerative mitral valve disease with ruptured chordae tendinae and vegetations at the posterior leaflet were found. He underwent successful robotically assisted mitral valve repair with a 33-mm Duran annuloplasty band (Figs. 7.1, 7.2, 7.3, 7.4, 7.5, and 7.6).

Video 7.1 Apical four-chamber transthoracic echocardiography (TTE) showing large vegetation attached to the posterior leaflet of the mitral valve (AVI 8904 kb)

Video 7.2 Color Doppler imaging of Fig. 7.1 demonstrated severe mitral regurgitation with an eccentric, anteriorly directed jet (AVI 2018 kb)

Video 7.3 Three-dimensional TTE showing vegetation at the posterior mitral leaflet (AVI 2539 kb)

Video 7.4 Four-chamber transesophageal echocardiography (TEE) showing flail of the P2 segment of the posterior mitral leaflet (AVI 6317 kb)

Video 7.5 Zoom view of mitral valve showing large vegetation at the posterior mitral leaflet (AVI 17801 kb)

7.1.1 Learning Points

For the diagnosis of infective endocarditis (IE), TTE is considered the first-line cardiac imaging modality to demonstrate valvular vegetation, leaflet destruction, and complications of IE. TTE has a sensitivity between 50 and 90 % and a specificity greater than 90 % for detection of vegetations in native valve endocarditis (NVE). Transesophageal echocardiography (TEE) has a sensitivity ranging from 90 to 100 % for detection of NVE. TEE is recommended for all patients with known or suspected IE when TTE is nondiagnostic, when complications have developed or are clinically suspected, or when intracardiac device leads are present [1].

Mitral valve vegetation typically is located on the upstream side of the leaflet (i.e., the atrial side) but also can be attached to the chordae or the posterior wall of the left atrium. Echocardiographic features to define vegetation include a highly mobile mass that is typically irregularly shaped and low-reflectant, with rapid independent motion, prolapse into the left atrium during systole, and functional evidence of valve destruction.

Combined TTE and TEE detect vegetations in 90 % of cases, valve regurgitation in 60 %, paravalvular abscess in 20 % [2, 3], and rarely, prosthetic valve dehiscence pseudoaneurysms and fistulas [4].

Electronic supplementary material The online version of this chapter (doi:10.1007/978-1-4471-6672-6_7) contains supplementary material, which is available to authorized users.

T. Yingchoncharoen
Department of Cardiovascular Medicine, Cleveland Clinic, 9500 Euclid Avenue, Cleveland, OH 44195, USA
e-mail: teerapatmdcu@gmail.com

M. Desai et al. (eds.), *An Atlas of Mitral Valve Imaging*, DOI 10.1007/978-1-4471-6672-6_7, © Springer-Verlag London 2015

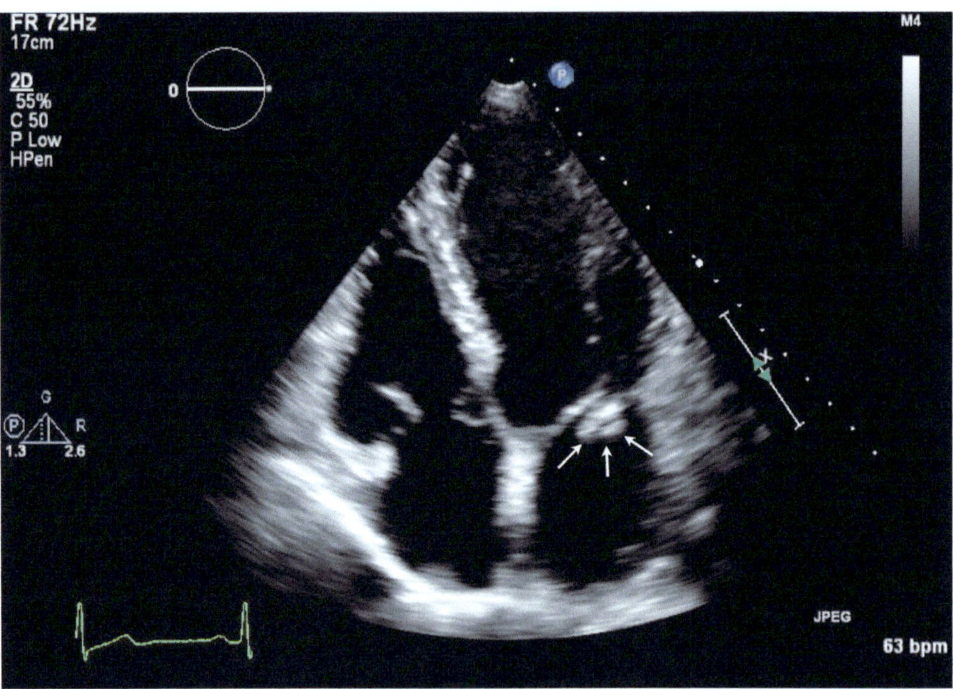

Fig. 7.1 Apical four-chamber transthoracic echocardiography (TTE) showing large vegetation attached to the posterior leaflet of the mitral valve (*arrows*)

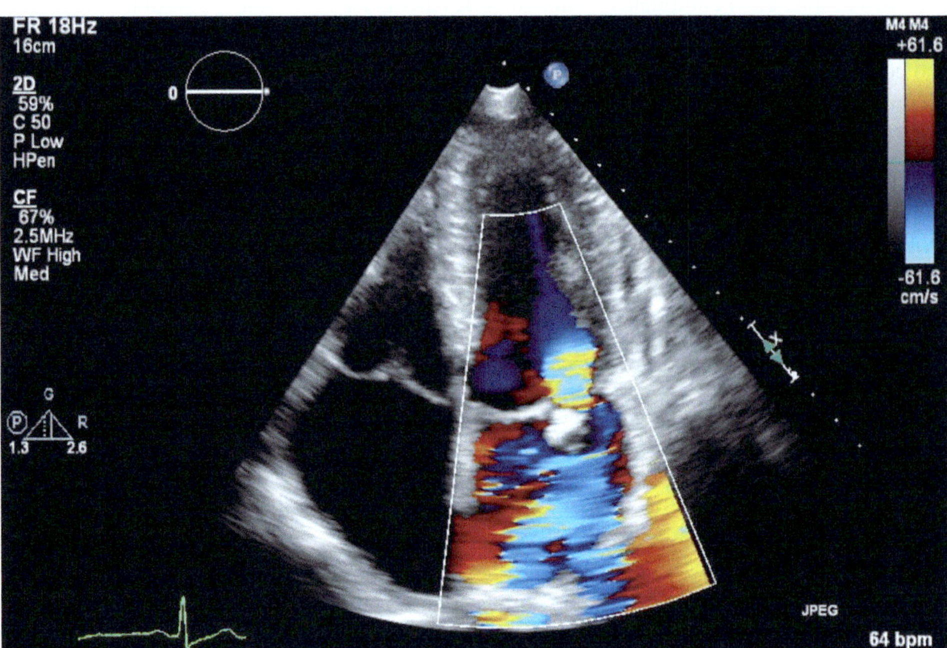

Fig. 7.2 Color Doppler imaging of Fig. 7.1 demonstrated severe mitral regurgitation with an eccentric, anteriorly directed jet

Fig. 7.3 Three-dimensional TTE showing vegetation at the posterior mitral leaflet (*arrows*). *Ao* aorta, *LA* left atrium, *LV* left ventricle

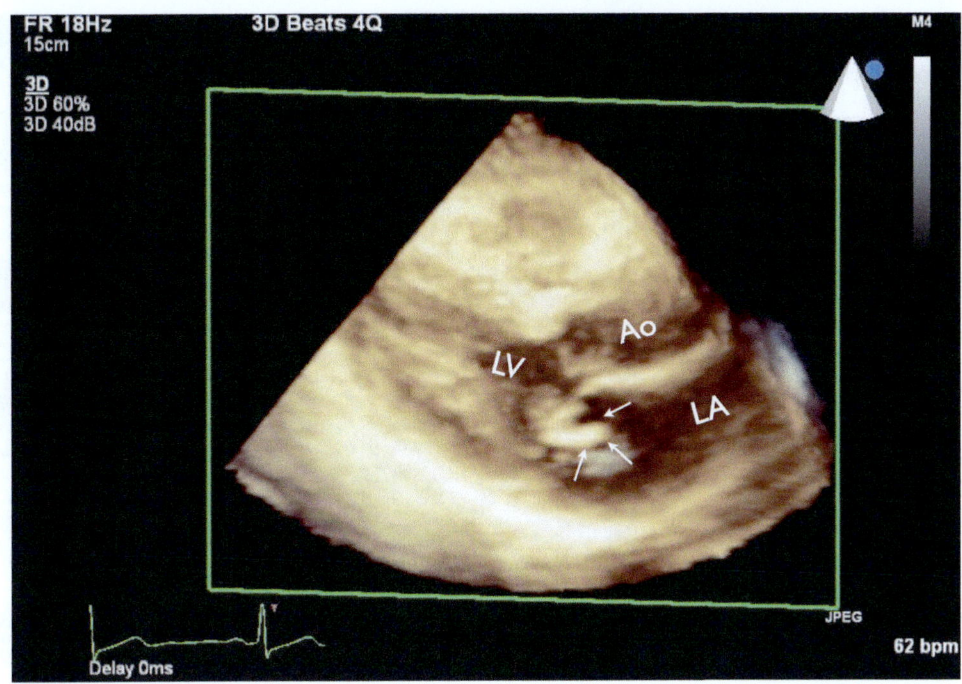

Fig. 7.4 Four-chamber transesophageal echocardiography (TEE) showing flail of the P2 segment of the posterior mitral leaflet (*arrow*). *RV* right ventricle

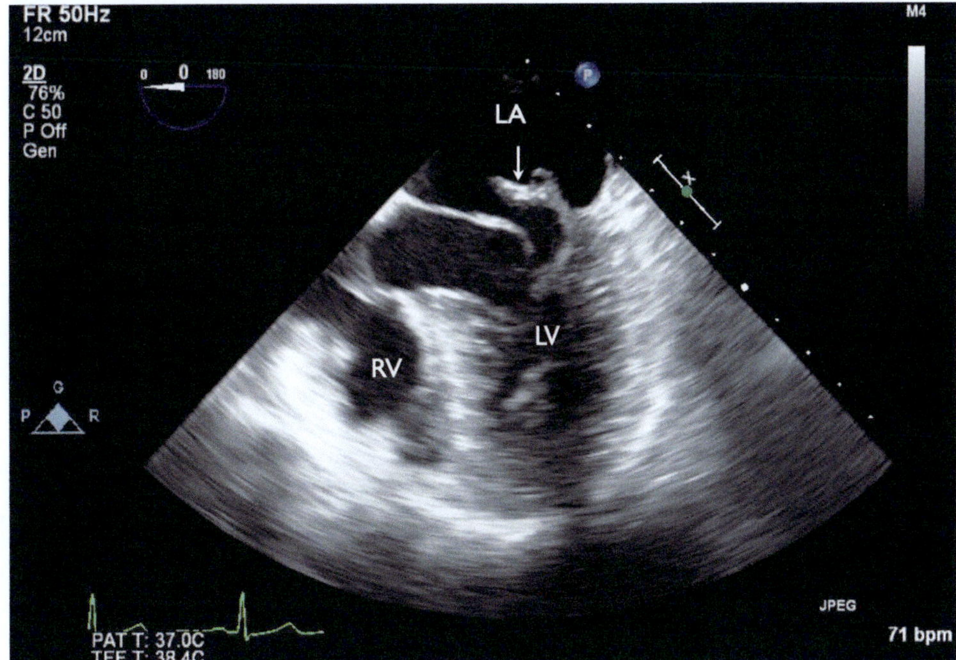

Fig. 7.5 Zoom view of mitral valve showing large vegetation at the posterior mitral leaflet (*arrows*)

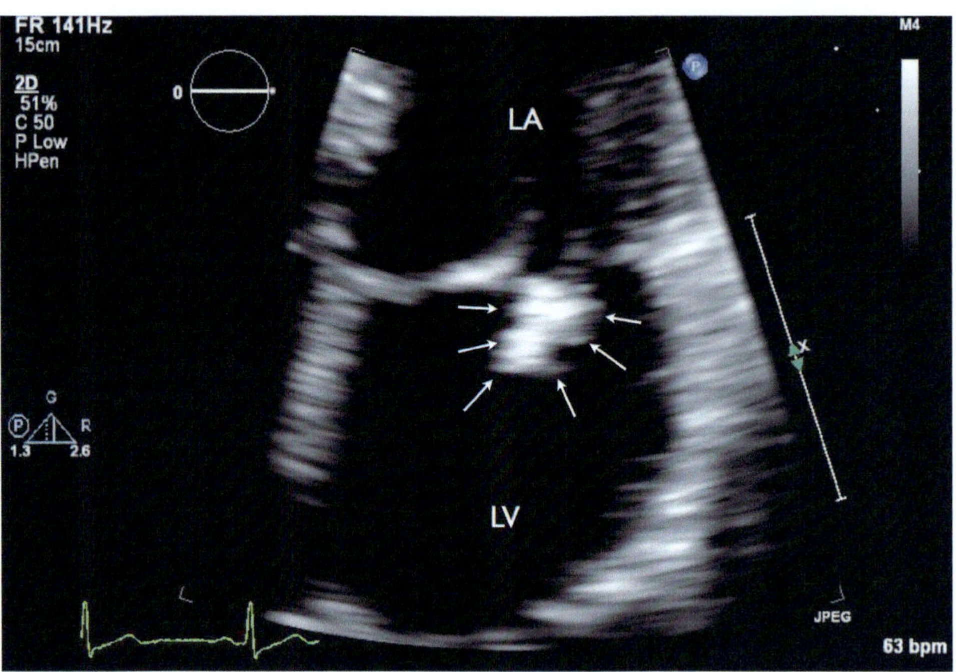

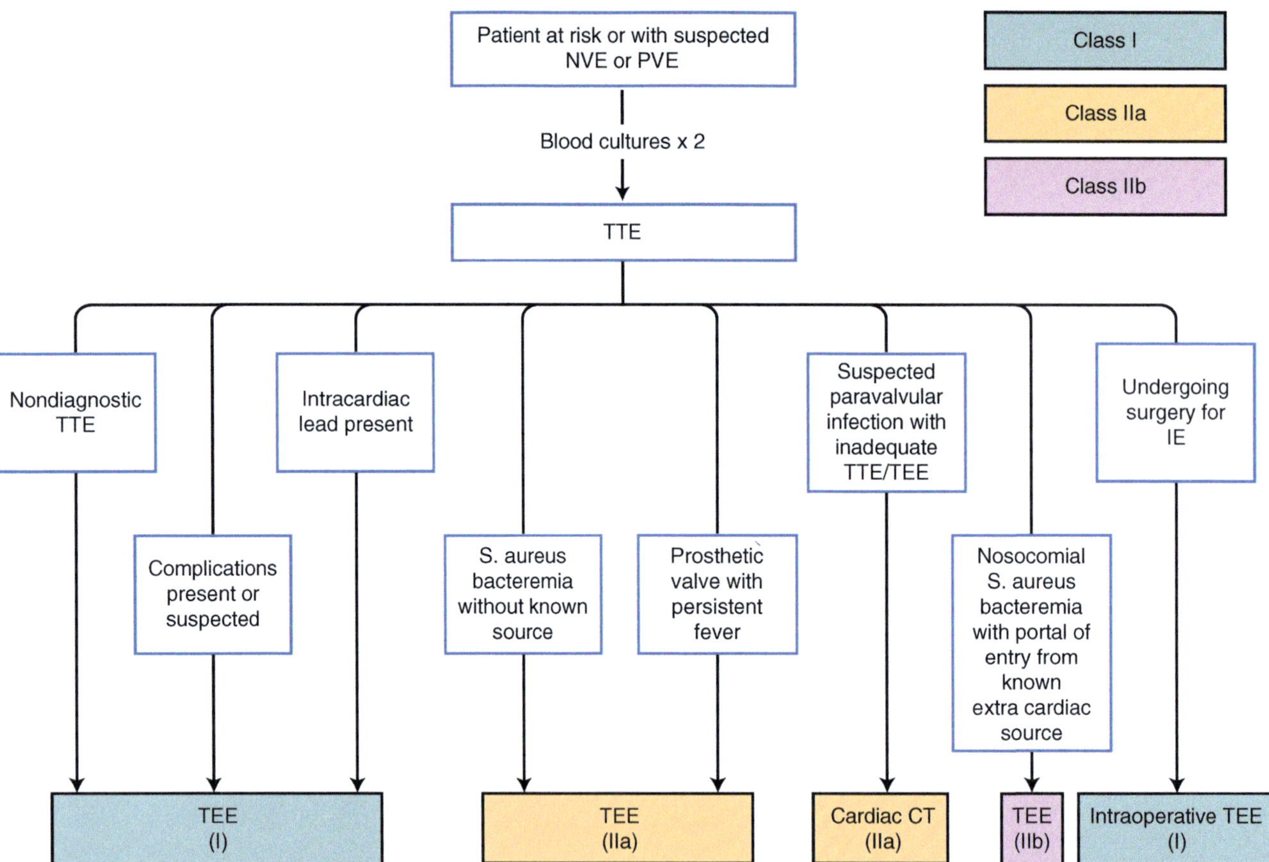

Fig. 7.6 Appropriate use of multimodality imaging in infective endocarditis according to 2014 ACC/AHA guidelines for management of valvular heart disease. *IE* infective endocarditis, *NVE* native valve endocarditis, *PVE* prosthetic valve endocarditis, *S. aureus staphylococcus aureus* (From Nishimura et al. [1])

7.2 Case 2. Native Valve Infective Endocarditis with Complications

A 60-year-old woman with a history of hypertension, intravenous drug abuse, and end-stage renal disease on hemodialysis was admitted to the hospital because of progressive dyspnea. Laboratory tests showed leukocytosis, and a chest x-ray showed diffuse bilateral pulmonary edema. Two sets of blood cultures grew methicillin-resistant *Staphylococcus aureus* (MRSA). TTE was performed and showed 60 % left ventricular ejection fraction with new, moderate mitral regurgitation and probable vegetation on the anterior mitral leaflet. She was treated with intravenous vancomycin for mitral valve IE.

Two days later, she developed acute-onset chest pain; electrocardiography showed diffuse ST segment elevations in the anterior, inferior, and lateral leads with elevated cardiac troponin T (TnT). She was transferred to our institute. Her cardiac catheterization revealed distal left anterior descending (LAD) embolism likely due to IE. She was supported on an intra-aortic balloon pump. She later developed first-degree AV block and disseminated intravascular coagulopathy (DIC), which required several vasopressors to maintain her hemodynamics. With her critically ill status and comorbidities, she was deemed too high-risk for open heart surgery and died a few days later (Figs. 7.7, 7.8, 7.9, 7.10, 7.11, 7.12, 7.13, and 7.14).

Video 7.6 Apical four-chamber TEE showing a large vegetation attached to the anterior and posterior leaflet of the mitral valve (AVI 4594 kb)

Video 7.7 Apical four-chamber TEE with color Doppler flow imaging showing severe mitral regurgitation (AVI 837 kb)

Video 7.8 Long-axis TEE demonstrated posterior mitral leaflet vegetation and mitral-aortic intervalvular fibrosa abscess and aneurysm (AVI 4764 kb)

Video 7.9 Long-axis TEE with color Doppler flow imaging showing mild aortic insufficiency and perforation of the anterior mitral leaflet. During diastole, a mild aortic insufficiency (AI) jet was seen, which was eccentric and anteriorly directed. During systole, there was mitral regurgitation caused by leaflet perforation from a "kissing lesion." (AVI 1713 kb)

Video 7.10 Three-dimensional (3D) TEE of the mitral valve (LA view) showing multiple vegetations (AVI 1022 kb)

Video 7.11 Coronary angiogram showing total occlusion of the distal left anterior descending artery. Given the angiographic features of acute cut-off appearance and the history of multiple vegetations, the finding is most likely consistent with coronary embolism from IE (AVI 5517 kb)

7.2.1 Learning Points

This case demonstrated two serious complications of mitral valve infective endocarditis: coronary embolism and pseudoaneurysm of the aortomitral curtain. Septic embolism leading to an acute myocardial infarction is rare, and balloon angioplasty with emergent cardiac surgery has been proposed as a treatment option. It can be argued that balloon dilation and stent implantation should be avoided, to prevent distal embolization and entrapment of septic embolism material in situ, which may affect vascular integrity in the long run [5, 6].

Because of the close anatomical relationship between the mitral and aortic valves, the infection can start from either valve and extend toward the other. There are two main mechanisms of extension of the infection from the aortic valve to the mitral valve: (1) aortic annular abscess that extends to the aortomitral curtain or intervalvular fibrous curtain and anterior mitral leaflet (Fig. 7.13), and (2) the aortic regurgitation caused by IE of the aortic valve, causing a "kissing lesion" on the secondarily infected anterior mitral leaflet. Various types of pseudoaneurysm of the aortomitral curtain are shown in Fig. 7.14. Endocarditis can also extend from the mitral to the aortic valve, by direct extension of a mitral annular abscess or as an isolated satellite lesion. The vegetation is usually small, typically located on the ventricular side of a leaflet, and does not result in aortic valve regurgitation. Comprehensive analysis of the aortic valve is mandatory in all patients with mitral valve endocarditis.

Fig. 7.7 Apical four-chamber TEE showing a large vegetation attached to the anterior and posterior leaflet of the mitral valve (*arrows*). *RA* right atrium

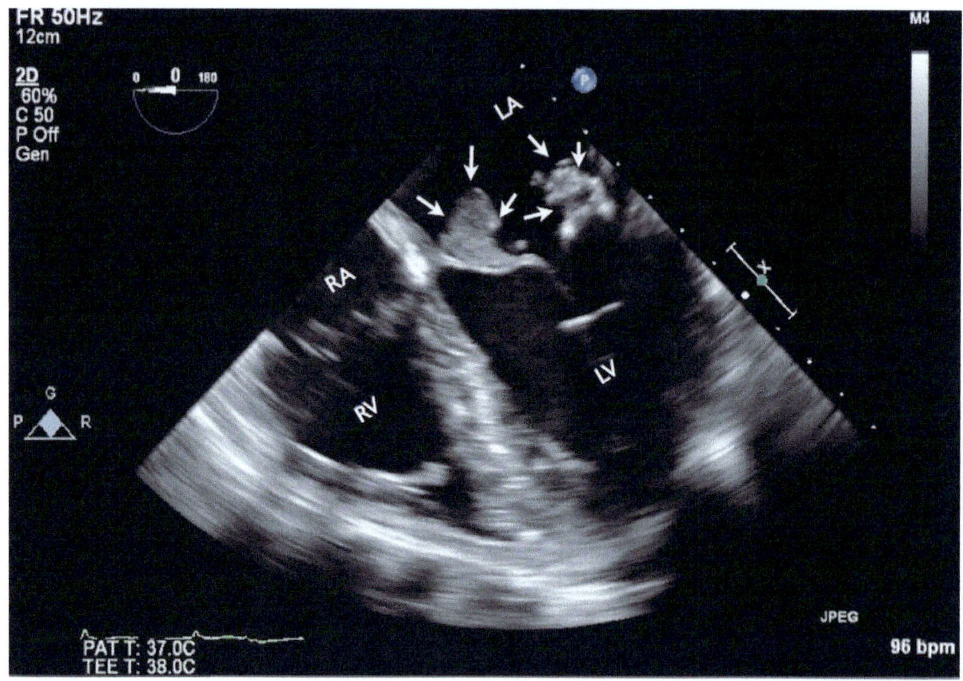

Fig. 7.8 Apical four-chamber TEE with color Doppler flow imaging showing severe mitral regurgitation

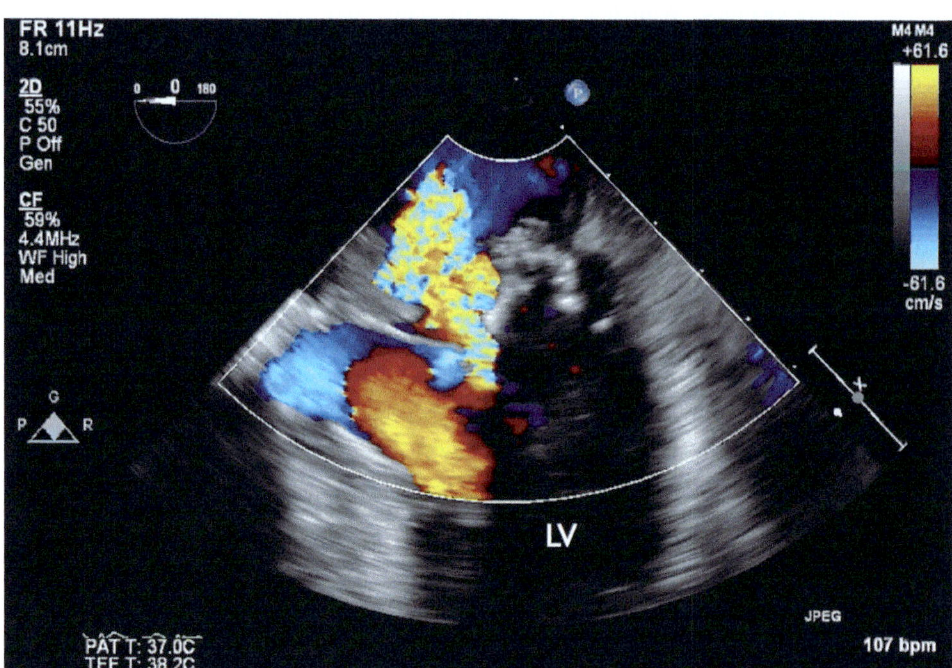

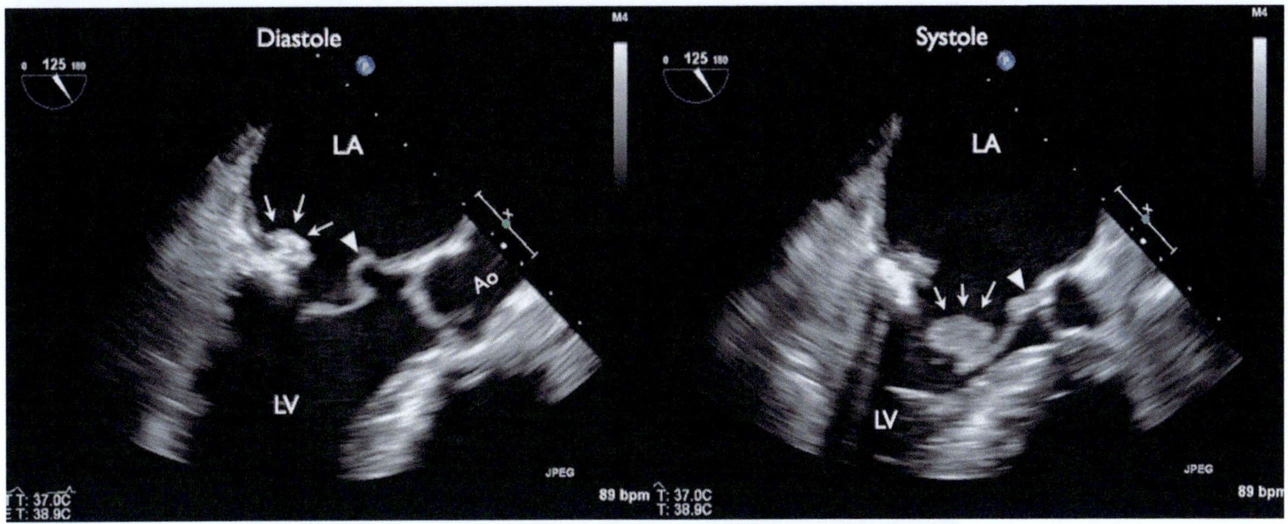

Fig. 7.9 Long-axis TEE demonstrated posterior mitral leaflet vegetation and mitral-aortic intervalvular fibrosa abscess and aneurysm. During diastole (*left panel*), vegetation was seen attached to the P2 segment of the posterior mitral leaflet (*arrows*), with outpouching of the proximal A2 segment of anterior mitral leaflet at the aortomitral curtain area, a finding consistent with mitral-aortic intervalvular fibrosa pseudoaneurysm (*arrowhead*). During systole (*right panel*), vegetation was seen attached to the P2 segment of the posterior mitral leaflets (*arrows*). There is a thickening of the aortomitral curtain area, with an area of hyperechodensity consistent with aortic abscess (*arrowhead*)

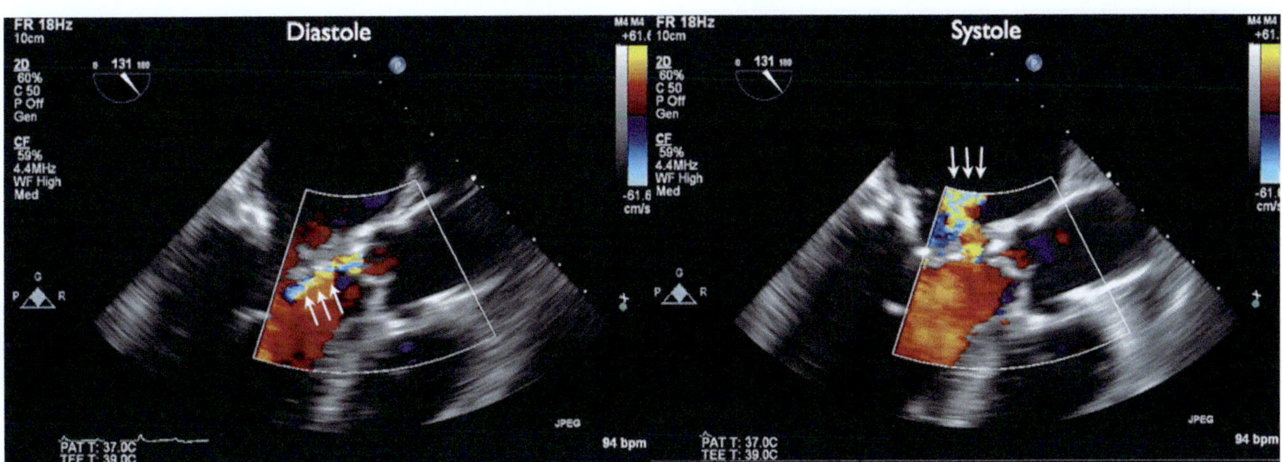

Fig. 7.10 Long-axis TEE with color Doppler flow imaging showing mild aortic insufficiency and perforation of the anterior mitral leaflet. During diastole (*left panel*), a mild aortic insufficiency (AI) jet was seen (*arrows*). The AI jet was eccentric and anteriorly directed. During systole (*right panel*), there was mitral regurgitation caused by leaflet perforation from a "kissing lesion."

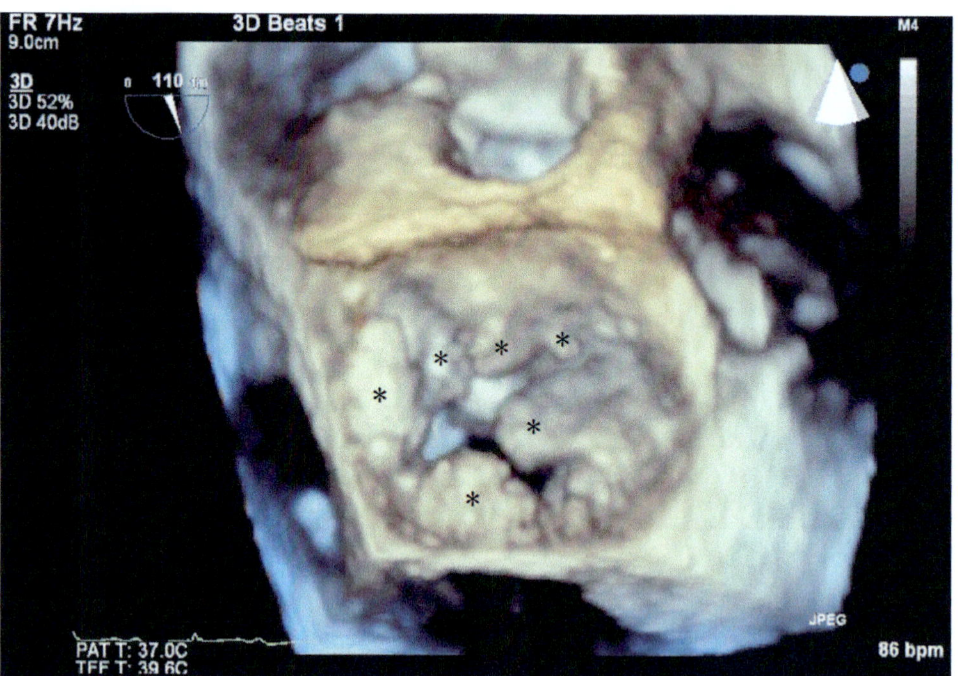

Fig. 7.11 Three-dimensional (3D) TEE of the mitral valve (LA view) showing multiple vegetations (*asterisks*)

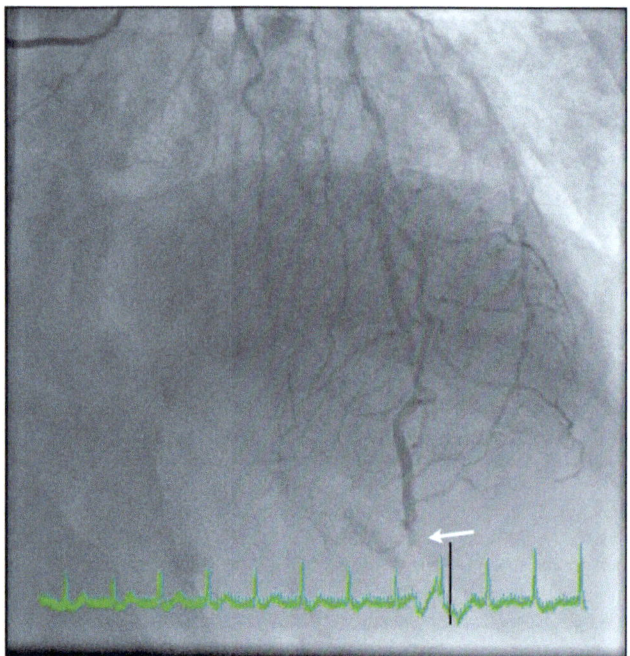

Fig. 7.12 Coronary angiogram showing total occlusion of the distal left anterior descending artery (LAD) (*arrow*). Given the angiographic features of acute cut-off appearance and the history of multiple vegetations, the finding is most likely consistent with coronary embolism from IE

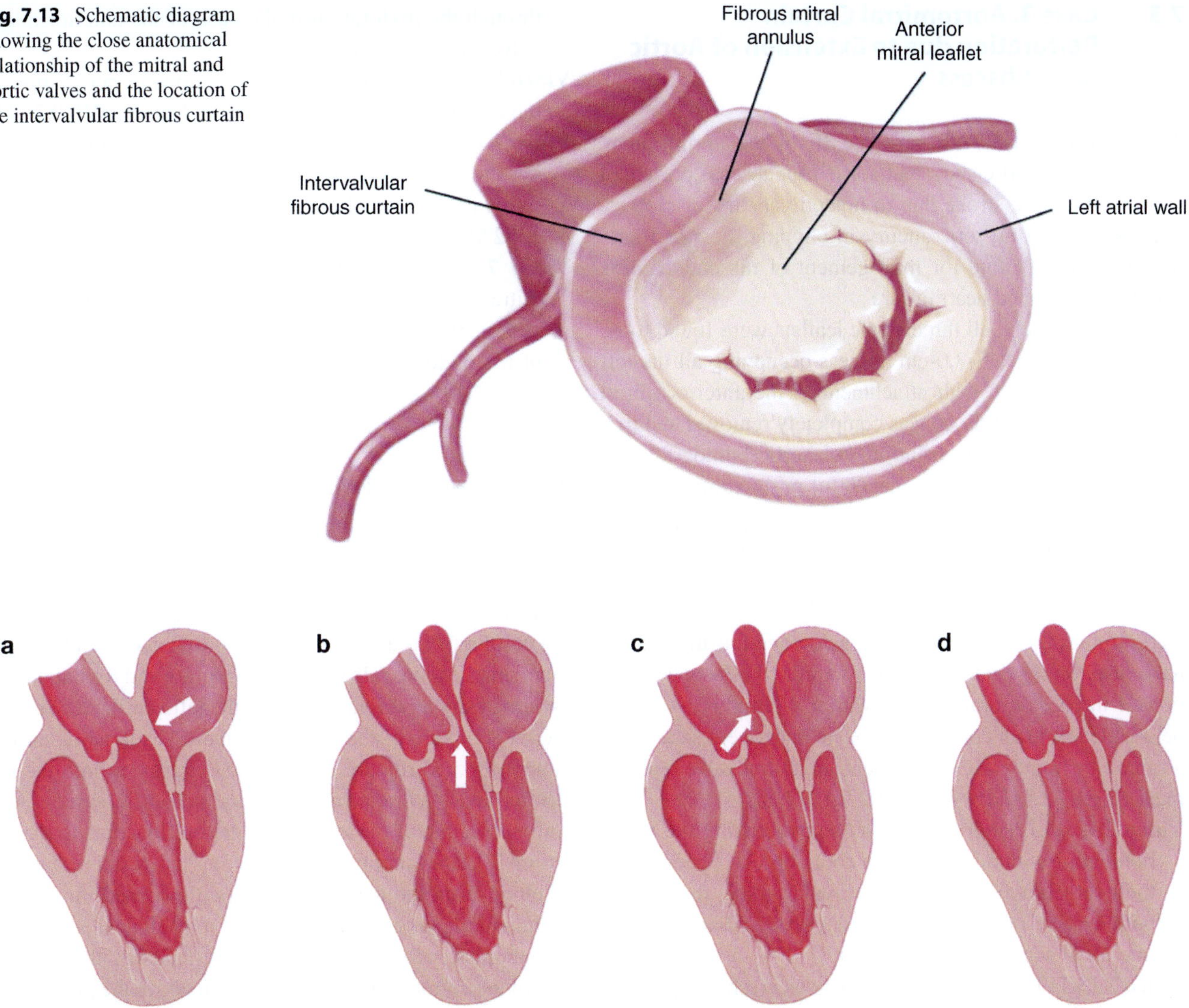

Fig. 7.13 Schematic diagram showing the close anatomical relationship of the mitral and aortic valves and the location of the intervalvular fibrous curtain

Fig. 7.14 The normal aortomitral curtain and several types of aortomitral curtain pseudoaneurysms. (**a**) Normal aortomitral curtain (*arrow*). (**b**) Aortomitral curtain pseudoaneurysm (*arrow*). (**c**) Aortomitral curtain pseudoaneurysm with fistula to the aorta (*arrow*). (**d**) Aortomitral curtain pseudoaneurysm with fistula to the left atrium

7.3   Case 3. Aortomitral Curtain Perforation due to Extension of Aortic Root Abscess

A 33-year-old man with subacute IE of the aortic valve, severe aortic insufficiency, and aortic root abscess presented with hemorrhagic stroke due to mycotic aneurysm rupture. After successful mycotic aneurysm clipping, he was transferred to our institute for management of his endocarditis and decompensated heart failure.

Intraoperatively, all three aortic leaflets were found to be destroyed, with a 1.5–3.0-cm abscess occupying all the left coronary cusp area, with attachment to the anterior mitral leaflet. The infected tissue was completely removed and irrigated with vancomycin solution. An aortic homograft was placed. The patient had an uneventful postoperative course and was discharged 1 week later.

Two months later, he developed acute decompensated heart failure and was found to have severe mitral regurgitation due to perforation of the anterior leaflet. The abscess at the aortomitral curtain, extending below the left main coronary cusp, was again seen. Surgery identified a 3-cm perforation of the aortomitral curtain, with a 3-cm abscess cavity below the left main coronary cusp. He underwent successful aortic valve homograft replacement and mitral valve replacement (Figs. 7.15, 7.16, 7.17, 7.18, 7.19, 7.20).

Video 7.12 TEE (short-axis view) demonstrating the aortic homograft with a paravalvular root abscess. Specifically, there is circumferential paravalvular issue thickening, with a more organized echolucent space adjacent to the interatrial septum (AVI 2916 kb)

Video 7.13 TEE (3-chamber, long-axis view) showing perforation of the base of the anterior mitral valve leaflet (AVI 2970 kb)

Video 7.14 TEE (3 chamber, long-axis view) with color Doppler imaging showing severe mitral regurgitation through the perforation in the base of the anterior mitral valve leaflet (AVI 1224 kb)

Video 7.15 TEE (4-chamber view) showing perforation of the base of the anterior mitral valve leaflet (AVI 2824 kb)

Video 7.16 TEE (4-chamber view) with color Doppler imaging showing severe mitral regurgitation through the perforation in the base of the anterior mitral valve leaflet (AVI 1302 kb)

Video 7.17 TEE three-dimensional reconstruction of the mitral valve (surgical view from the left atrium) demonstrating well-circumscribed perforation in the basal aspect of the middle scallop of the anterior mitral valve leaflet (A2) (AVI 426 kb)

7.3.1   Learning Points

New mitral regurgitation or progression of pre-existing mitral regurgitation after aortic valve replacement is uncommon, occurring in 4–14 % of patients [7]. Infection of the aortomitral curtain forms a subaortic abscess that may lead to one of four complications: (1) incomplete rupture and formation of a pseudoaneurysm originating from the left ventricular outflow tract; (2) rupture of the pseudoaneurysm resulting in cardiac tamponade; (3) rupture of the pseudoaneurysm into the left atrium, and (4) direct rupture of the subaortic abscess with communication of the left ventricular outflow tract to the left atrium [8]. The latter two complications can result in shunting of blood from the left ventricular outflow tract into the left atrium, mimicking mitral regurgitation by clinical and routine transthoracic echocardiography. Anatomically, the perforation of the aortomitral curtain is located above the plane of the mitral annulus and below the aortic annulus. This complication should be differentiated from mitral regurgitation caused by a perforation of the anterior mitral leaflet, in which the defect is below the mitral annulus.

Fig. 7.15 TEE (short-axis view) demonstrating the aortic homograft with a paravalvular root abscess. Specifically, there is circumferential paravalvular issue thickening, with a more organized echolucent space adjacent to the interatrial septum

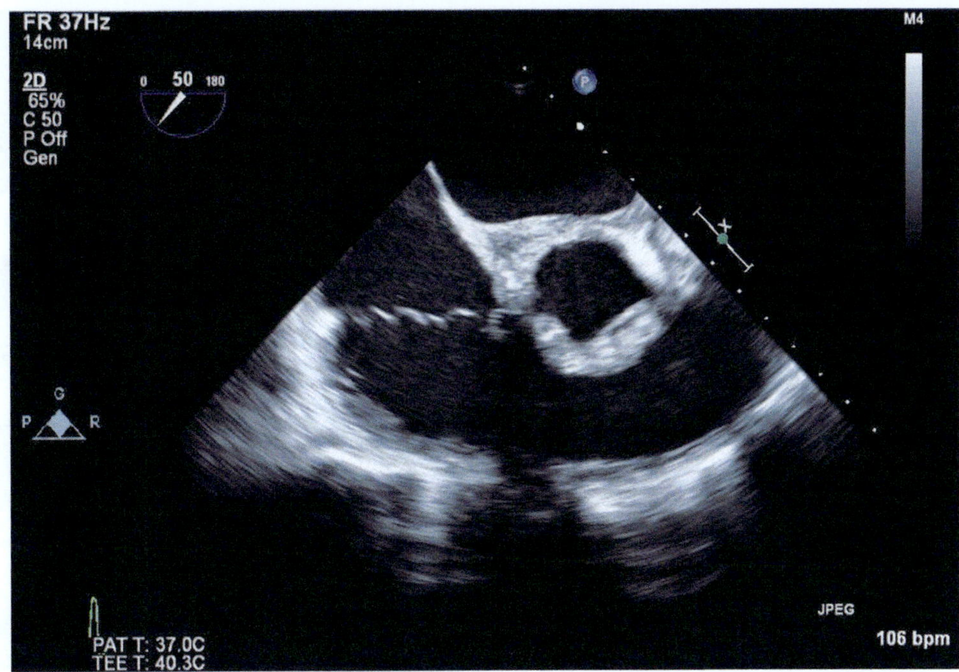

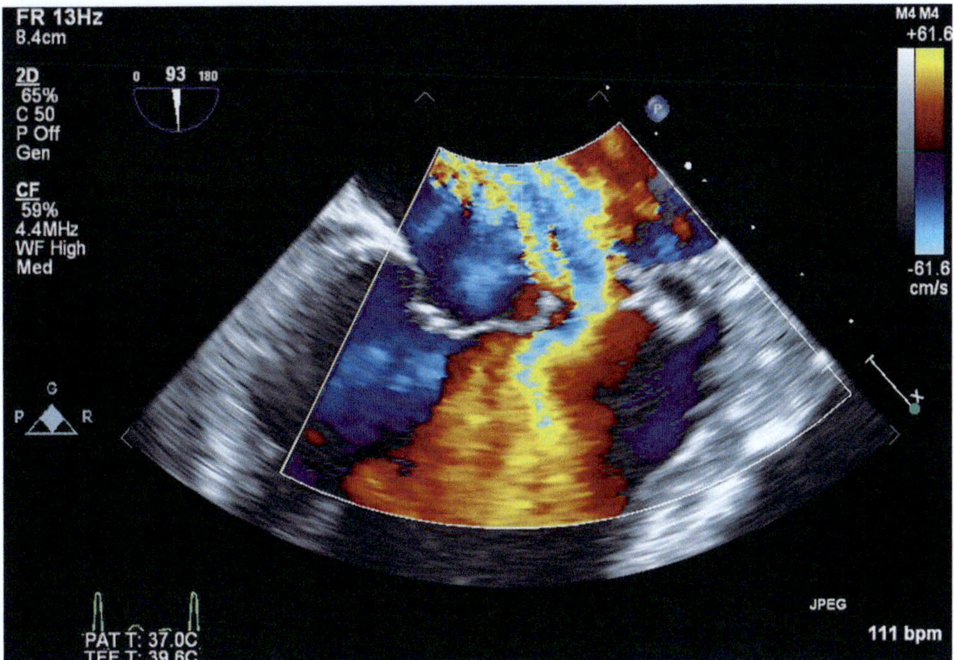

Fig. 7.16 TEE (2 chamber view) showing perforation of the base of the anterior mitral valve leaflet

Fig. 7.17 TEE (3-chamber, long-axis view) with color Doppler imaging showing perforation in the base of the anterior mitral valve leaflet

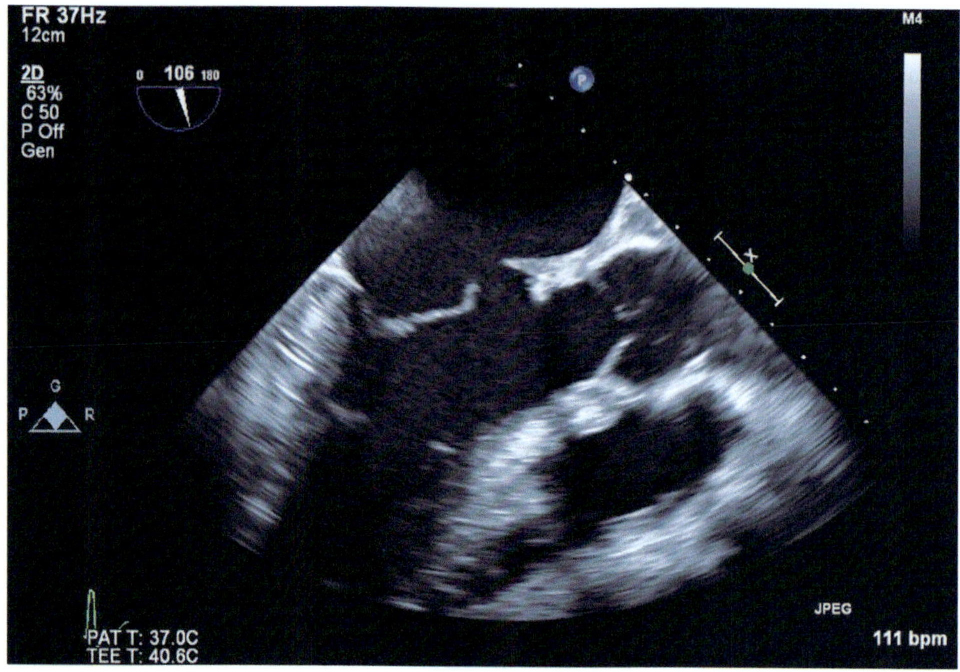

Fig. 7.18 TEE (4-chamber view) showing perforation of the base of the anterior mitral valve leaflet

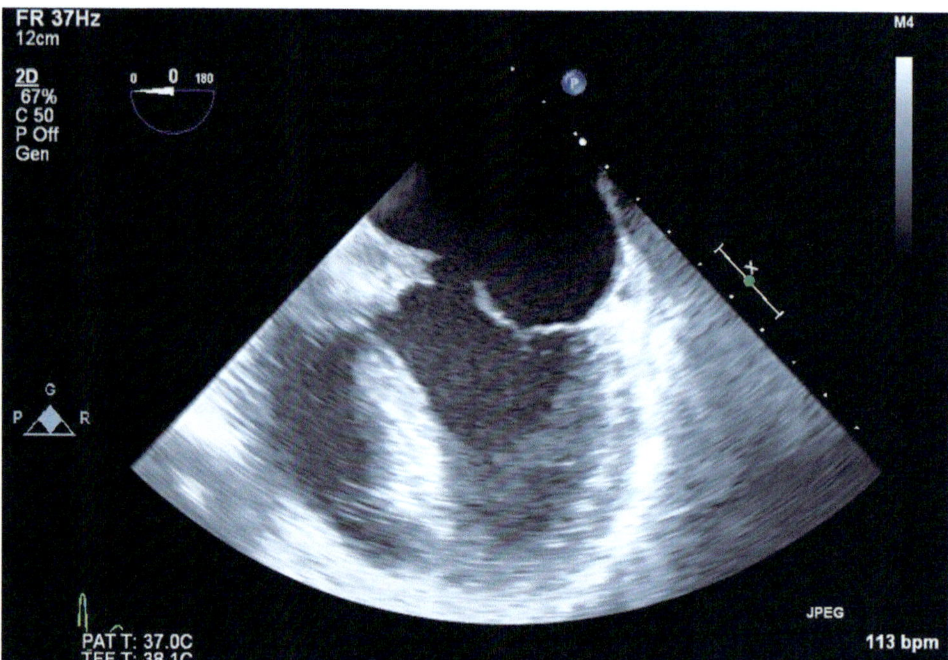

Fig. 7.19 TEE (4-chamber view) with color Doppler imaging showing severe mitral regurgitation through the perforation in the base of the anterior mitral valve leaflet

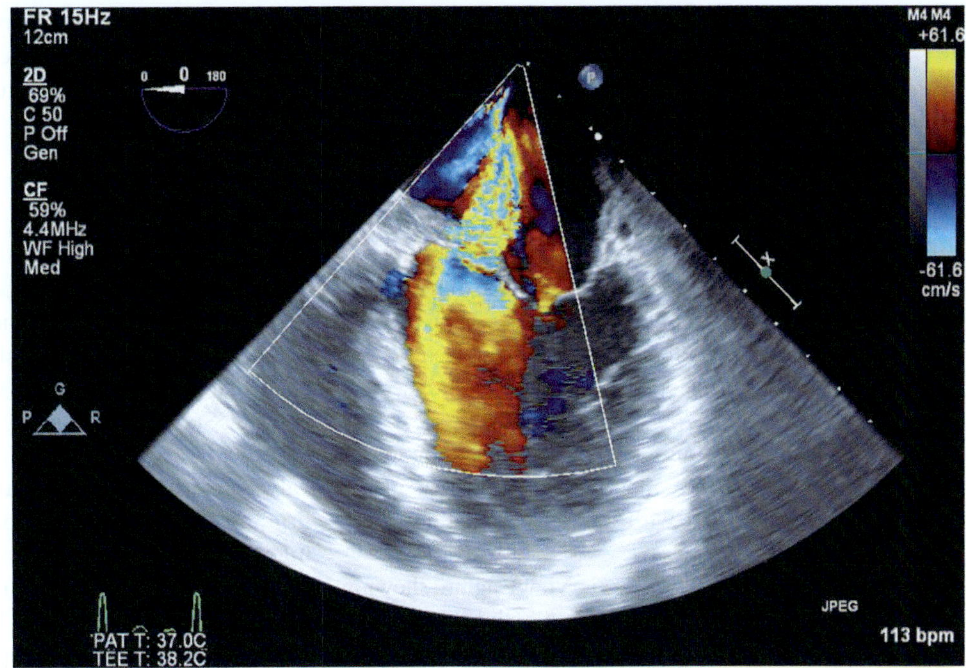

Fig. 7.20 TEE three-dimensional reconstruction of the mitral valve (surgical view from the left atrium) demonstrating well-circumscribed perforation in the basal aspect of the middle scallop of the anterior mitral valve leaflet (A2)

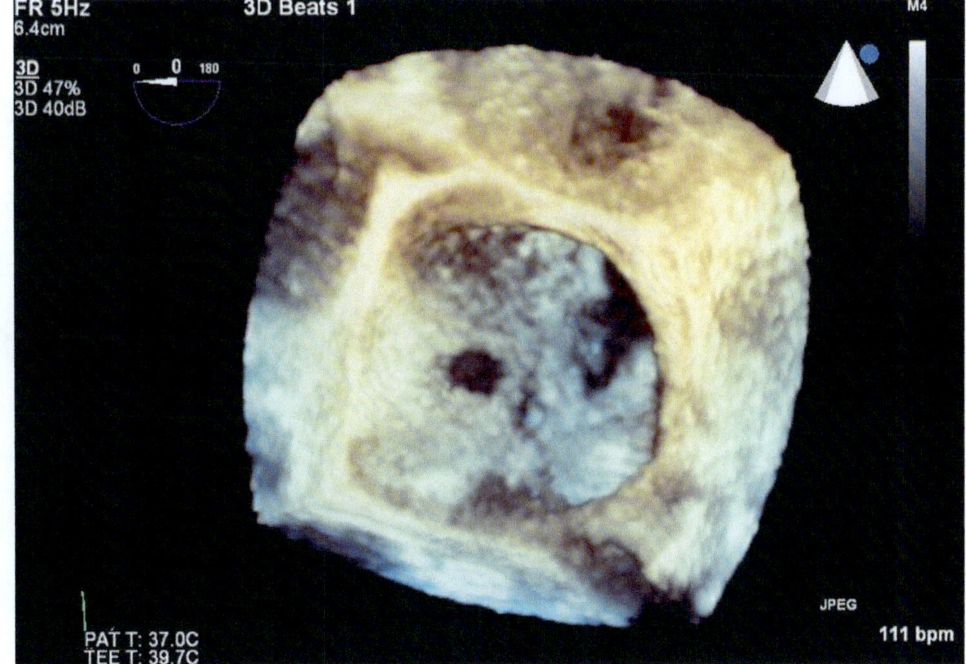

7.4 Case 4. Endocarditis with Gerbode Defect

A 60-year-old woman was referred to our institution for evaluation of postoperative heart murmur. Severe symptomatic mitral regurgitation due to mitral prolapse was diagnosed a year ago, and she underwent mitral valve repair with a mitral valve ring a few months ago at another hospital. She was undertaking cardiac rehabilitation when cardiac murmur was noted. She subsequently underwent TEE, which demonstrated ventricular septal defect, and she was advised to have the defect closed percutaneously. She then sought a second opinion (Figs. 7.21, 7.22, 7.23, 7.24, and 7.25).

Video 7.18 TEE image (four-chamber view) showing multiple mobile echodensities attached to both leaflets of the mitral valve, consistent with multiple vegetations (AVI 6108 kb)

Video 7.19 TEE images (long-axis view) again showing multiple mobile echodensities seen at both leaflets of the mitral valve, consistent with multiple vegetations (AVI 2617 kb)

Video 7.20 3D-TEE images of the surgical view of the mitral valve showing multiple vegetations (AVI 2074 kb)

Video 7.21 TEE images (four-chamber view) showing LV to RA shunts (just above the septal leaflet of the tricuspid valve) during systole, features consistent with a Gerbode defect (AVI 1880 kb)

7.4.1 Learning Points

The Gerbode defect is a type of communication between the left ventricle (LV) and the right atrium (RA). The congenital form of the LV-RA shunt is very rare and was first classified in 1958 by Frank Gerbode, a noted cardiac surgeon at Stanford University. Acquired causes have been described secondary to IE, trauma, and aortic or mitral valve surgery. TEE is the main diagnostic modality to confirm the diagnosis and the location of the LV-RA shunt. A high Doppler gradient across the defect is one of the hallmarks of the Gerbode ventriculoatrial defect because of the difference between the left ventricular systolic pressure and the low right atrial pressure. The echocardiogram typically shows a dilated right atrium in patients with a significant Gerbode defect. Surgical correction is the definitive treatment.

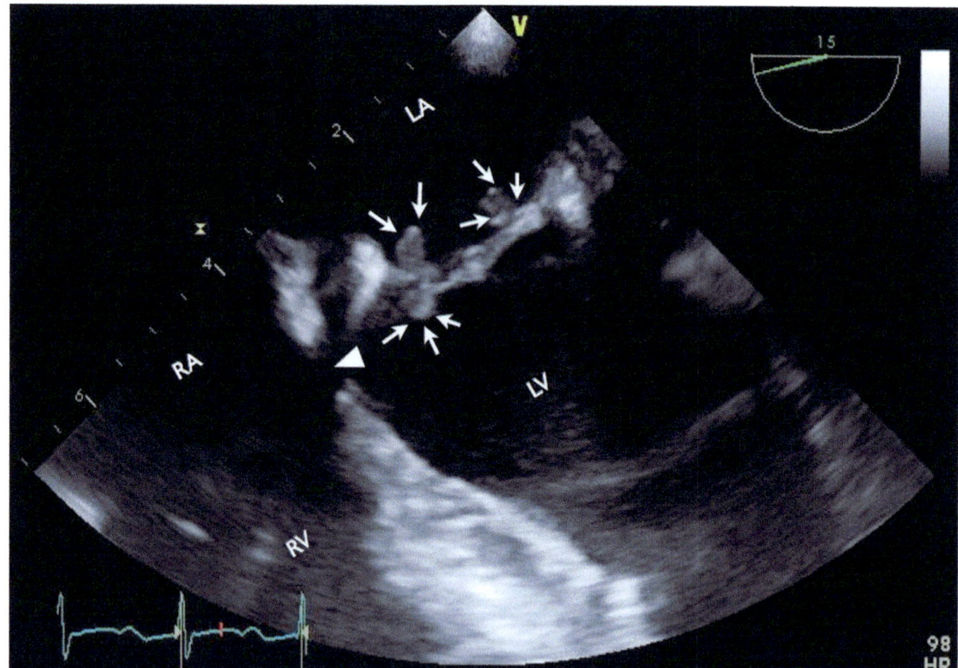

Fig. 7.21 TEE image (four-chamber view) showing multiple mobile echodensities attached to both leaflets of the mitral valve (*arrows*), consistent with multiple vegetations and echo drop-out at the interventricular septum area (*arrowhead*)

Fig. 7.22 TEE images (long-axis view) again showing multiple mobile echodensities (*arrows*) seen at both leaflets of the mitral valve, consistent with multiple vegetations

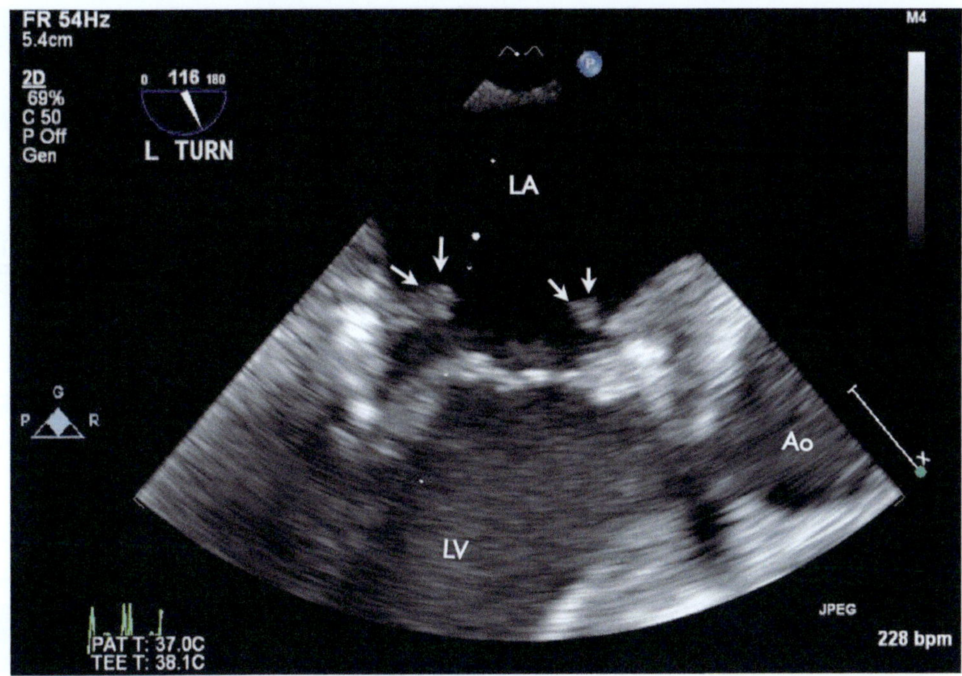

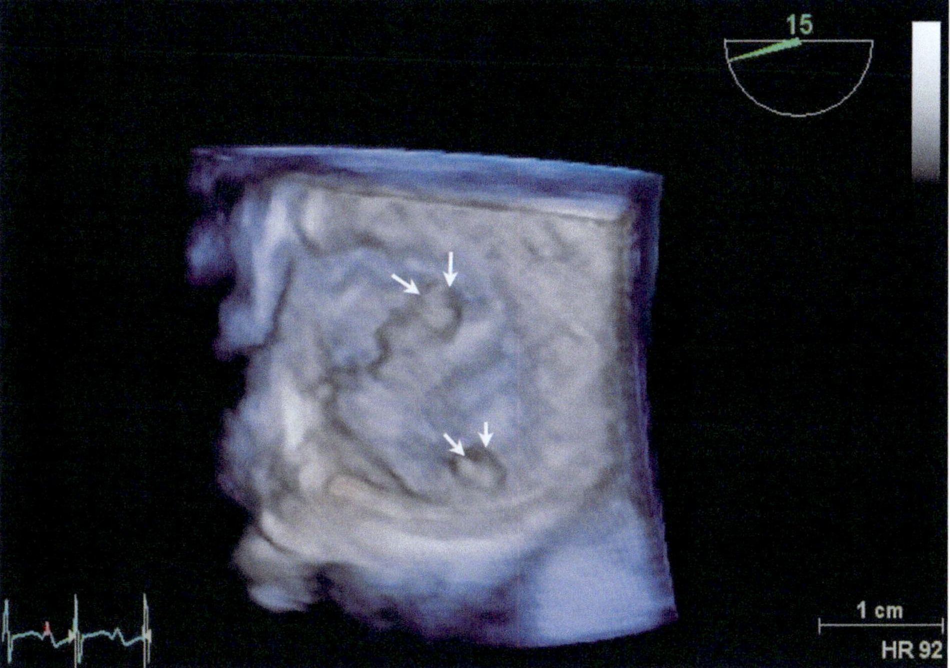

Fig. 7.23 3D-TEE images of the surgical view of the mitral valve showing multiple vegetations (*arrows*)

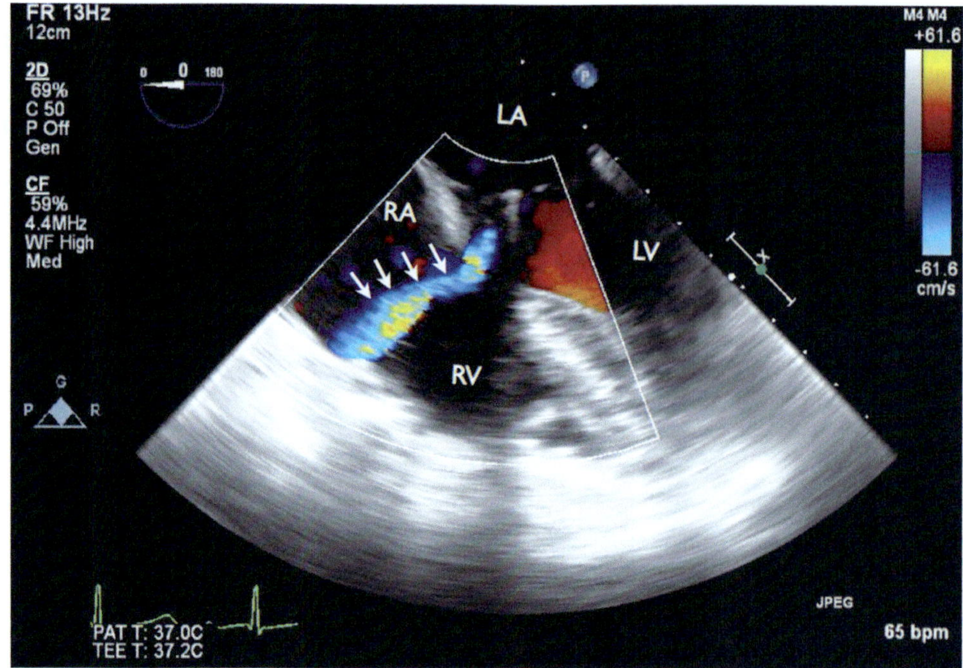

Fig. 7.24 TEE images (four-chamber view) showing LV to RA shunts (just above the septal leaflet of the tricuspid valve) during systole, features consistent with a Gerbode defect (*arrows*)

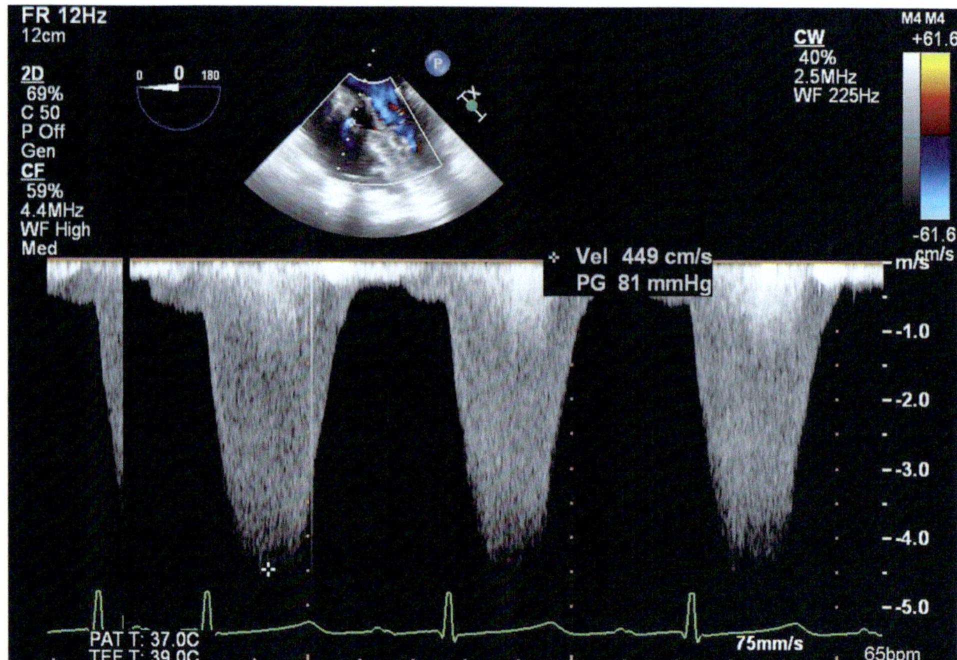

Fig. 7.25 Doppler envelope of the ventricular septal defect showing that the maximum peak instantaneous gradient in this patient was 81 mmHg

7.5 Case 5. Mechanical Valve Infective Endocarditis with Submitral Left Ventricular Pseudoaneurysm

A 55-year-old woman had a past medical history significant for rheumatic heart disease and chronic anemia due to colonic arteriovenous malformation (AVM). She had undergone aortic and mitral valve replacement 12 years previously. She had a left chest mediport for her chronic blood transfusion, and 2 weeks ago was found to have *S. epidermiditis* bacteremia, which was treated with intravenous vancomycin and then switched to oxacillin, gentamicin, and rifampin. She now presented with shortness of breath and fever (Figs. 7.26, 7.27, 7.28, 7.29, 7.30, 7.31, and 7.32).

Video 7.22 TTE, parasternal view, showing expansile submitral echolucent space consistent with ventricular pseudoaneurysm (AVI 5261 kb)

Video 7.23 TTE, apical four-chamber view, showing rocking motion of the prosthetic mitral valve consistent with prosthetic dehiscence. There is an expansile echolucent space consistent with ventricular pseudoaneurysm (AVI 4559 kb)

Video 7.24 TTE, apical two-chamber view, showing rocking motion of the prosthetic mitral valve consistent with prosthetic dehiscence. There is an expansile echolucent space consistent with ventricular pseudoaneurysm (AVI 5034 kb)

Video 7.25 TTE, subcostal view, showing mitral prosthetic dehiscence and ventricular pseudoaneurysm (AVI 2774 kb)

7.5.1 Learning Points

Submitral left ventricular pseudoaneurysm, a very rare condition caused by disruption of the posterior mitral annulus, occurs in 0.02–2 % of mitral valve replacement operations. The major risk factors are removal of excess leaflet and annular tissue, previous mitral valve replacement, and a mitral prosthesis that is too large [9]. Surgical repair is the definitive treatment; it can be done by an internal approach (from inside the left atrium) or an external approach. The external repair approach is typically advocated for small defects limited to myocardium.

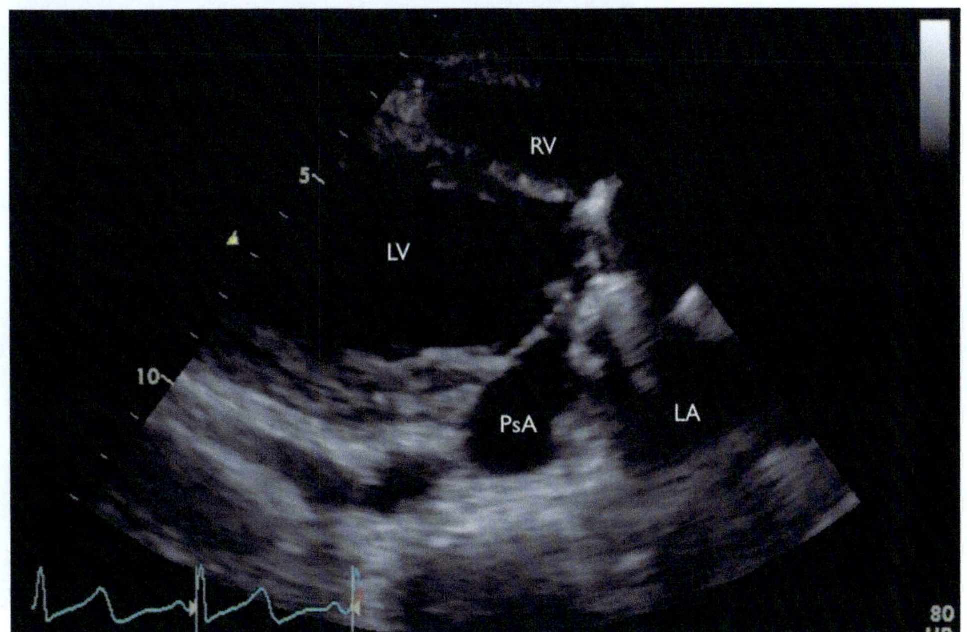

Fig. 7.26 TTE, parasternal view, showing expansile submitral echolucent space consistent with ventricular pseudoaneurysm (*PsA*)

Fig. 7.27 TTE, apical four-chamber view, showing rocking motion of the prosthetic mitral valve (*arrows*) consistent with prosthetic dehiscence. There is an expansile echolucent space consistent with ventricular PsA

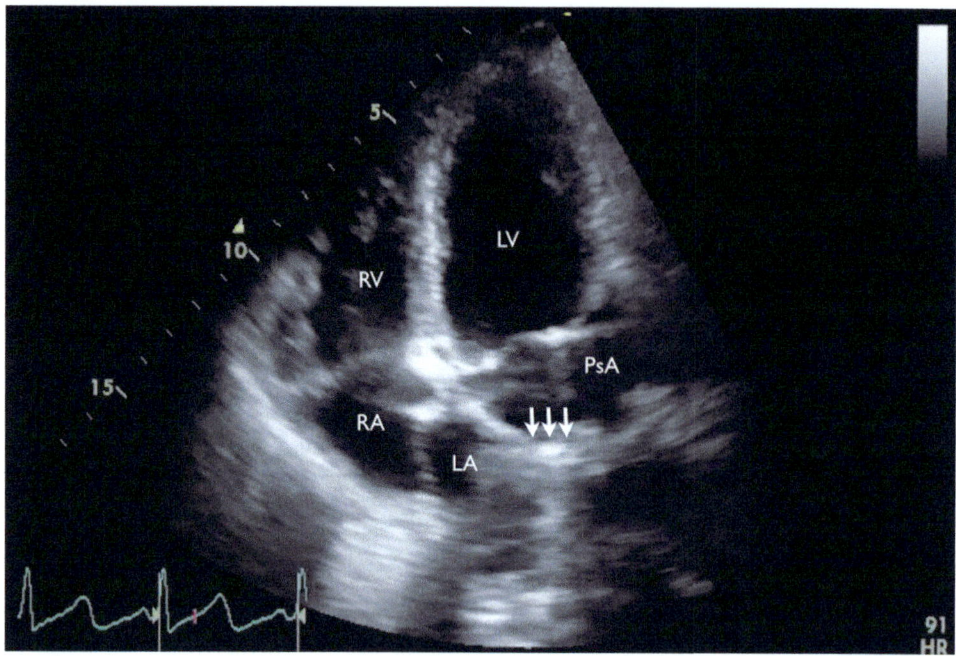

Fig. 7.28 TTE, apical two-chamber view, showing rocking motion of the prosthetic mitral valve (*arrows*) consistent with prosthetic dehiscence. There is an expansile echolucent space consistent with ventricular PsA

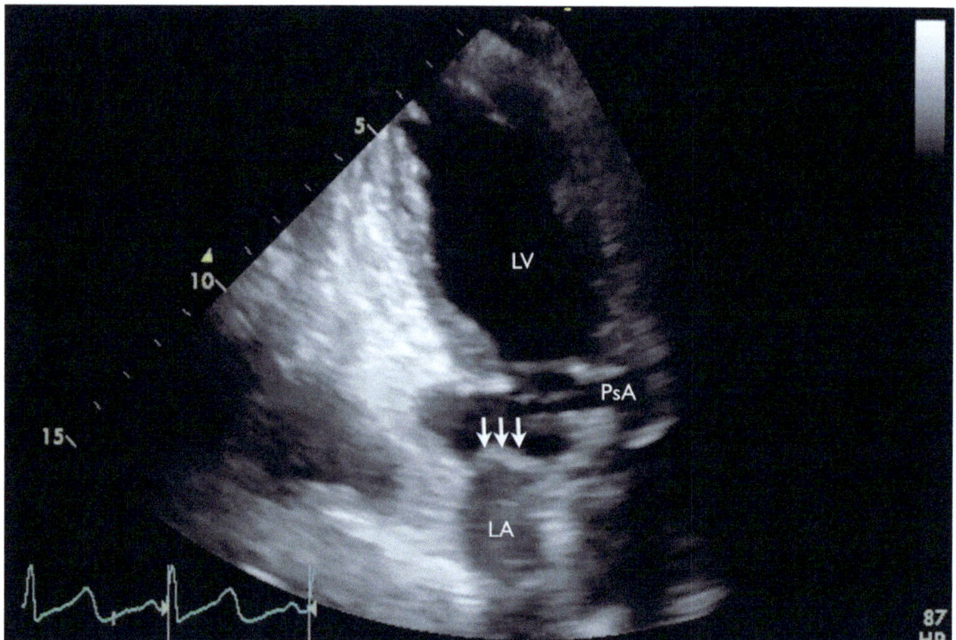

Fig. 7.29 TTE, subcostal view, showing mitral prosthetic dehiscence (*arrow*) and ventricular PsA

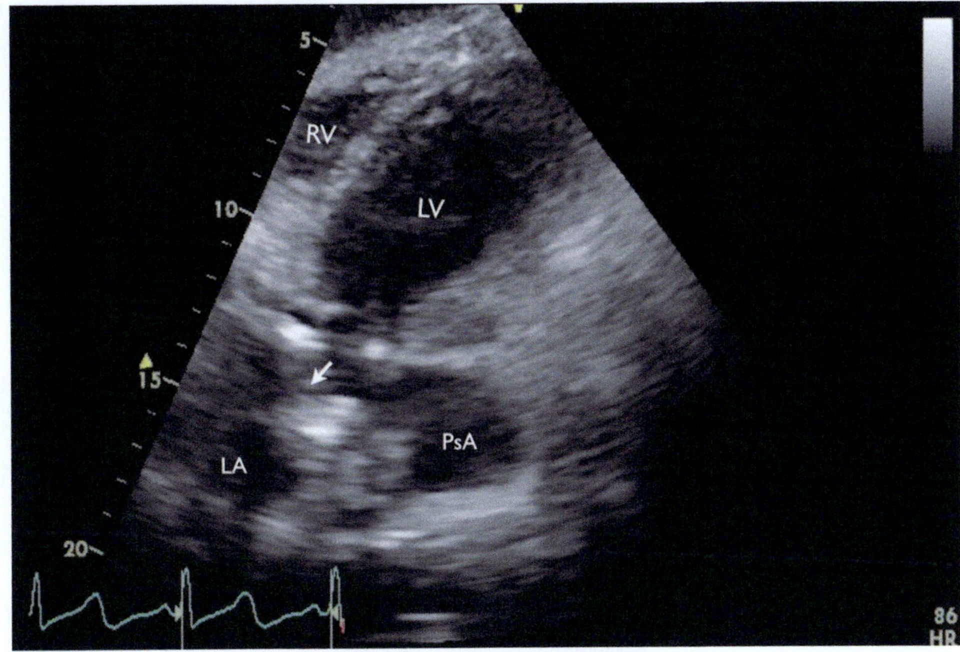

Fig. 7.30 TEE, two-chamber view with zoom at the mitral valve level, showing two vegetations (*arrows*) attached to the mechanical bileaflet mitral prosthesis

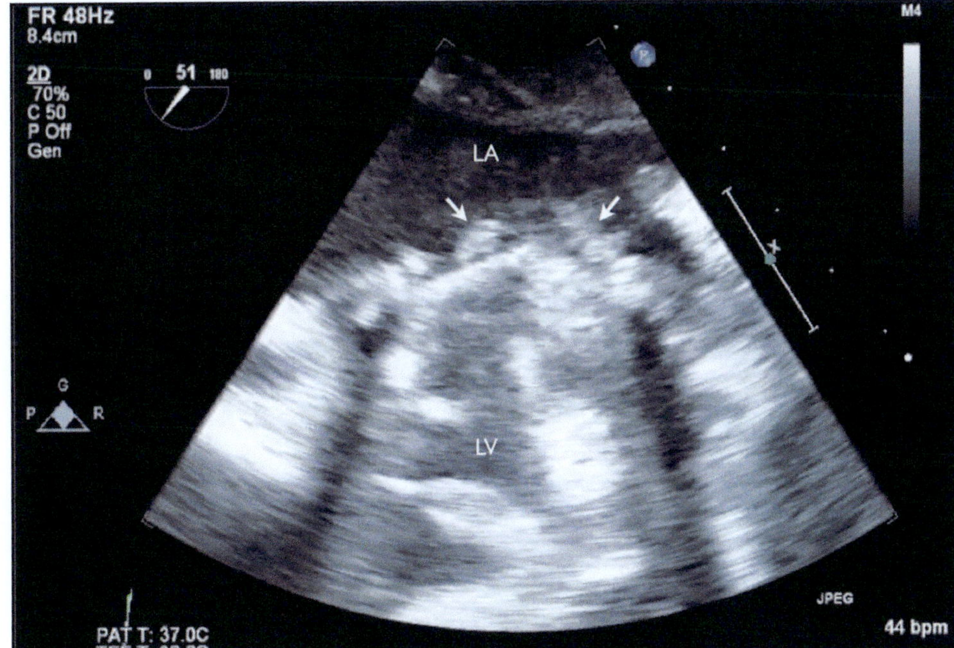

Fig. 7.31 Cardiac CT scan demonstrating mitral prosthesis dehiscence into the left atrium (*arrow*) and multiple submitral PsA

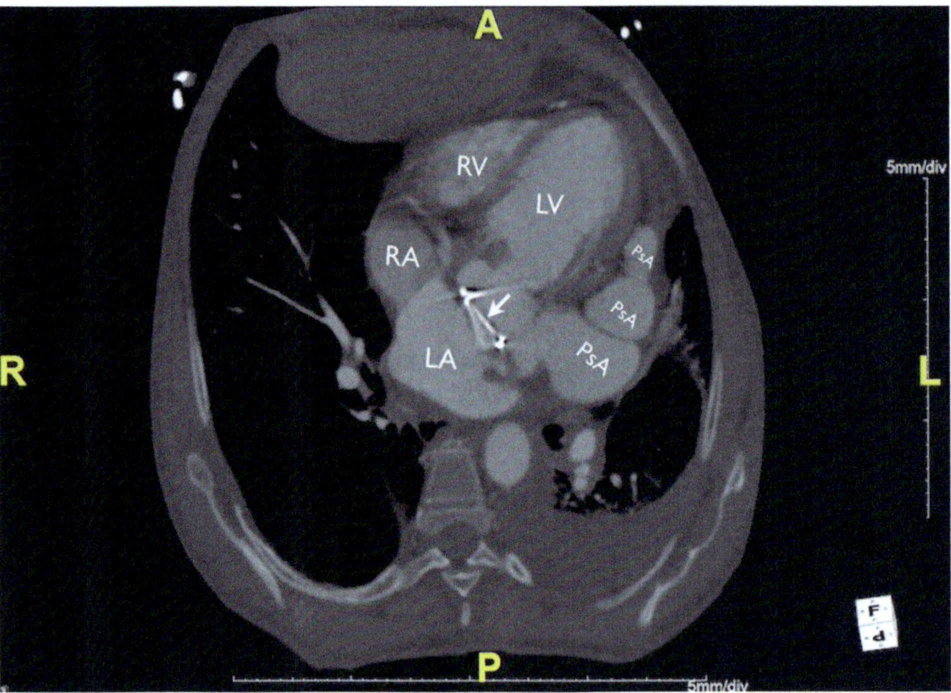

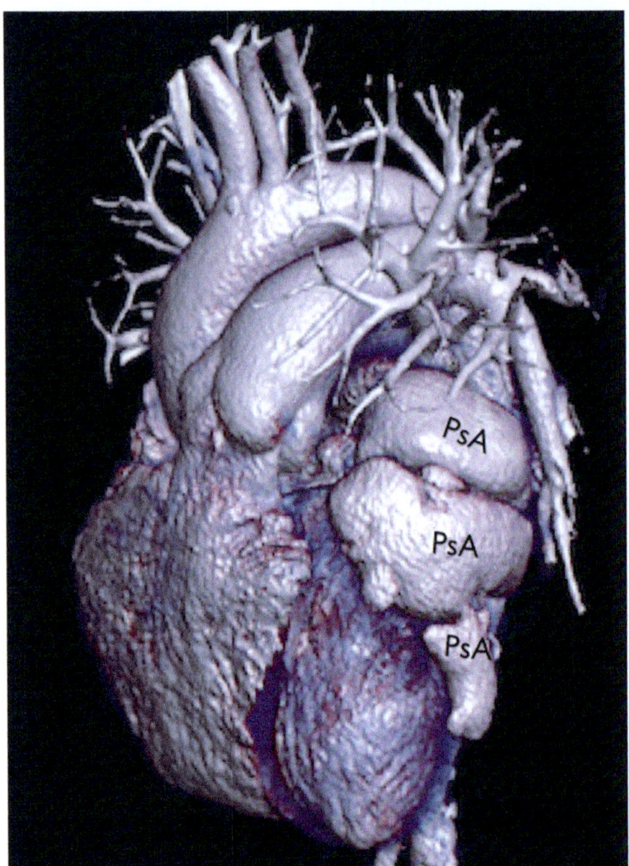

Fig. 7.32 Cardiac CT with 3D reconstruction demonstrating multiple PsA

7.6 Case 6. Cardiac Crux Abscess and Mitral Inflow Obstruction

A 59-year-old man with a past medical history significant for aortic insufficiency underwent aortic valve replacement with aortic aneurysm repair and mitral valve repair 6 months previously. He presented to another hospital with new-onset dyspnea and dry cough, which progressed to hemoptysis in a few days. He had leukocytosis, elevated BNP, and hypoxemia requiring a nonrebreather mask. TTE showed a mobile mass (about 1 cm) on the aortic valve, suspicious for vegetation. He was treated with cefepime, vancomycin, and ceftriaxone and transferred to our institution. He had pulmonary edema on arrival and went into severe bradycardia and cardiac arrest shortly after arrival. He was successfully resuscitated and a temporary pacemaker was placed (Figs. 7.33, 7.34, 7.35, 7.36, and 7.37).

Video 7.26 TEE, four-chamber view, showing mobile echodensity at the cardiac crux, extending over the mitral and tricuspid annulus, as well as a central, echolucent area consistent with cardiac crux abscess (AVI 7362 kb)

Video 7.27 TEE, two-chamber view, showing extensive vegetation obstructing mitral inflow (AVI 7370 kb)

Video 7.28 TEE, short-axis view at the aortic valve level, showing communicating flow between the proximal aorta and the right ventricle, with systolic and diastolic flow consistent with an aortic-ventricular fistula (AVI 1448 kb)

Video 7.29 TEE, short-axis view at the aortic valve level, showing prosthetic aortic valve dehiscence along the posterior aspect. There are vegetations involving the aortic valve and the tricuspid valve (AVI 7312 kb)

7.6.1 Learning Points

Conduction abnormalities are commonly associated with aortic paravalvular abscess extension due to anatomical proximity of the aortic valve to the His bundle. This case also demonstrated extension of aortic paravalvular abscess to the cardiac crux, causing mitral inflow obstruction. The decompensation in this case was most likely due to worsening rupture of the aortic valve and fistulous connection with the right ventricle.

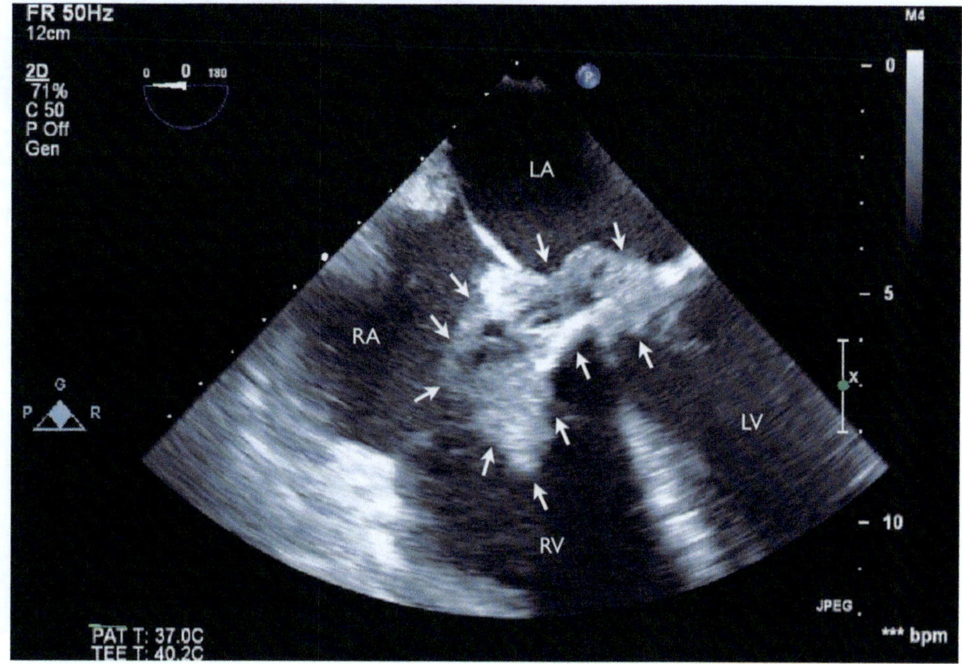

Fig. 7.33 TEE, four-chamber view, showing mobile echodensity at the cardiac crux, extending over the mitral and tricuspid annulus (*arrows*), as well as a central, echolucent area consistent with cardiac crux abscess

Fig. 7.34 TEE, two-chamber view, showing extensive vegetation obstructing mitral inflow (*arrows*)

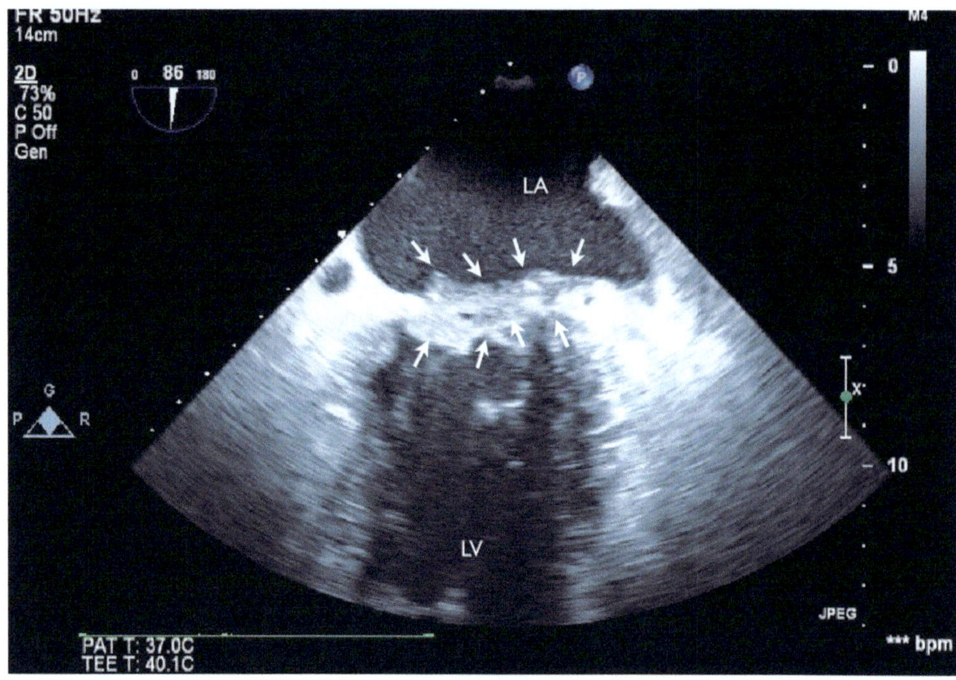

Fig. 7.35 Transmitral Doppler flow imaging showing significant mitral inflow obstruction (mean pressure gradient 17 mmHg)

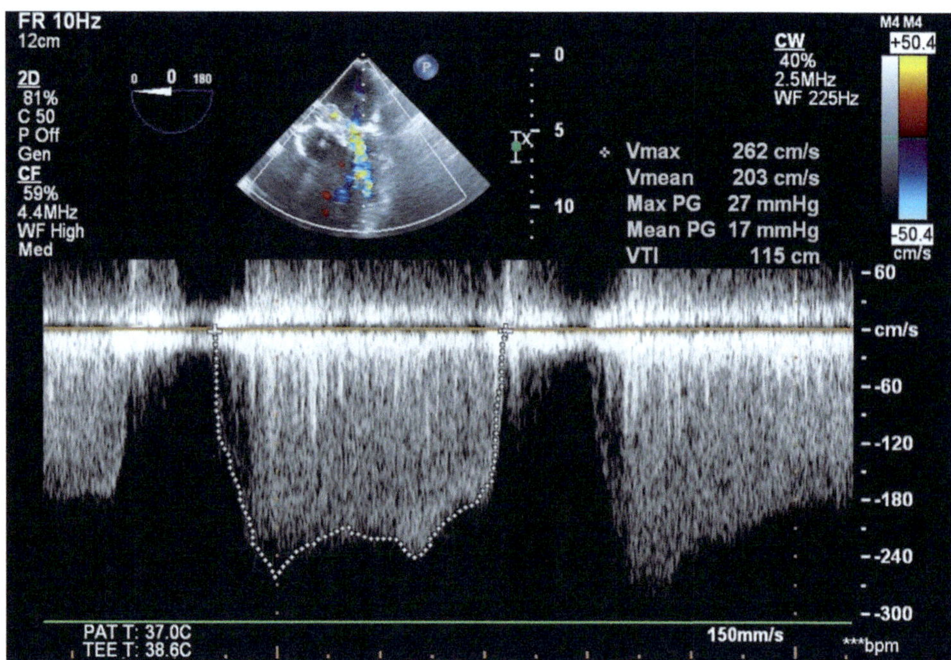

Fig. 7.36 TEE, short-axis view at the aortic valve level, showing communicating flow between the proximal aorta and the right ventricle, with systolic and diastolic flow (*arrows*) consistent with an aortic-ventricular fistula

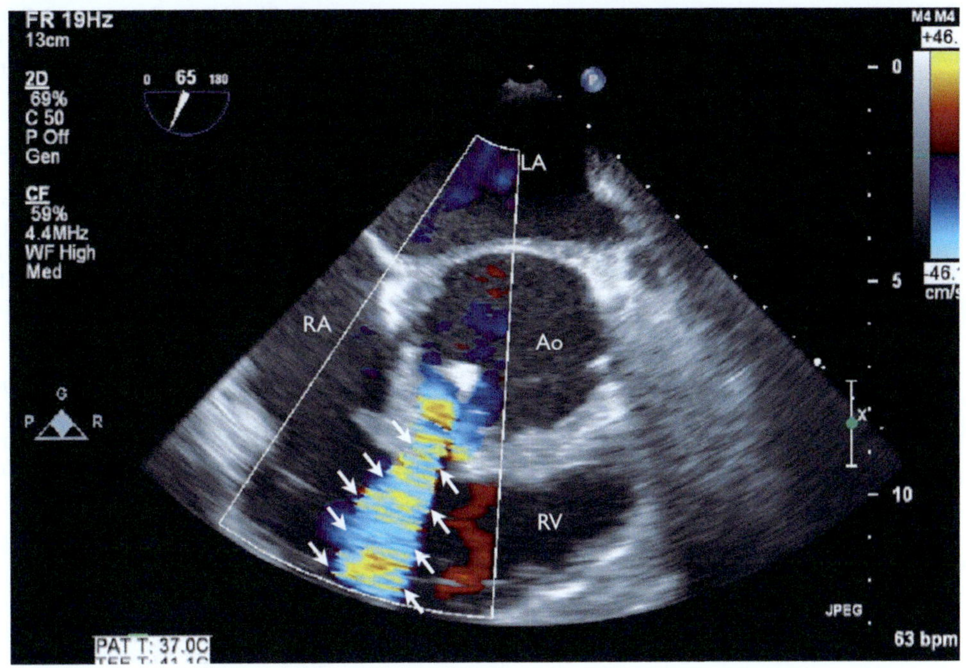

Fig. 7.37 TEE, short-axis view at the aortic valve level, showing prosthetic aortic valve dehiscence along the posterior aspect. There is vegetation involving the aortic valve (*arrow*) and the tricuspid valve (*arrowhead*)

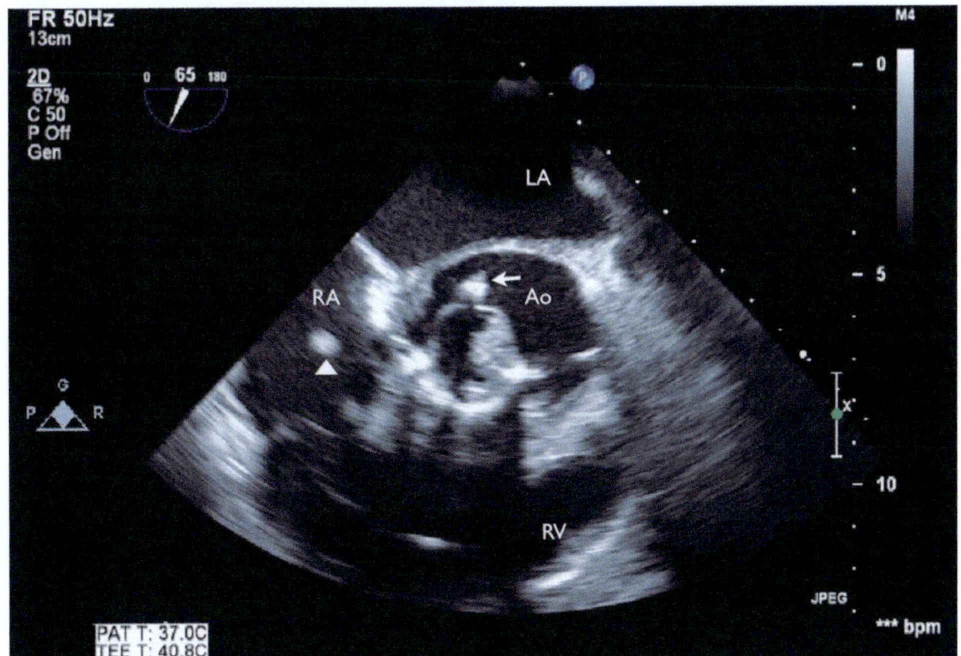

References

1. Nishimura RA, Otto CM, Bonow RO, Carabello BA, Erwin JP, Guyton RA, et al. 2014 AHA/ACC guideline for the management of patients with valvular heart disease: a report of the American College of Cardiology/American Heart Association Task Force on Practice Guidelines. J Am Coll Cardiol. 2014;63:e57–185.
2. Murdoch DR, Corey GR, Hoen B, Miro JM, Fowler Jr VG, Bayer AS, et al. Clinical presentation, etiology, and outcome of infective endocarditis in the 21st century: the International Collaboration on Endocarditis-Prospective Cohort Study. Arch Intern Med. 2009;169:463–73.
3. Selton-Suty C, Celard M, Le Moing V, Doco-Lecompte T, Chirouze C, Iung B, et al. Preeminence of Staphylococcus aureus in infective endocarditis: a 1-year population-based survey. Clin Infect Dis. 2012;54:1230–9.
4. Hoen B, Duval X. Clinical practice. Infective endocarditis. N Engl J Med. 2013;368:1425–33.
5. Bloechlinger S, Nebiker M, Windecker S. Unusual cause of myocardial infarction and congestive heart failure in a patient with prosthetic valve endocarditis. Catheter Cardiovasc Interv. 2014;83: E69–72.
6. Khan F, Khakoo R, Failinger C. Managing embolic myocardial infarction in infective endocarditis: current options. J Infect. 2005;51:e101–5.
7. Unger P, Dedobbeleer C, Van Camp G, Plein D, Cosyns B, Lancellotti P. Mitral regurgitation in patients with aortic stenosis undergoing valve replacement. Heart. 2010;96:9–14.
8. Bansal RC, Graham BM, Jutzy KR, Shakudo M, Shah PM. Left ventricular outflow tract to left atrial communication secondary to rupture of mitral-aortic intervalvular fibrosa in infective endocarditis: diagnosis by transesophageal echocardiography and color flow imaging. J Am Coll Cardiol. 1990;15:499–504.
9. Carlson EB, Wolfe WG, Kisslo J. Subvalvular left ventricular pseudoaneurysm after mitral valve replacement: two-dimensional echocardiographic findings. J Am Coll Cardiol. 1985;6:1164–6.

Hypertrophic Cardiomyopathy and Mitral Valve Disease

8

Milind Desai

8.1 Case 1. Familial Hypertrophic Obstructive Cardiomyopathy

A 38-year-old man presented with progressively worse exertional dyspnea, effort-related chest tightness, and one episode of exertional syncope. He had a strong history of multiple family members dying suddenly. He also reported intermittent palpitations over the years. On examination, he was found to have a harsh systolic ejection murmur at left upper sternal border that increased with Valsalva and reduced with squatting. Patient also had a moderate intensity systolic precordial murmur. Electrocardiogram revealed normal sinus rhythm with severe left ventricular hypertrophy (LVH) and strain pattern. He was found to have hypertrophic obstructive cardiomyopathy (HOCM) with severe left ventricular outflow tract (LVOT) obstruction. He underwent surgical myectomy with complete relief of symptoms.

Video 8.1 Two-dimensional transthoracic echo in the parasternal view demonstrating severely hypertrophied basal interventricular septum with systolic anterior motion (SAM) of the mitral valve. The patient has a characteristic "reverse septal curvature" pattern, which is frequently seen in patients with a genetically transmitted mode of disease (AVI 5952 kb)

Video 8.2 Two-dimensional transthoracic echo with color Doppler in the parasternal view demonstrating severe turbulence of blood flow across the LVOT, due to a combination of SAM of the anterior mitral leaflet and severely hypertrophied basal interventricular septum. Notice the characteristic SAM-related posteriorly directed jet of mitral regurgitation (MR) in the left atrium (AVI 3537 kb)

Video 8.3 Four-chamber balanced steady-state free precession (b-SSFP) cine cardiac magnetic resonance (CMR) image of the same patient confirming severe basal septal hypertrophy, LVOT obstruction, and posteriorly directed jet of MR. Again, notice the characteristic reverse septal curvature pattern (AVI 1425 kb)

Electronic supplementary material The online version of this chapter (doi:10.1007/978-1-4471-6672-6_8) contains supplementary material, which is available to authorized users.

M. Desai
Department of Cardiovascular Medicine, Cleveland Clinic,
9500 Euclid Avenue, Cleveland, OH 44195, USA
e-mail: desaim2@ccf.org

M. Desai et al. (eds.), *An Atlas of Mitral Valve Imaging*,
DOI 10.1007/978-1-4471-6672-6_8, © Springer-Verlag London 2015

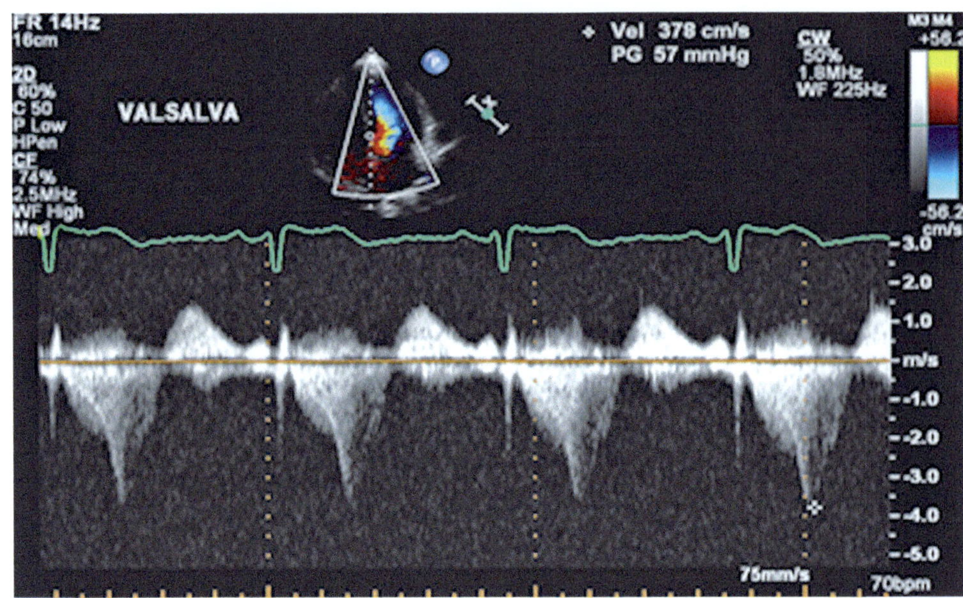

Fig. 8.1 Spectral Doppler echocardiographic image across the LVOT after Valsalva maneuver demonstrating a characteristic late-peaking "dagger-shaped" signal suggestive of severe dynamic LVOT obstruction, characteristic of HOCM

8.2   Case 2. Hypertensive Heart Disease of Elderly with Severe LVOT Obstruction

A 78-year-old woman presented with progressively worse exertional dyspnea. She had a long-strong history hypertension, that was not well controlled. On examination, she was found to have a harsh systolic ejection murmur at left upper sternal border that increased with Valsalva and reduced with squatting. Electrocardiogram revealed normal sinus rhythm with severe LVH. She was diagnosed with hypertensive heart disease of elderly and severe LVOT obstruction. She underwent surgical myectomy with complete relief of symptoms.

Video 8.4 Two-dimensional transthoracic echocardiogram in the parasternal view demonstrating a severely hypertrophied focal segment of the basal interventricular septum with systolic anterior motion (SAM) of the mitral valve. The patient has a characteristic "sigmoid" pattern, which is frequently seen in elderly patients with long-standing history of uncontrolled hypertension (AVI 6144 kb)

Video 8.5 Two-dimensional transthoracic echocardiogram in the apical 5-chamber view again demonstrating the characteristic sigmoid-shaped interventricular septum with systolic anterior motion (SAM) of the mitral valve (AVI 2502 kb)

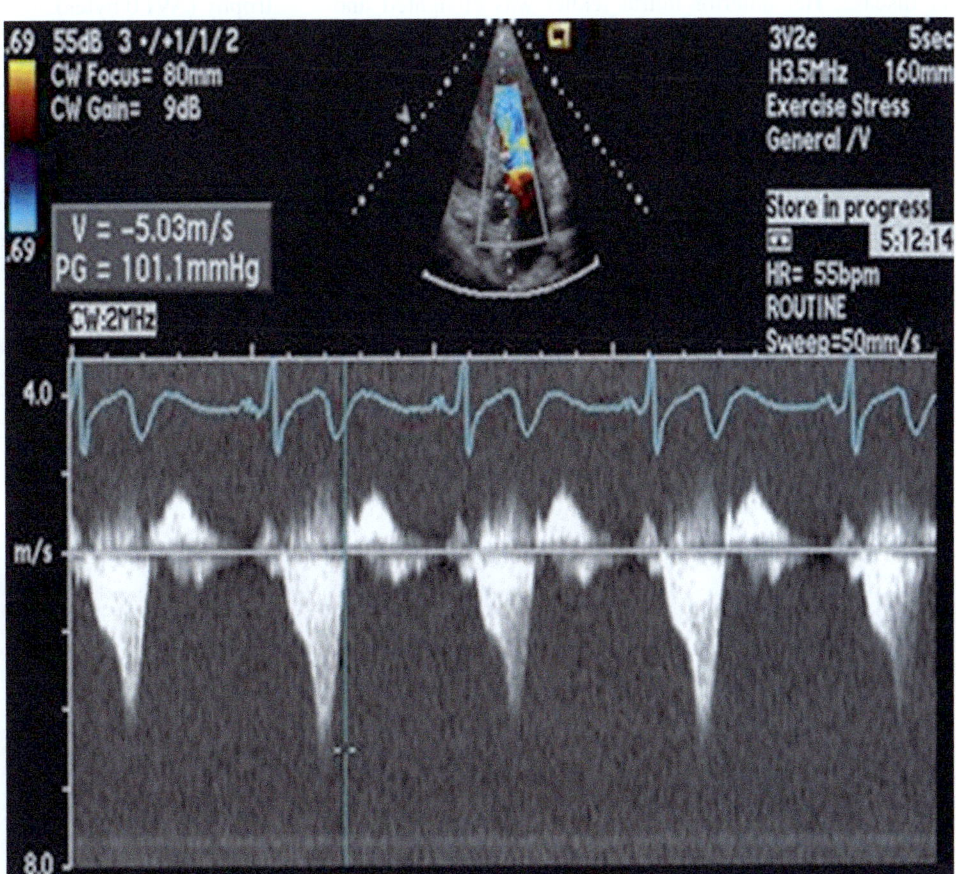

Fig. 8.2 Post-exercise spectral Doppler echocardiographic image across the LVOT in the same patient, demonstrating a characteristic late-peaking "dagger-shaped" signal, suggestive of severe dynamic LVOT obstruction

8.3 Case 3. Obstructive Cardiomyopathy Without Overt Basal Septal Hypertrophy: Intrinsic Mitral Calve Pathology

A 55-year-old woman presented with positional dizziness and progressive exertional dyspnea. She had a known history of mitral valve abnormality. On examination, she was found to have a harsh systolic ejection murmur at left upper sternal border that increased with Valsalva and reduced with squatting. She also had a loud systolic precordial murmur. Electrocardiogram revealed normal sinus rhythm. She was diagnosed with obstructive cardiomyopathy without overt basal septal hypertrophy, due to intrinsic anterior mitral leaflet disease. Her anterior mitral leaflet was elongated and resulted in systolic anterior motion (SAM) and symptomatic LVOT obstruction. She underwent anterior mitral valve repair (without a myectomy) with complete relief of symptoms.

Video 8.6 Two-dimensional transthoracic echocardiogram in the apical 3-chamber view demonstrating a long anterior mitral leaflet with obstructive SAM. Notice that the basal interventricular septum is normal in thickness (AVI 1709 kb)

Video 8.7 Two-dimensional transthoracic echocardiogram with color Doppler in the same apical 3-chamber view demonstrating severe turbulence of blood flow across the LVOT and characteristic severe posteriorly-directed jet of MR. However, there is no evidence of basal septal hypertrophy (AVI 0 bytes)

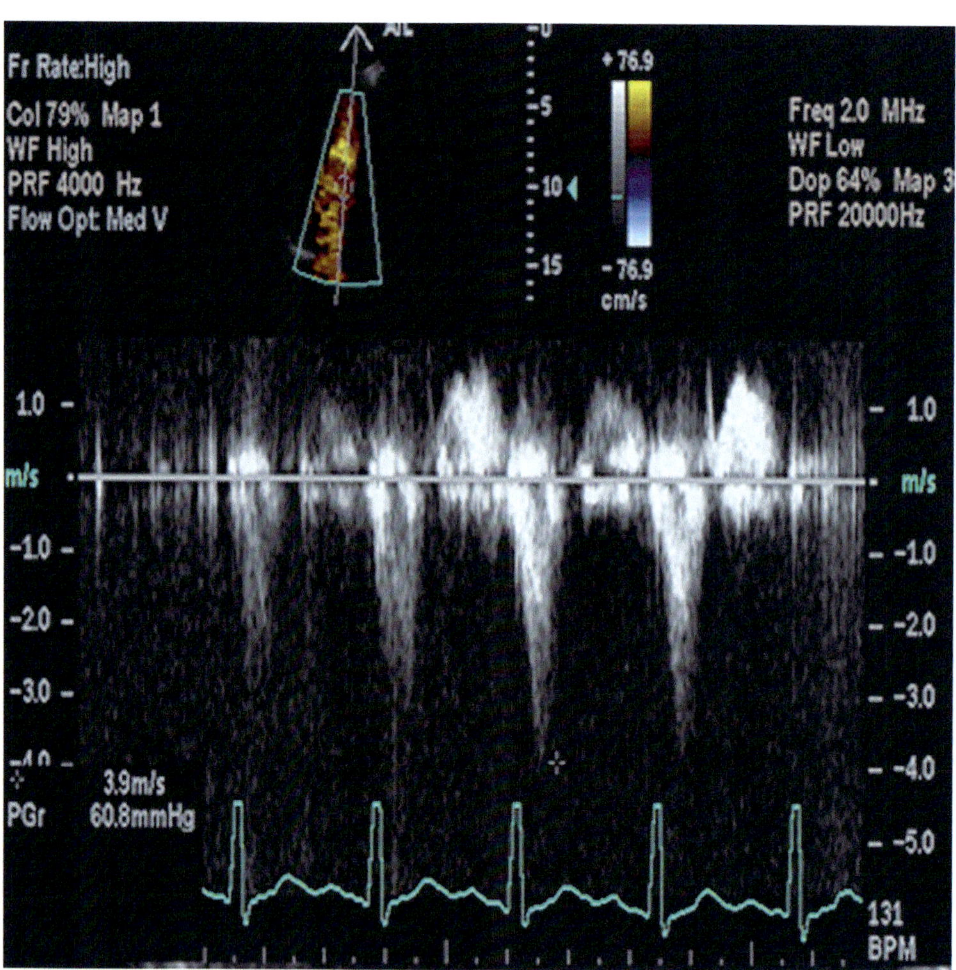

Fig. 8.3 Spectral Doppler echocardiographic image across the LVOT in the same patient, demonstrating a characteristic late-peaking "dagger-shaped" signal, suggestive of severe dynamic LVOT obstruction

8.4   Case 4. Obstructive Cardiomyopathy Without Overt Basal Septal Hypertrophy: Intrinsic Mitral Valve Pathology

A 48-year-old man presented with progressive exertional dyspnea. He had a known history of mitral valve abnormality. On examination, he was found to have a harsh systolic ejection murmur at left upper sternal border that increased with Valsalva and reduced with squatting. Patient also had a loud systolic precordial murmur. Electrocardiography revealed normal sinus rhythm. He was diagnosed with obstructive cardiomyopathy without overt basal septal hypertrophy, due to intrinsic posterior mitral leaflet disease. His posterior mitral leaflet was very elongated and resulted in SAM and symptomatic LVOT obstruction. He underwent posterior mitral valve repair (without a myectomy) with complete relief of symptoms.

Video 8.8 Two-dimensional transthoracic echocardiogram in the apical 2-chamber view demonstrating a long posterior mitral leaflet with SAM. Notice that the basal interventricular septum is normal in thickness (AVI 2035 kb)

Video 8.9 Two-dimensional transthoracic echocardiogram in the same apical 2-chamber view demonstrating severe SAM with septal contact, following inhalation of amyl nitrite (AVI 128 kb)

Video 8.10 Two-dimensional transthoracic echo with color Doppler in the parasternal long-axis view, demonstrating flow turbulence across LVOT suggestive of significant LVOT obstruction. Additionally, there is an anteriorly directed jet of MR, which is atypical for being SAM-related. In HOCM patients, presence of an anteriorly directed jet of MR should always raise a suspicion of intrinsic mitral valve (especially posterior leaflet) pathology (AVI 1459 kb)

8.5   Case 5. Obstructive Cardiomyopathy Without Overt Basal Septal Hypertrophy: Mitral Subvalvular (Papillary Muscle) Pathology

An 18-year-old man presented with recent onset of recurrent extreme fatigue after eating a large meal. In addition, he also had exertional palpitations and dizziness. His workup thus far was negative. He was told he was anxious. On examination, he had no murmur and electrocardiogram revealed normal sinus rhythm. His workup at our institution included resting echocardiography, echocardiography with provocation, upright bike echocardiography, transesophageal echocardiogram, and cardiovascular magnetic resonance imaging (CMR).

He also underwent genetic testing and was found positive for myosin-binding protein C mutation, consistent with hypertrophic cardiomyopathy (HCM). He was diagnosed with obstructive cardiomyopathy without overt basal septal hypertrophy, due to an abnormally hypertrophied papillary muscle. He underwent papillary muscle reorientation with complete relief of LVOT obstruction and symptoms.

Video 8.11 Two-dimensional transthoracic echocardiogram in the apical 3-chamber view demonstrating a very hypertrophied anterolateral papillary muscle. Notice that the mitral leaflet lengths are normal and the basal interventricular septum is normal in thickness (AVI 5927 kb)

Video 8.12 Two-dimensional transthoracic echocardiogram in the apical 3-chamber view in the same patient following inhalation of amyl nitrite. Notice severe SAM with septal contact (AVI 0 bytes)

Video 8.13 Two-dimensional transthoracic echocardiogram in the apical 3-chamber view at peak upright bicycle exercise in the same patient, demonstrating severe SAM with septal contact (AVI 1847 kb)

Video 8.14 Two-dimensional transesophageal images (mid-esophageal view) in the same patient after administration of intravenous Isoprenaline, demonstrating severe SAM with septal contact (AVI 7703 kb)

Video 8.15 Two-dimensional Color Doppler transesophageal images (mid-esophageal view) in the same patient after administration of intravenous Isoprenaline demonstrating severe posteriorly directed SAM-related MR and turbulence across the LVOT suggestive of LVOT obstruction (AVI 3759 kb)

Video 8.16 Four-chamber b-SSFP cine CMR image of the same patient confirming a very hypertrophied anterolateral papillary muscle and absence of basal septal hypertrophy (AVI 1290 kb)

Video 8.17 Two-dimensional transthoracic echocardiogram in the apical 3-chamber view obtained following surgical correction of LVOT obstruction (papillary muscle reorientation). Notice the bright suture material in the mid portion of the LV cavity. Also there is no LVOT obstruction (AVI 10920 kb)

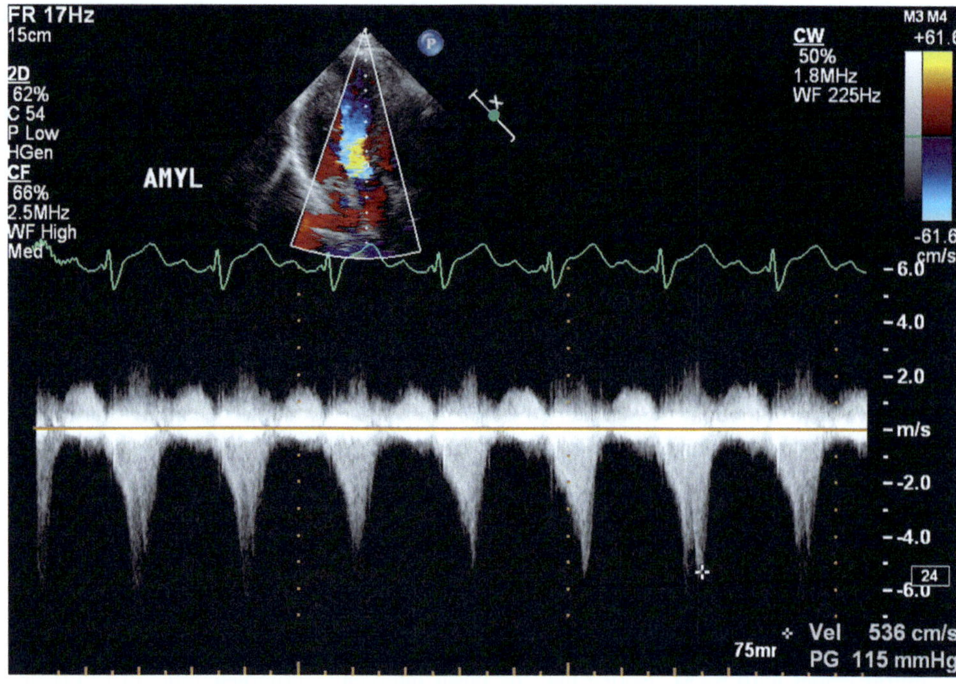

Fig. 8.4 Spectral Doppler echocardiographic image across the LVOT in the same patient, following amyl nitrite administration, demonstrating a characteristic late-peaking "dagger-shaped" signal, suggestive of severe dynamic LVOT obstruction

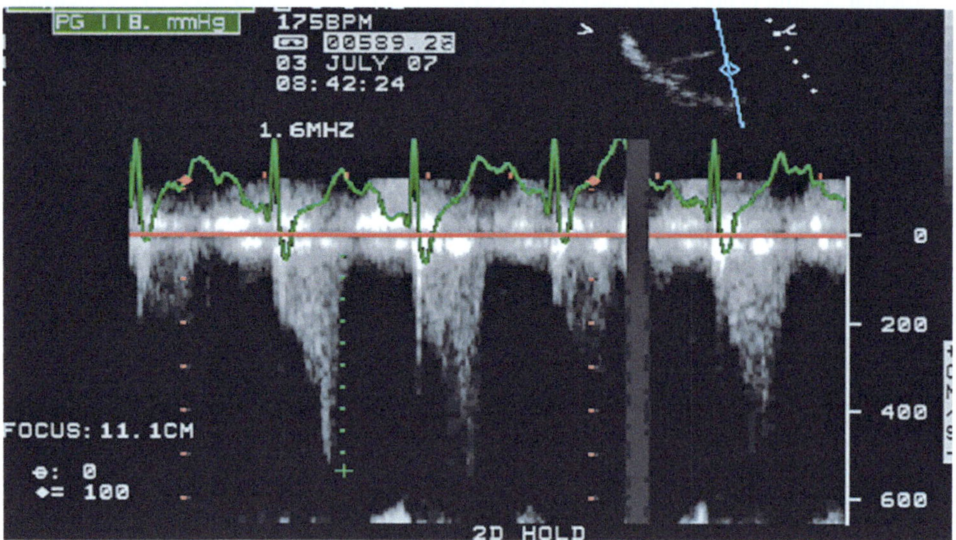

Fig. 8.5 Spectral Doppler echocardiographic image across the LVOT in the same patient, at peak upright bicycle exercise, demonstrating a characteristic late-peaking "dagger-shaped" signal, suggestive of severe dynamic LVOT obstruction

8.6 Case 6. Obstructive Cardiomyopathy Without Overt Basal Septal Hypertrophy: Mitral Subvalvular (Papillary Muscle) Pathology

An 18-year-old man with one episode of syncope. His workup thus far had been negative. He had been told he was anxious. On examination, he had no murmur and electrocardiography revealed normal sinus rhythm. He also underwent genetic testing and was found to have an R1036C variant in myosin-binding protein C gene.

Video 8.18 Two-dimensional transthoracic echocardiogram in the apical 3-chamber view demonstrating a bifid and hypermobile anterolateral papillary muscle. Notice that the mitral leaflet lengths are normal and the basal interventricular septum is normal in thickness (AVI 2290 kb)

Video 8.19 Two-dimensional transthoracic echocardiogram in the apical 3-chamber view at peak treadmill exercise, demonstrating severe SAM (AVI 0 bytes)

Video 8.20 Three-chamber b-SSFP cine CMR image of the same patient confirming a bifid and hypermobile anterolateral papillary muscle and absence of basal septal hypertrophy (AVI 0 bytes)

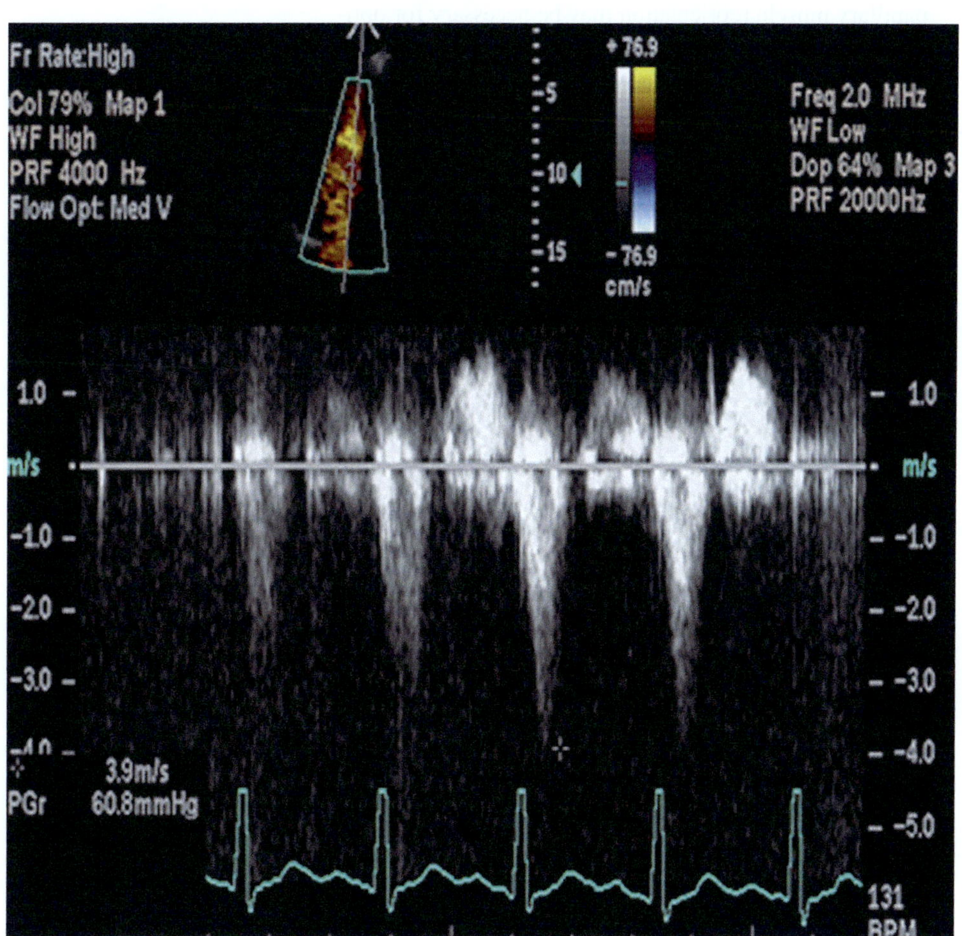

Fig. 8.6 Spectral Doppler echocardiographic image across the LVOT in the same patient, at peak-exercise, demonstrating a characteristic late-peaking "dagger-shaped" signal, suggestive of severe dynamic LVOT obstruction

8.7 Teaching Points

- Involvement of the mitral valve is intrinsic to the pathophysiology of obstructive HCM. When evaluated carefully, ~70 % patients with HCM have resting or provocable LVOT obstruction, related to SAM
- Not all patients with LVOT obstruction have basal septal hypertrophy. Approximately 15–20 % of patients have abnormal mitral valve or subvalvular (papillary muscle) abnormality resulting in LVOT obstruction
- In many instances, surgical myectomy or alcohol septal ablation are not sufficient to relieve LVOT obstruction. In these situations, mitral valve repair/replacement and/or papillary muscle reorientation may be necessary for optimal relief of LVOT obstruction
- A detailed multimodality imaging evaluation might be necessary in many instances to come to an accurate diagnosis and develop an optimal therapeutic plan

Suggested Reading

Desai MY, Ommen SR, McKenna WJ, Lever HM, Elliott PM. Imaging phenotype versus genotype in hypertrophic cardiomyopathy. Circ Cardiovasc Imaging. 2011;4(2):156–68.

Gersh BJ, Maron BJ, Bonow RO, Dearani JA, Fifer MA, Link MS, et al. 2011 ACCF/AHA Guideline for the Diagnosis and Treatment of Hypertrophic Cardiomyopathy: a report of the American College of Cardiology Foundation/American Heart Association Task Force on Practice Guidelines. Developed in collaboration with the American Association for Thoracic Surgery, American Society of Echocardiography, American Society of Nuclear Cardiology, Heart Failure Society of America, Heart Rhythm Society, Society for Cardiovascular Angiography and Interventions, and Society of Thoracic Surgeons. J Am Coll Cardiol. 2011;58(25):e212–60.

Teerapat Yingchoncharoen

9.1 Case 1. Primum Atrial Septal Defect with Mitral Valve Cleft

A 66-year-old woman has a history of coronary artery bypass grafting in 1987, when she had left main stenosis and underwent bypass with anastomosis of the left internal mammary artery to the left anterior descending artery and a saphenous vein graft to the obtuse marginal branch. The patient now returns with symptoms of congestive heart failure. She is found to have an atrioventricular canal defect including mitral valve regurgitation with mitral valve cleft, primum atrial septal defect, and severe tricuspid regurgitation. She also has a left-sided superior vena cava, into which she has an anomalous left upper pulmonary vein. She has recently noticed a significant decline and can now walk only half a block at a slow pace before having to stop. She was referred to our institute for surgical correction of her complex congenital heart disease (Figs. 9.1, 9.2, 9.3, 9.4, 9.5, 9.6, 9.7, 9.8, 9.9, and 9.10).

Video 9.1 Transthoracic echocardiography (TTE), parasternal long-axis view, showing dilatation of the coronary sinus in the setting of persistent left superior vena cava and mitral regurgitation (AVI 1923 kb)

Video 9.2 TTE, parasternal short-axis view, showing atrial septal defect with left-to-right shunt (AVI 2013 kb)

Video 9.3 Three-dimensional (3D) TTE short-axis view at the aortic valve level showing the bicuspid aortic valve. The aortic valve orifice appears to have a "fish-mouth" appearance (AVI 1832 kb)

Video 9.4 TTE X-plane imaging showing two orthogonal views showing an anterior mitral valve cleft (AVI 3804 kb)

Video 9.5 TTE parasternal short-axis view of the mitral valve with color Doppler imaging showing anterior mitral valve cleft with corresponding mitral regurgitation (AVI 1818 kb)

Video 9.6 TTE four-chamber view showing dilated right-sided cardiac chambers with a ventricular upper septal aneurysm (AVI 5815 kb)

Video 9.7 TTE four-chamber view with color Doppler imaging showed atrial septal defect with left-to-right shunt at the level close to the cardiac crux, consistent with primum atrial septal defect. Also seen are mitral and tricuspid regurgitation (AVI 2320 kb)

Video 9.8 Transesophageal echocardiography (TEE) four-chamber view showed primum atrial septal defect (AVI 6583 kb)

Video 9.9 TEE short axis view at aortic valve level showed bicuspid aortic valve (AVI 6459 kb)

Video 9.10 3D TEE of mitral valve (surgical view) showed anterior mitral valve cleft (AVI 218 kb)

Electronic supplementary material The online version of this chapter (doi:10.1007/978-1-4471-6672-6_9) contains supplementary material, which is available to authorized users.

T. Yingchoncharoen
Department of Cardiovascular Medicine, Cleveland Clinic, 9500 Euclid Avenue, Cleveland, OH 44195, USA
e-mail: teerapatmdcu@gmail.com

M. Desai et al. (eds.), *An Atlas of Mitral Valve Imaging*, DOI 10.1007/978-1-4471-6672-6_9, © Springer-Verlag London 2015

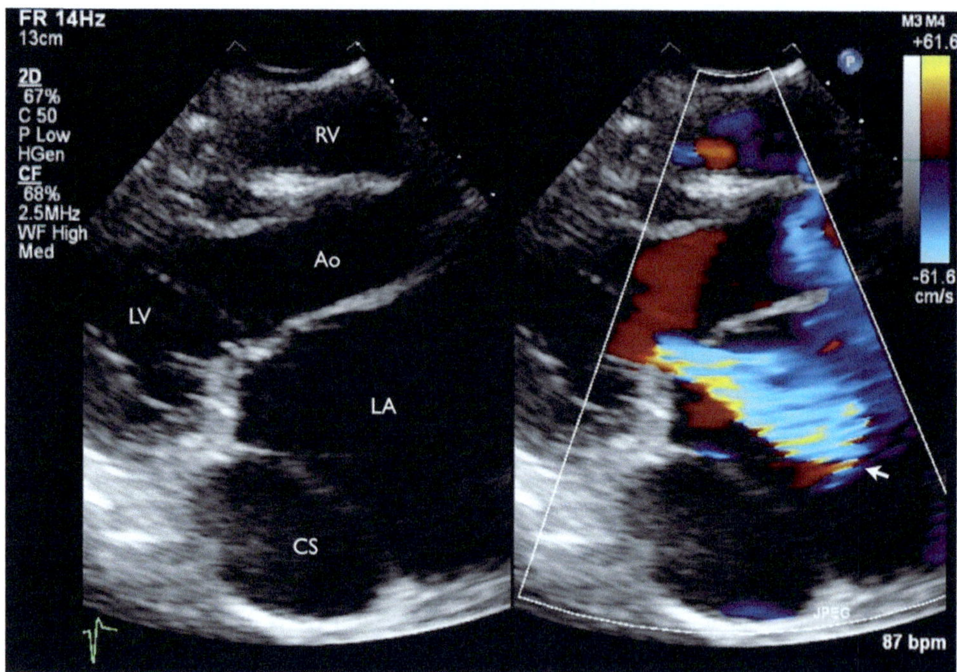

Fig. 9.1 Transthoracic echocardiography (TTE) parasternal long-axis view showing dilatation of the coronary sinus (CS) in the setting of persistent left superior vena cava and mitral regurgitation (*arrow*). *Ao* aorta, *LA* left atrium, *LV* left ventricle, *RV* right ventricle

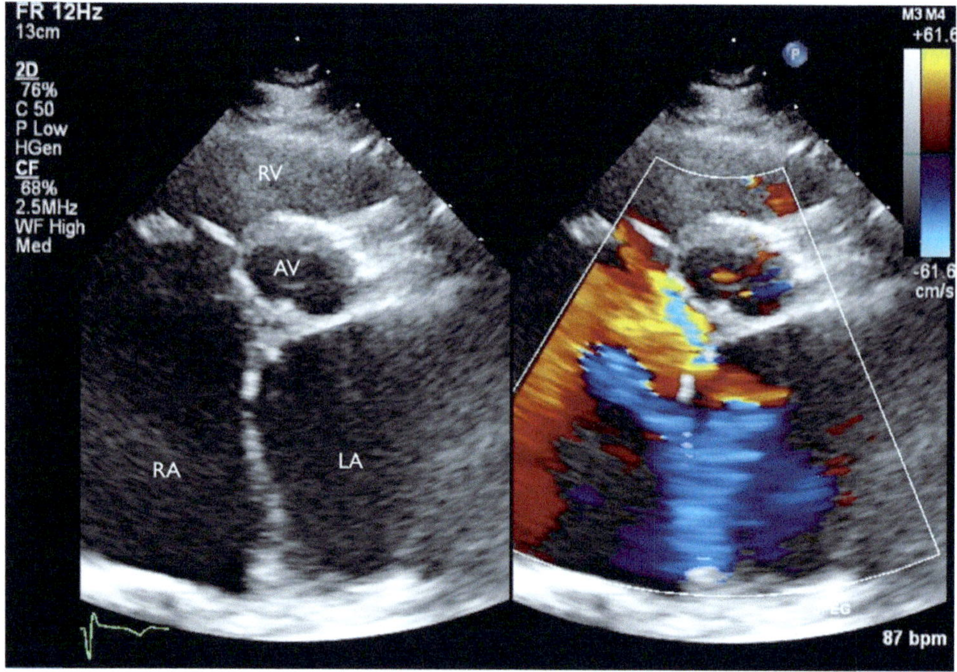

Fig. 9.2 TTE parasternal short-axis view showing atrial septal defect with left-to-right shunt. *AV* aortic valve, *RA* right atrium, *RV* right ventricle

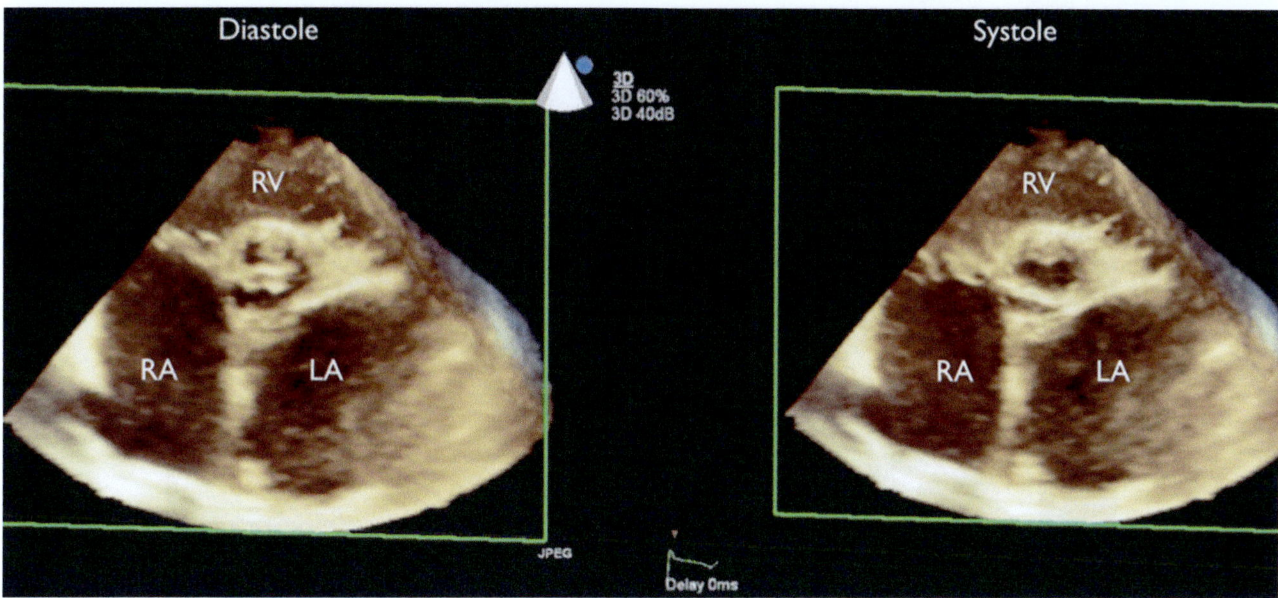

Fig. 9.3 Three-dimensional (3D) TTE short-axis view at the aortic valve level showing the bicuspid aortic valve. The aortic valve orifice appears to have a "fish-mouth" appearance. *LA* left atrium, *RA* right atrium, *RV* right ventricle

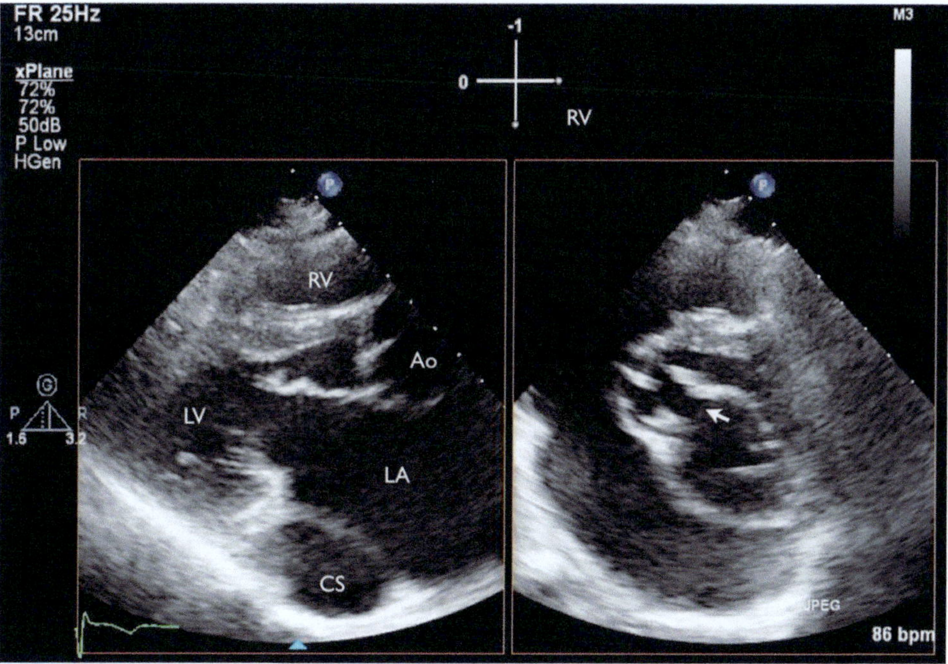

Fig. 9.4 TTE X-plane imaging showing two orthogonal views showing an anterior mitral valve cleft (*arrow*). *Ao* aorta, *CS* coronary sinus, *LA* left atrium, *LV* left ventricle, *RV* right ventricle

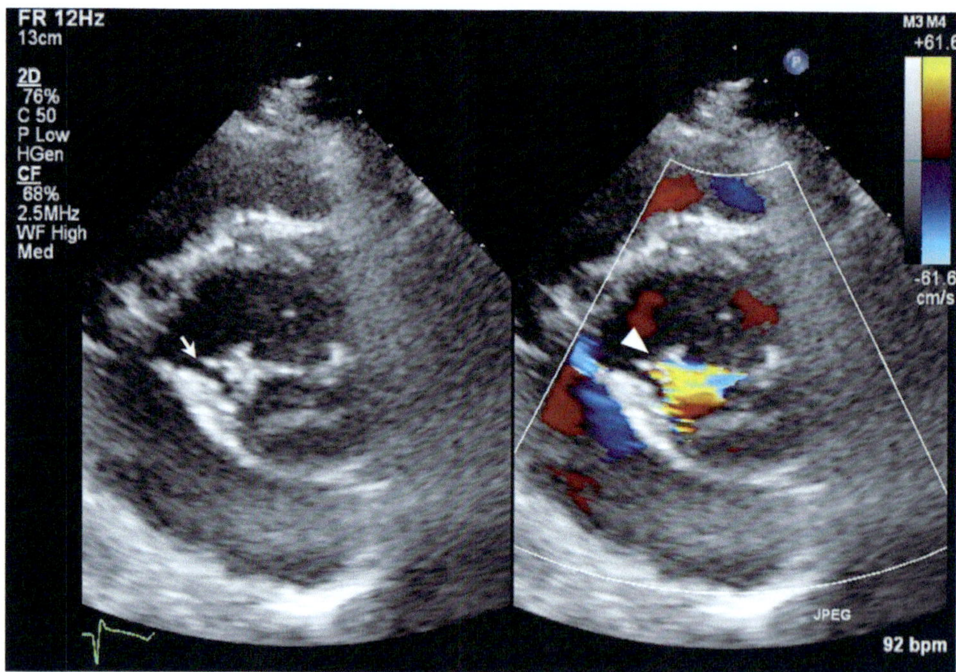

Fig. 9.5 TTE parasternal short-axis view of the mitral valve with color Doppler imaging showing anterior mitral valve cleft (*arrow*) with corresponding mitral regurgitation (*arrowhead*)

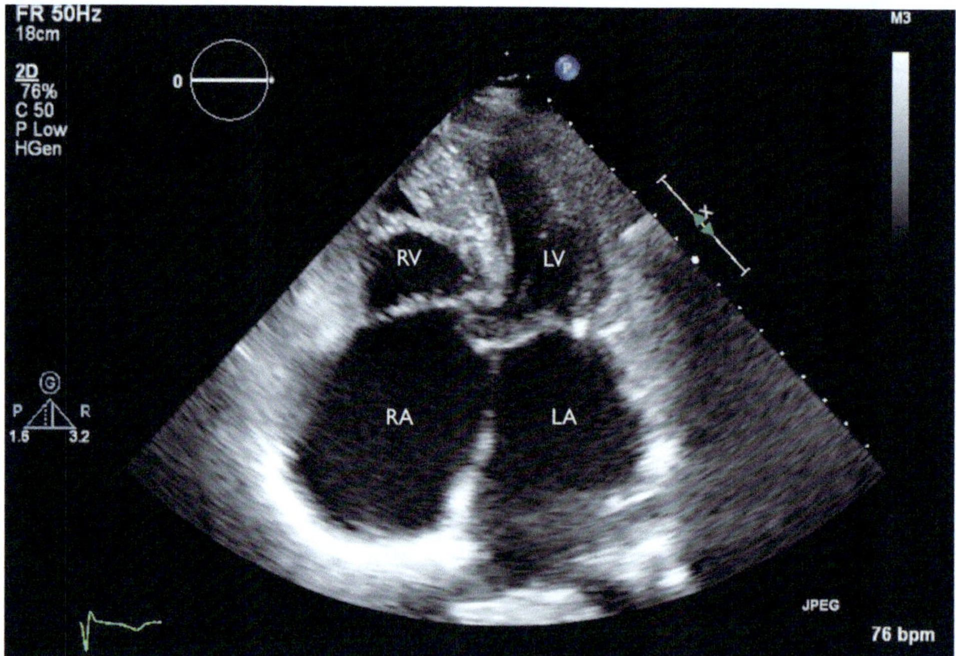

Fig. 9.6 TTE four-chamber view showing dilated right-sided cardiac chambers with a ventricular upper septal aneurysm. *LA* left atrium, *LV* left ventricle, *RA* right atrium, *RV* right ventricle

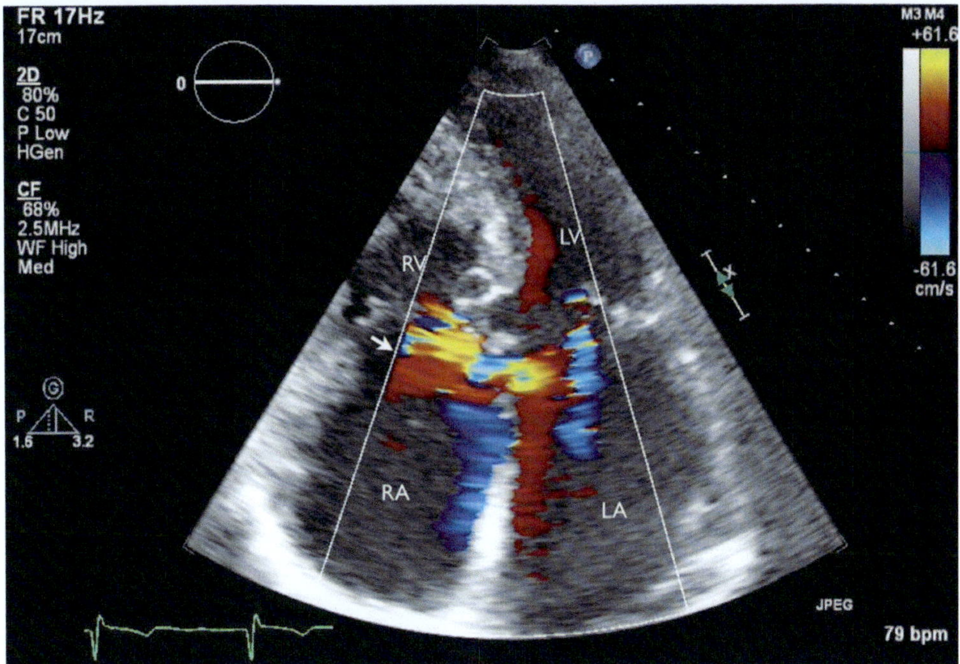

Fig. 9.7 TTE four-chamber view with color Doppler imaging showed atrial septal defect with left-to-right shunt (*arrow*) at the level close to the cardiac crux, consistent with primum atrial septal defect. Also seen are mitral and tricuspid regurgitation. *LA* left atrium, *LV* left ventricle, *RA* right atrium, *RV* right ventricle

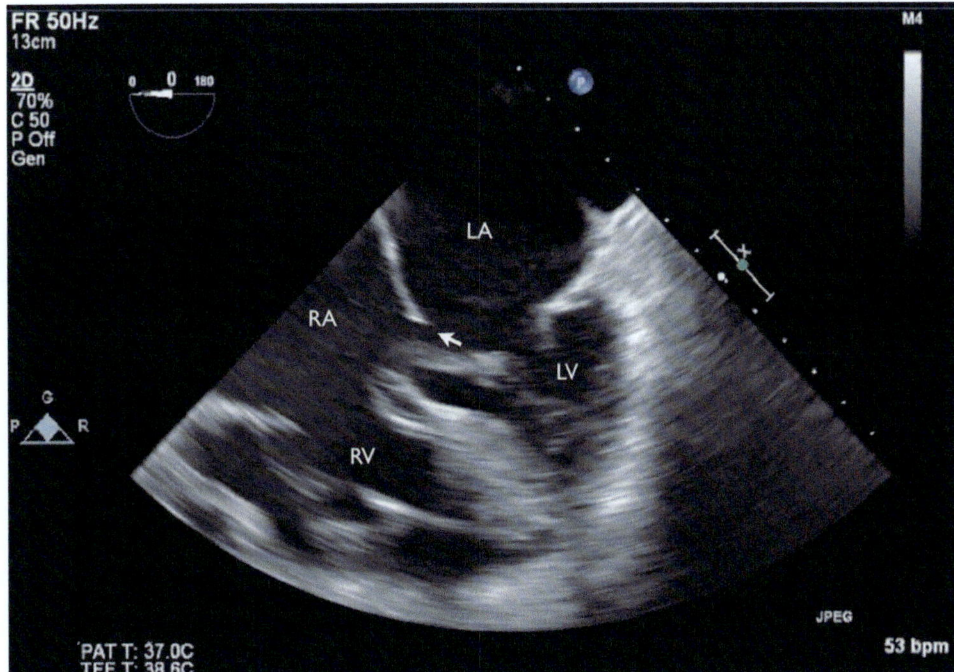

Fig. 9.8 Transesophageal echocardiography (TEE) four-chamber view showed primum atrial septal defect (*arrow*). *LA* left atrium, *LV* left ventricle, *RA* right atrium, *RV* right ventricle

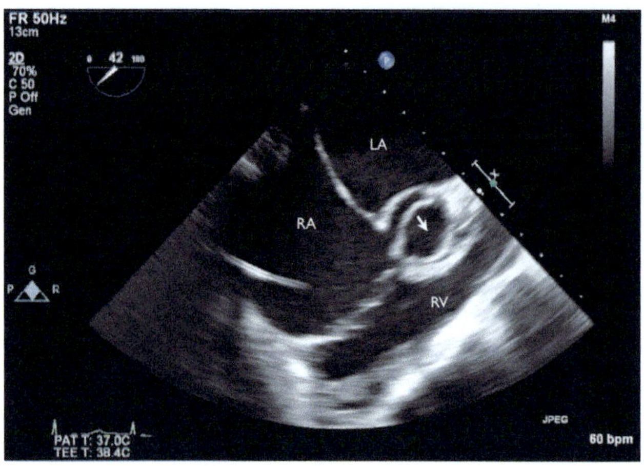

Fig. 9.9 TEE short-axis view at aortic valve level showed bicuspid aortic valve (*arrow*). *LA* left atrium, *RA* right atrium, *RV* right ventricle

9.1.1 Learning Points

In ostium primum atrial septal defect, absence of the membranous septum and a cleft in the anterior mitral leaflet are the characteristic features resulting from maldevelopment of the endocardial cushions [1]. The echocardiographic features of mitral valve cleft include the separation of the anterior mitral leaflets during diastole, typically with accessory chordae seen as thin linear echoes between the ridges of both parts of the anterior leaflet and the ventricular septum.

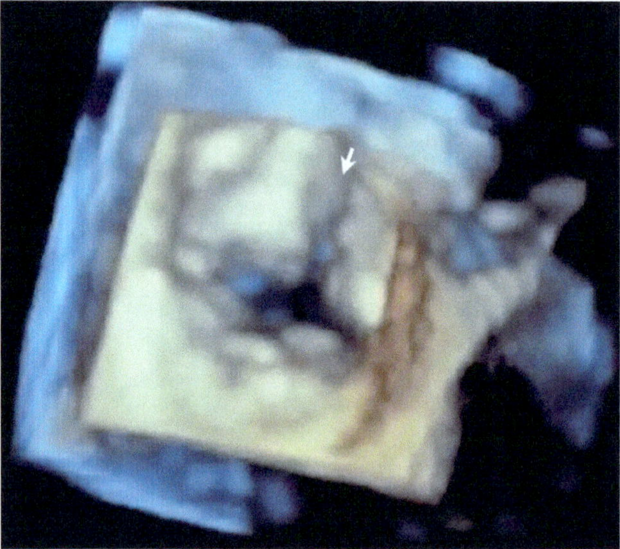

Fig. 9.10 3D TEE of mitral valve (surgical view) showed anterior mitral valve cleft (*arrow*)

9.2   Case 2. Parachute Mitral Valve

A 27-year-old woman has a history of Shone complex, which includes coarctation of the aorta, a bicuspid aortic valve, and a parachute-variant mitral valve with supramitral ring status post multiple previous operative repairs, including patch arterioplasty, a supramitral ring resection, and subaortic stenosis resection, as well as a Konno procedure with implantation of a #19 St. Jude aortic valve replacement. She is here for routine follow-up. She has remained asymptomatic and continues to exercise vigorously several times per week (Figs. 9.11, 9.12, 9.13, 9.14, and 9.15).

Video 9.11 TTE parasternal long-axis view showed an elongated anterior mitral leaflet with parachute mitral valve with a unifocal attachment of the mitral valve chordae to a single papillary muscle (AVI 7949 kb)

Video 9.12 TTE parasternal long-axis view with color Doppler imaging showed turbulent flow across the mitral valve during diastole (AVI 3947 kb)

Video 9.13 TTE apical four-chamber view showed mitral valve opening during diastole. The valve opening was restricted because of abnormal chordal attachment, giving the appearance of the parachute mitral valve (AVI 6701 kb)

Video 9.14 TTE apical four-chamber view with color Doppler flow showed diastolic flow acceleration across the mitral valve, consistent with mitral stenosis, as well as mild mitral regurgitation (AVI 1969 kb)

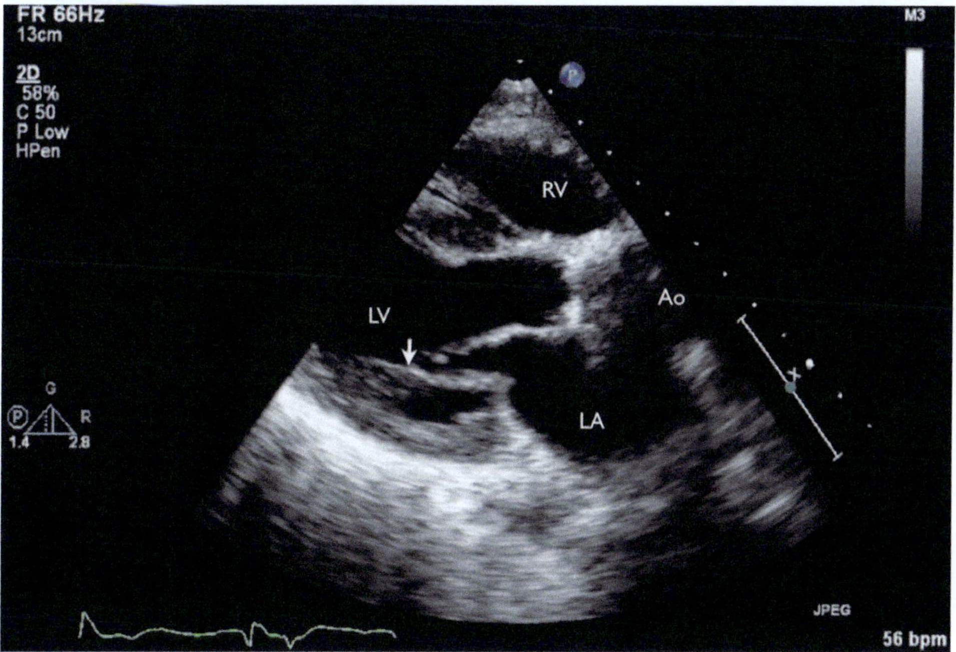

Fig. 9.11 TTE parasternal long-axis view showed an elongated anterior mitral leaflet with parachute mitral valve with a unifocal attachment of the mitral valve chordae to a single papillary muscle (*arrow*)

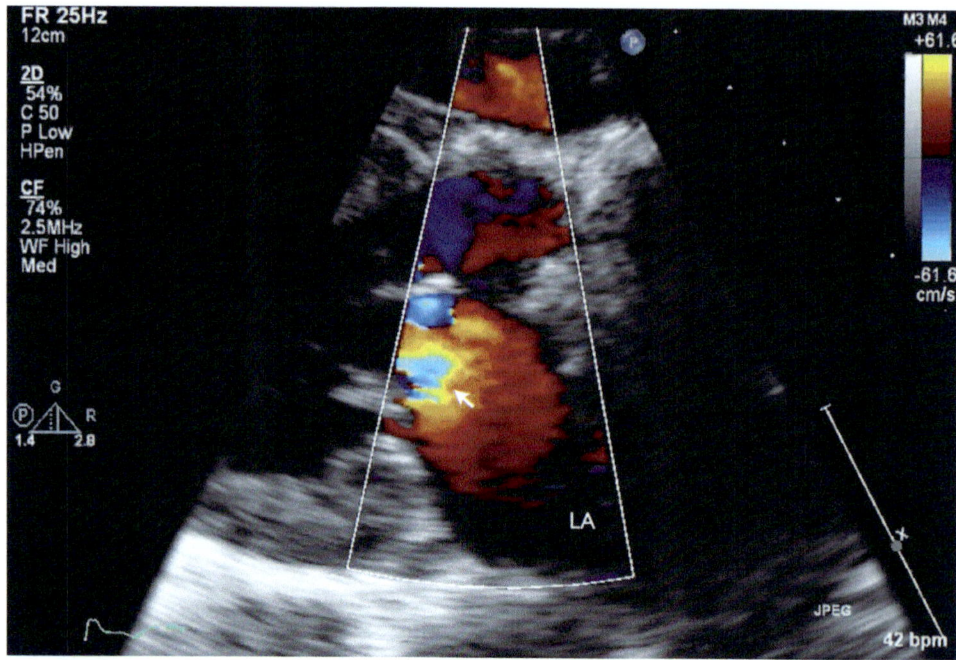

Fig. 9.12 TTE parasternal long-axis view with color Doppler imaging showed turbulent flow across the mitral valve during diastole (*arrow*). *LA* left atrium

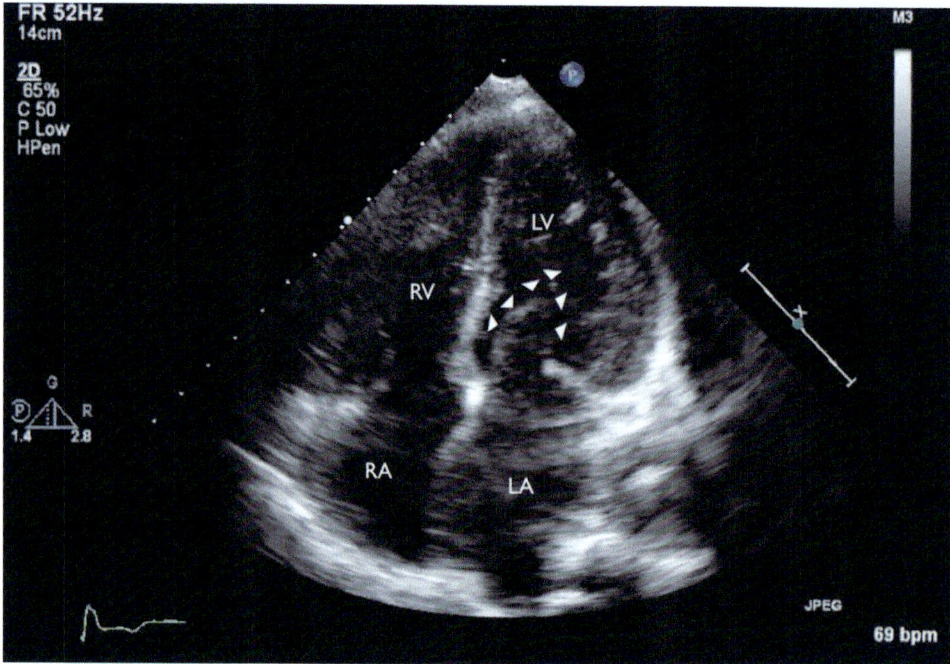

Fig. 9.13 TTE apical four-chamber view showed mitral valve opening during diastole. The valve opening was restricted because of abnormal chordal attachment, giving the appearance of the parachute mitral valve (*arrowheads*). *LA* left atrium, *LV* left ventricle, *RA* right atrium, *RV* right ventricle

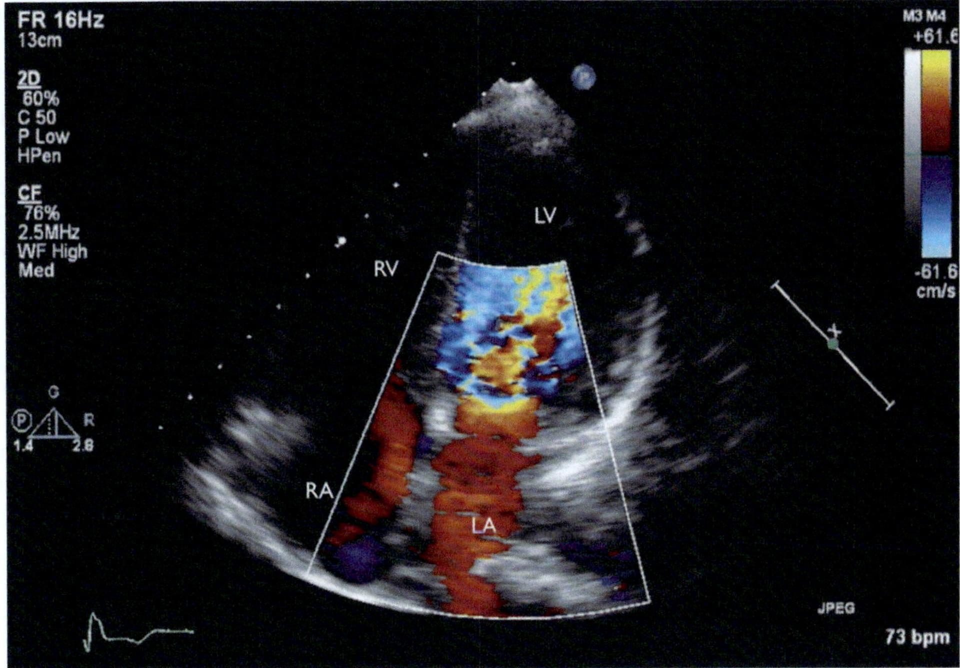

Fig. 9.14 TTE apical four-chamber view with color Doppler flow showed diastolic flow acceleration across the mitral valve, consistent with mitral stenosis, as well as mild mitral regurgitation. *LA* left atrium, *LV* left ventricle, *RA* right atrium, *RV* right ventricle

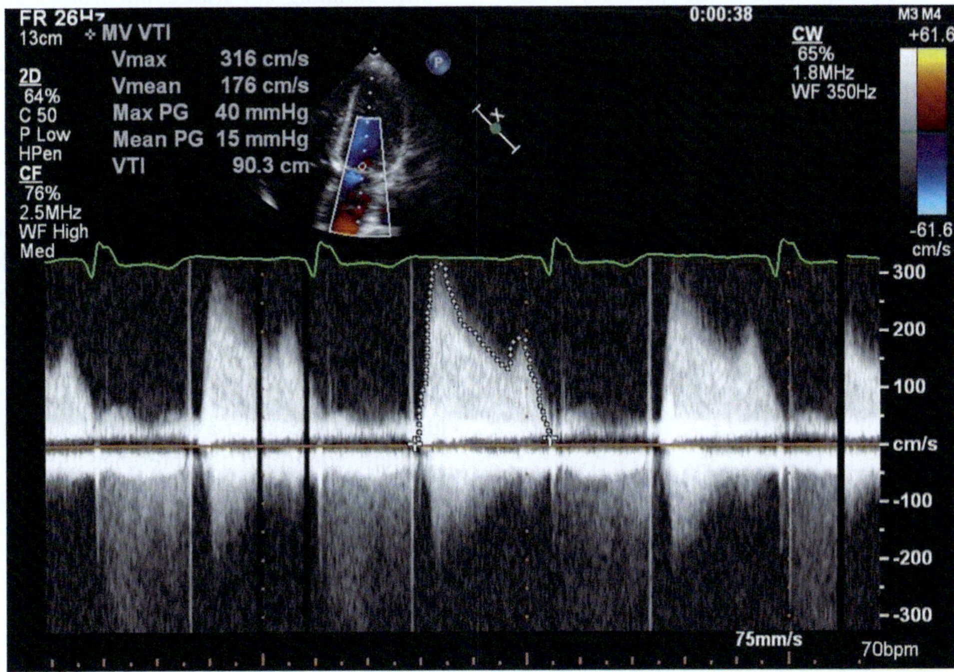

Fig. 9.15 Continuous-wave Doppler imaging across the mitral valve showed severe mitral stenosis (mean pressure gradient 15 mmHg)

9.2.1 Learning Points

In 1963, Shone et al. [2] described a developmental complex in which four obstructive anomalies of the left side of the heart and aorta coexist. Most patients with Shone's Anomaly are diagnosed in childhood. The complex includes a parachute mitral valve and aortic coarctation (68 % of patients), atrial septal defect (54 % of patients), ventricular septal defect (46 % of patients), aortic valve stenosis (32 % of patients), subaortic stenosis (20 % of patients), and left ventricular hypoplasia (19 % of patients) [3]. The primary morphological feature of parachute mitral valve is the unifocal attachment of chordae tendineae. "True" parachute mitral valve is characterized by attachment of the chordae to a single or fused papillary muscle, whereas in "parachute-like asymmetric mitral valve" the mitral valve can be asymmetrical, having two papillary muscles, one of which is dominant and elongated, with its tip reaching to the valve leaflets. It is believed embryologically that the development of the anterolateral and posteromedial papillary muscles was disrupted between the 5th and 19th weeks of gestation, thereby forcing the embryonic predecessors of the papillary muscles to condense into a single muscle [4]. Survival for patients with parachute mitral valve is dependent on the spectrum of associated cardiac lesions (left ventricular hypoplasia and atrial septal defect). The degree of mitral valve obstruction remains stable, and most patients do not require valvotomy [3].

9.3 Case 3. Cor Triatriatum Sinister with Atrial Septal Defect

A 56-year-old woman has a history of heart murmur noted during childhood, with exertional dyspnea, frequent light-headedness, and presyncope, especially after exertion. She was recently diagnosed with cor triatriatum sinister and a secundum atrial septal defect and was referred to our institute for further evaluation and possible surgical correction (Figs. 9.16, 9.17, 9.18, 9.19, 9.20, and 9.21).

Video 9.15 TTE parasternal long-axis view showing a thin membrane separating the left atrium into two chambers. The proximal or superior chamber drains the pulmonary venous blood, and the distal inferior chamber (or true atrium) is in contact with the atrioventricular valve (AVI 954 kb)

Video 9.16 TTE apical four-chamber view showing a thin membrane separating the left atrium into two chambers, a finding consistent with cor triatriatum sinister (AVI 1141 kb)

Video 9.17 TTE apical two-chamber view showed that the left atrial appendage and the foramen ovale are distal to the cor triatriatum membrane. This feature is important in differentiating cor triatriatum from a supramitral valve ring, which tends to attach to the base of the mitral valve, past the left atrial appendage and the foramen ovale (AVI 1095 kb)

Video 9.18 TTE subcostal view zoomed at the interatrial septum, demonstrating atrial septal defect with left-to-right shunt (AVI 1582 kb)

Video 9.19 TTE apical four-chamber view with color Doppler flow imaging showed nonturbulent flow across the cor triatriatum membrane. This finding was confirmed by pulsed-wave Doppler and cardiac cathetherization showing a nonobstructive cor triatriatum membrane (AVI 1502 kb)

Video 9.20 TEE short-axis view zoomed at the interatrial septum confirmed the presence of the cor triatriatum membrane. The color Doppler flow imaging showed nonturbulent flow across the membrane (AVI 2049 kb)

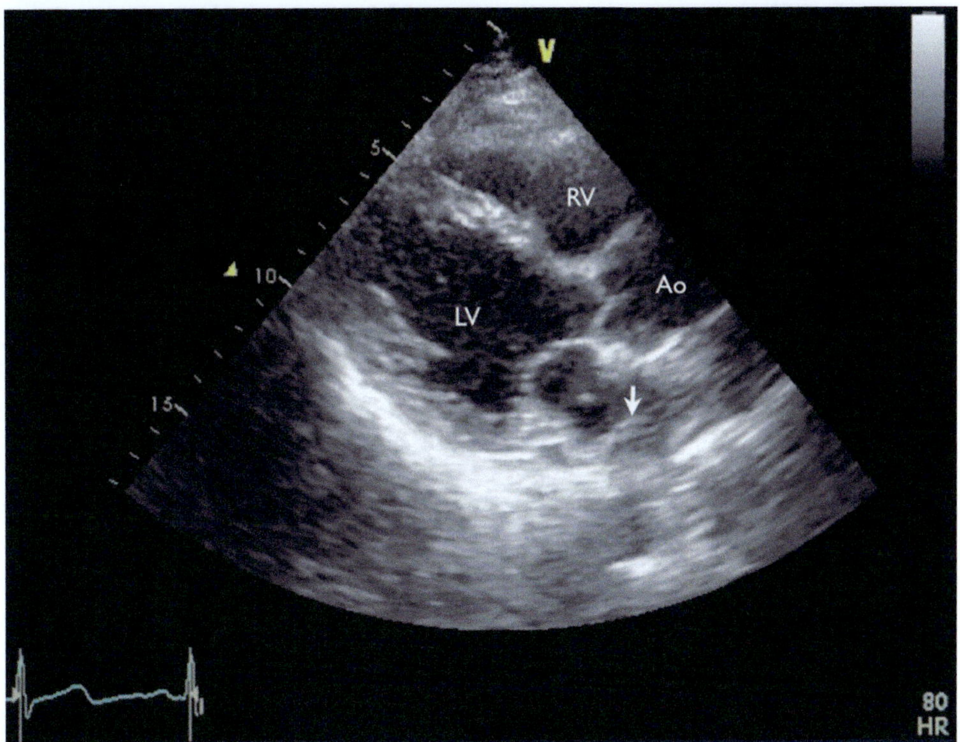

Fig. 9.16 TTE parasternal long-axis view showed a thin membrane (*arrow*) separating the left atrium into two chambers. The proximal or superior chamber drains the pulmonary venous blood, and the distal inferior chamber (or true atrium) is in contact with the atrioventricular valve. *Ao* aorta, *LV* left ventricle, *RV* right ventricle

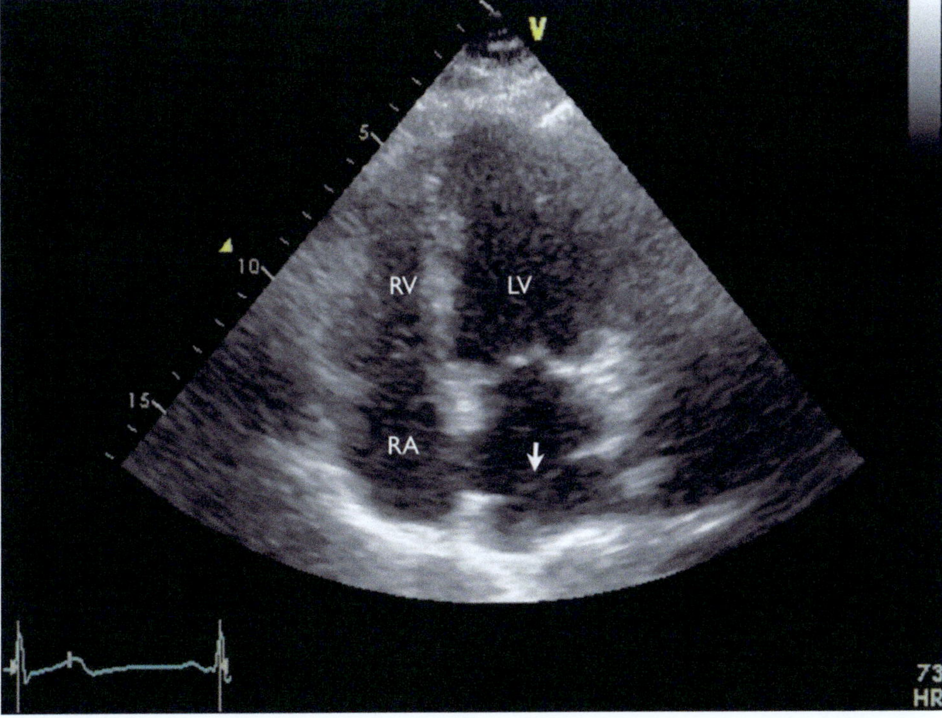

Fig. 9.17 TTE apical four-chamber view showed a thin membrane separating the left atrium into two chambers (*arrow*), a finding consistent with cor triatriatum sinister. *LV* left ventricle, *RA* right atrium, *RV* right ventricle

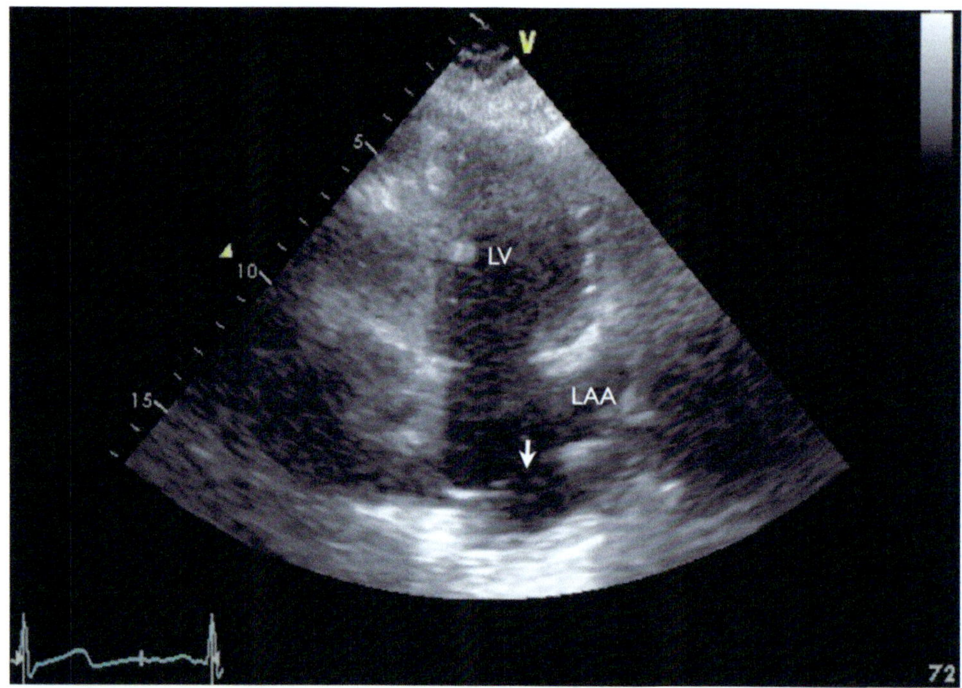

Fig. 9.18 TTE apical two-chamber view showed that the left atrial appendage (*LAA*) and the foramen ovale are distal to the cor triatriatum membrane (*arrow*). This feature is important in differentiating cor tria-triatum from a supramitral valve ring, which tends to attach to the base of the mitral valve, past the LAA and the foramen ovale. *LV* left ventricle

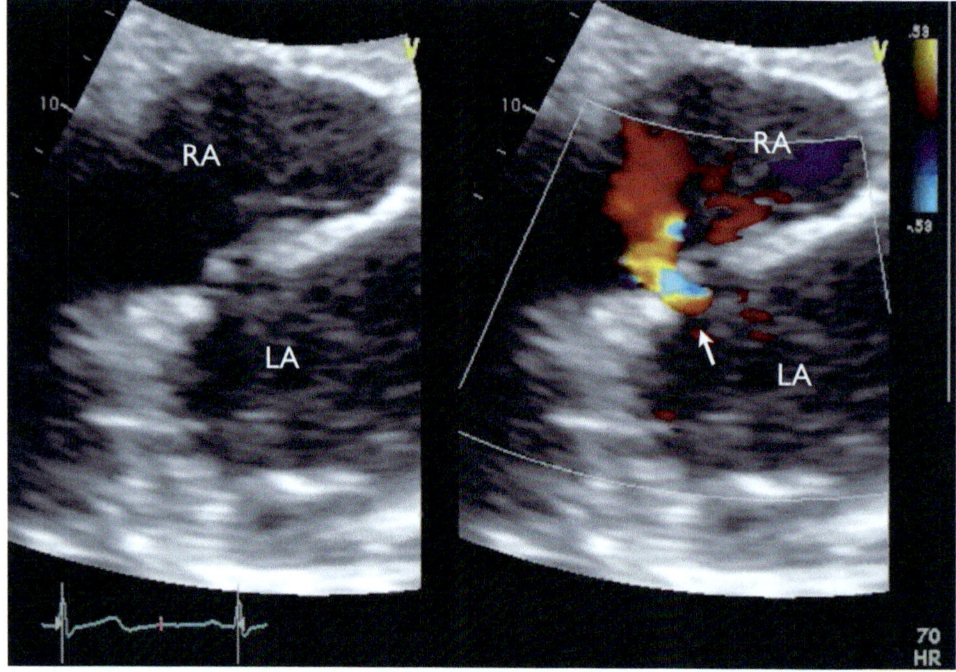

Fig. 9.19 TTE subcostal view zoomed at the interatrial septum, demonstrating atrial septal defect with left-to-right shunt (*arrow*). *LA* left atrium, *RA* right atrium

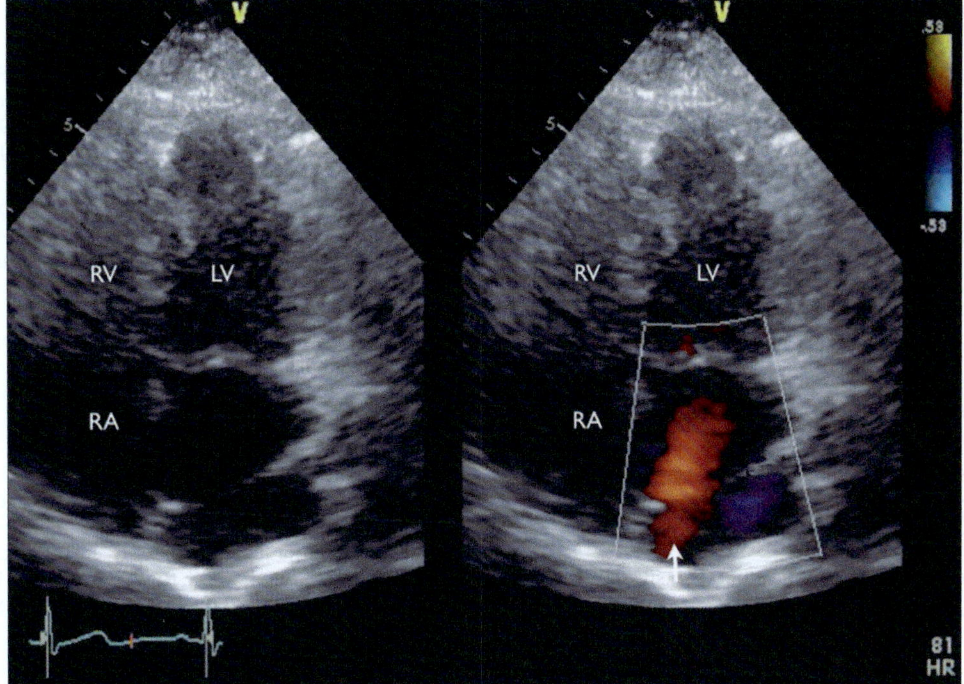

Fig. 9.20 TTE apical four-chamber view with color Doppler flow imaging showed nonturbulent flow across the cor triatriatum membrane (*arrow*). This finding was confirmed by pulsed-wave Doppler and cardiac cathetherization showing a nonobstructive cor triatriatum membrane. *LV* left ventricle, *RA* right atrium, *RV* right ventricle

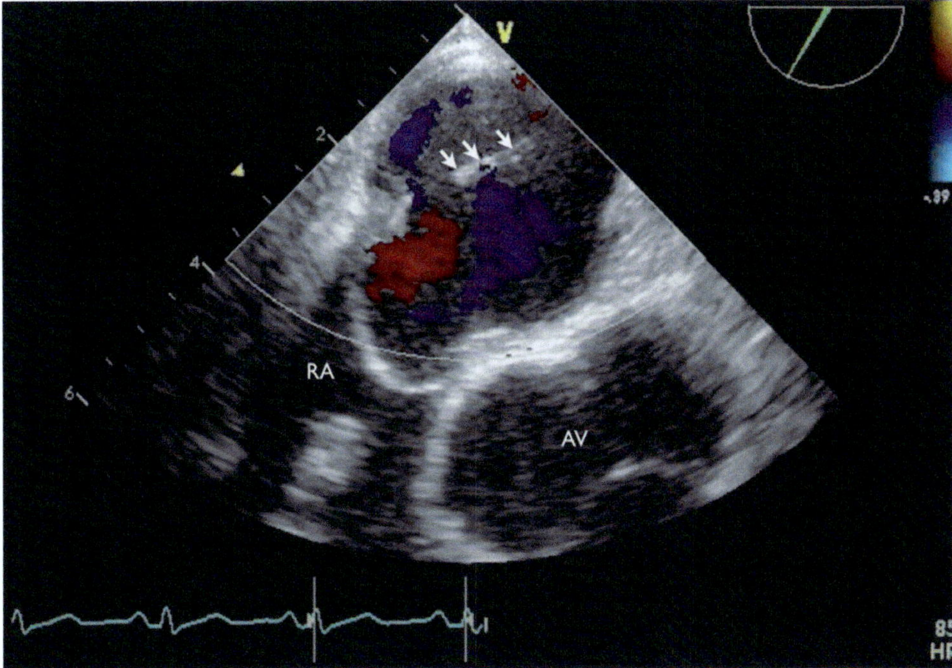

Fig. 9.21 TEE short-axis view zoomed at the interatrial septum confirmed the presence of the cor triatriatum membrane (*arrows*). The color Doppler flow imaging showed nonturbulent flow across the membrane. *AV* aortic valve, *RA* right atrium

9.3.1 Learning Points

Cor triatriatum sinister is a rare congenital abnormality reported in 0.4 % of patients with congenital heart disease at autopsy [5]. In cor triatriatum sinister, the left atrium is divided into two chambers by a thick, fibromuscular, membranous septum, which can have a transverse or horizontal orientation or can be bandlike or funnel-shaped. The proximal or superior chamber drains the pulmonary venous blood, whereas the distal inferior chamber (or true atrium) is in contact with the atrioventricular valve and contains the atrial appendage and the true atrial septum [6]. Echocardiography of cor triatriatum sinister shows a thin, linear structure bisecting the atrium on a four-chamber view, distal to the mitral valve and the left atrial appendage. In the long-axis view, the superior part of the membrane is usually parallel to the aortic wall and its inferior part connects to the left atrial posterior wall. Color Doppler flow imaging and measurement of the transmembrane maximal pressure gradient differentiates obstructive cor triatriatum from the nonobstructive group. A maximal Doppler velocity greater than 2 m/s indicates severe obstruction [7].

References

1. Beppu S, Nimura Y, Sakakibara H, Nagata S, Park YD, Baba K, et al. Mitral cleft in ostium primum atrial septal defect assessed by cross-sectional echocardiography. Circulation. 1980;62:1099–107.
2. Shone JD, Sellers RD, Anderson RC, Adams Jr P, Lillehei CW, Edwards JE. The developmental complex of "parachute mitral valve," supravalvular ring of left atrium, subaortic stenosis, and coarctation of aorta. Am J Cardiol. 1963;11:714–25.
3. Schaverien MV, Freedom RM, McCrindle BW. Independent factors associated with outcomes of parachute mitral valve in 84 patients. Circulation. 2004;109:2309–13.
4. Oosthoek PW, Wenink AC, Wisse LJ, Gittenberger-de Groot AC. Development of the papillary muscles of the mitral valve: morphogenetic background of parachute-like asymmetric mitral valves and other mitral valve anomalies. J Thorac Cardiovasc Surg. 1998;116:36–46.
5. Jegier W, Gibbons JE, Wiglesworth FW. Cortriatriatum: clinical, hemodynamic and pathological studies surgical correction in early life. Pediatrics. 1963;31:255–67.
6. Niwayama G. Cor triatriatum. Am Heart J. 1960;59:291–317.
7. Houston A, Hillis S, Lilley S, Richens T, Swan L. Echocardiography in adult congenital heart disease. Heart. 1998;80 Suppl 1:S12–26.

Teerapat Yingchoncharoen

10.1 Case 1. Inferior Wall Myocardial Infarction Complicated by Ruptured Papillary Muscle

A 78-year-old woman had a past medical history of atrial fibrillation and acute ST-elevation inferior wall myocardial infarction 2 weeks prior to presentation. Her hospital course was complicated by ventricular tachycardia, cardiac arrest, and cardiogenic shock. After discharge to a rehabilitation facility, she was readmitted because of acute decompensated congestive heart failure. She successfully underwent mitral valve repair with coronary artery bypass grafting (Figs. 10.1, 10.2, 10.3, 10.4, 10.5, 10.6, and 10.7).

Video 10.1 Transesophageal echocardiography (TEE) four-chamber view showed ruptured chordae tendineae of the posterior leaflet. The ruptured chordae are seen as a freely moving structure from the left ventricle to the left atrium during the cardiac cycle (AVI 5505 kb)

Video 10.2 A TEE zoom view of the mitral valve demonstrating flail of the posterior mitral leaflet with ruptured chordae (AVI 12633 kb)

Video 10.3 TEE zoom view of the mitral valve with color flow Doppler imaging demonstrating anteriorly directed mitral regurgitation jet (AVI 3203 kb)

Video 10.4 TEE at 60° showed ruptured chordae with papillary muscle head moving freely into the left atrium (AVI 9826 kb)

Video 10.5 TEE at 120° showed ruptured chordae with papillary muscle head moving freely into the left atrium (AVI 10014 kb)

Video 10.6 TEE at 120° with color flow Doppler imaging demonstrating anteriorly directed mitral regurgitation jet (AVI 1972 kb)

Video 10.7 Three-dimensional (3D) reconstruction imaging of the mitral valve (surgical view) showing flail P3 segment of the mitral valve with ruptured papillary muscle (AVI 2454 kb)

Electronic supplementary material The online version of this chapter (doi:10.1007/978-1-4471-6672-6_10) contains supplementary material, which is available to authorized users.

T. Yingchoncharoen
Department of Cardiovascular Medicine, Cleveland Clinic, 9500 Euclid Avenue, Cleveland, OH 44195, USA
e-mail: teerapatmdcu@gmail.com

M. Desai et al. (eds.), *An Atlas of Mitral Valve Imaging*, DOI 10.1007/978-1-4471-6672-6_10, © Springer-Verlag London 2015

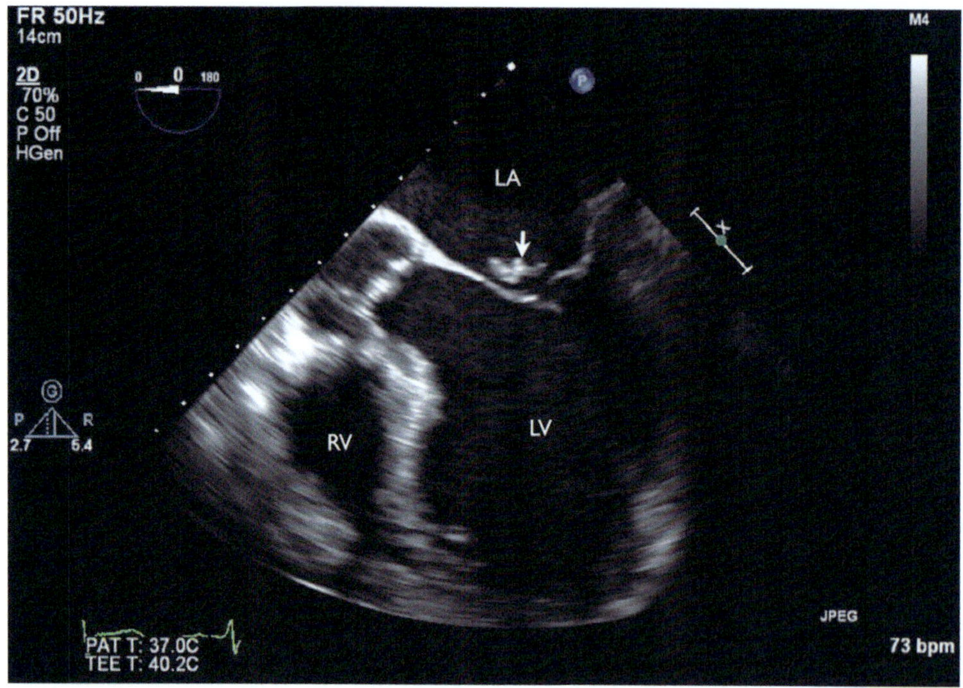

Fig. 10.1 Transesophageal echocardiography (TEE) four-chamber view showing ruptured chordae tendineae of the posterior leaflet. The ruptured chordae (*arrow*) are seen as a freely moving structure from the left ventricle to the left atrium during the cardiac cycle. *LA* left atrium, *LV* left ventricle, *RV* right ventricle

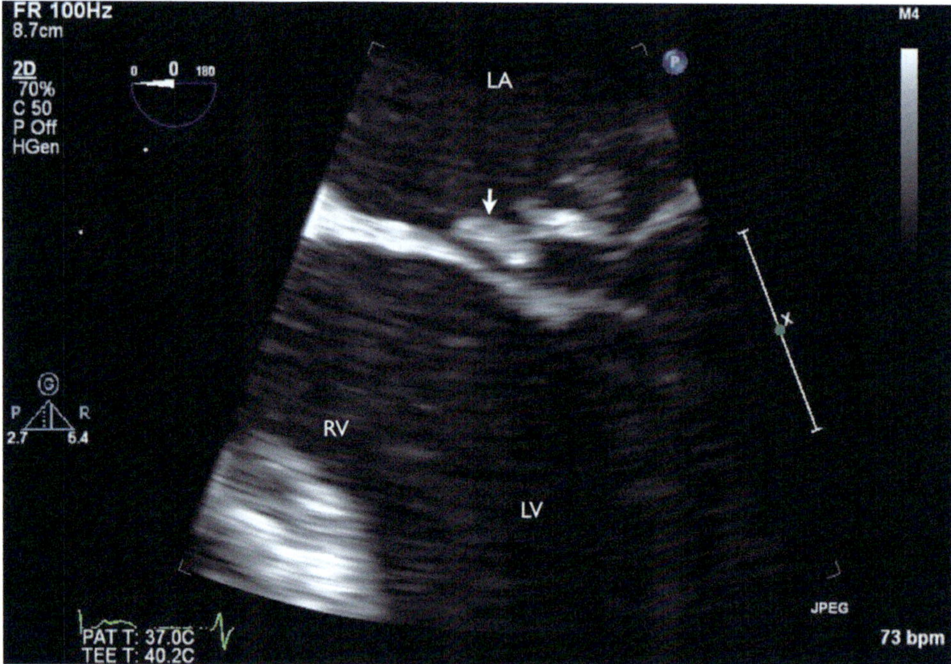

Fig. 10.2 A TEE zoom view of the mitral valve demonstrating flail of the posterior mitral leaflet with ruptured chordae (*arrow*). *LA* left atrium, *LV* left ventricle, *RV* right ventricle

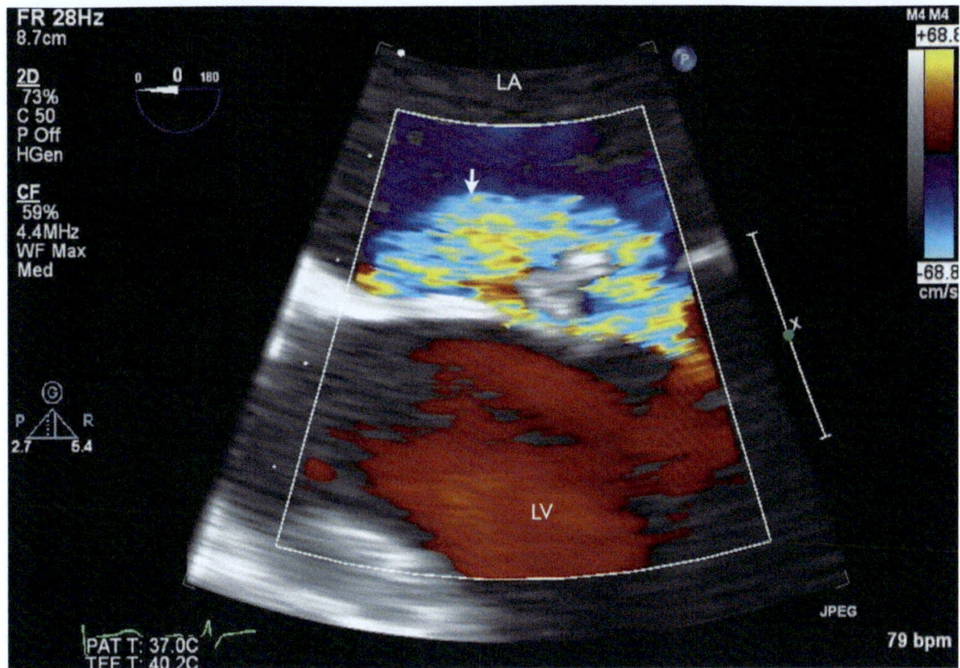

Fig. 10.3 TEE zoom view of the mitral valve with color flow Doppler imaging demonstrating anteriorly directed mitral regurgitation jet (*arrow*). *LA* left atrium, *LV* left ventricle

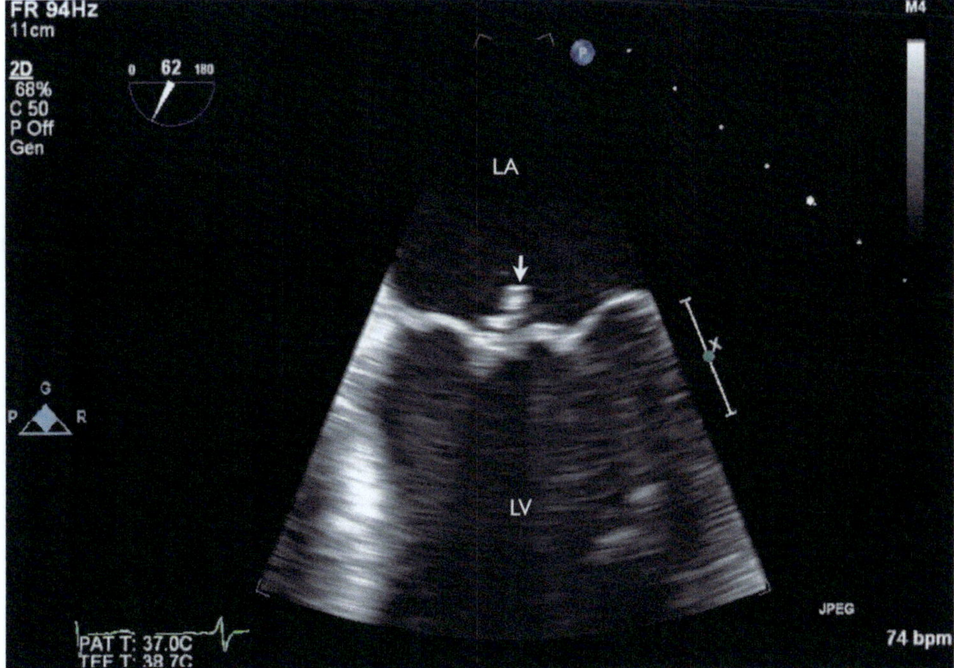

Fig. 10.4 TEE at 60° showed ruptured chordae with papillary muscle head moving freely into the left atrium (*arrow*). *LA* left atrium, *LV* left ventricle

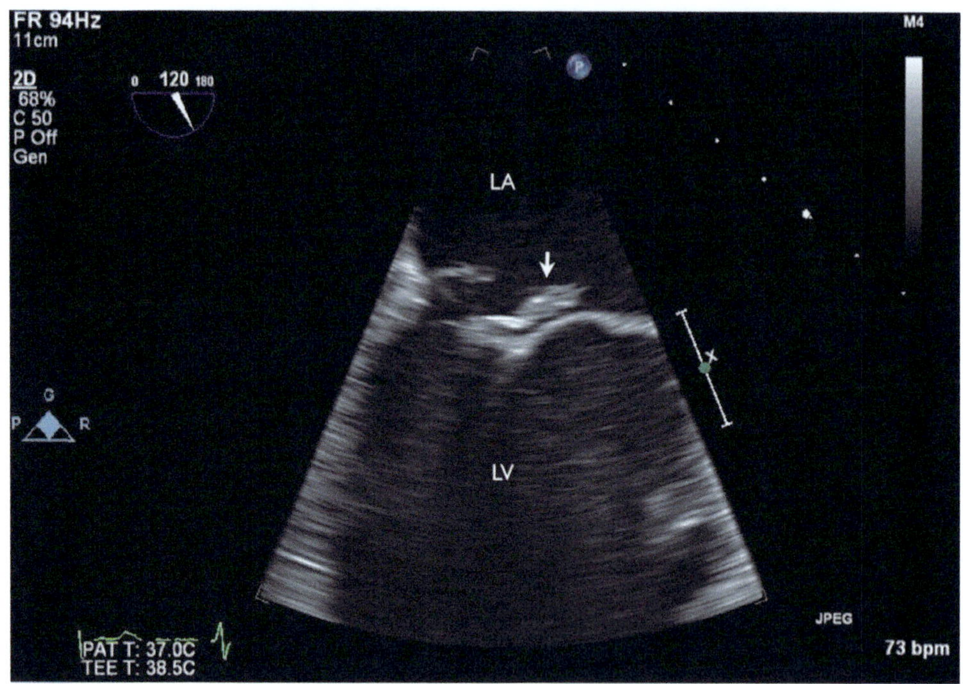

Fig. 10.5 TEE at 120° showed ruptured chordae with papillary muscle head moving freely into the left atrium (*arrow*). *LA* left atrium, *LV* left ventricle

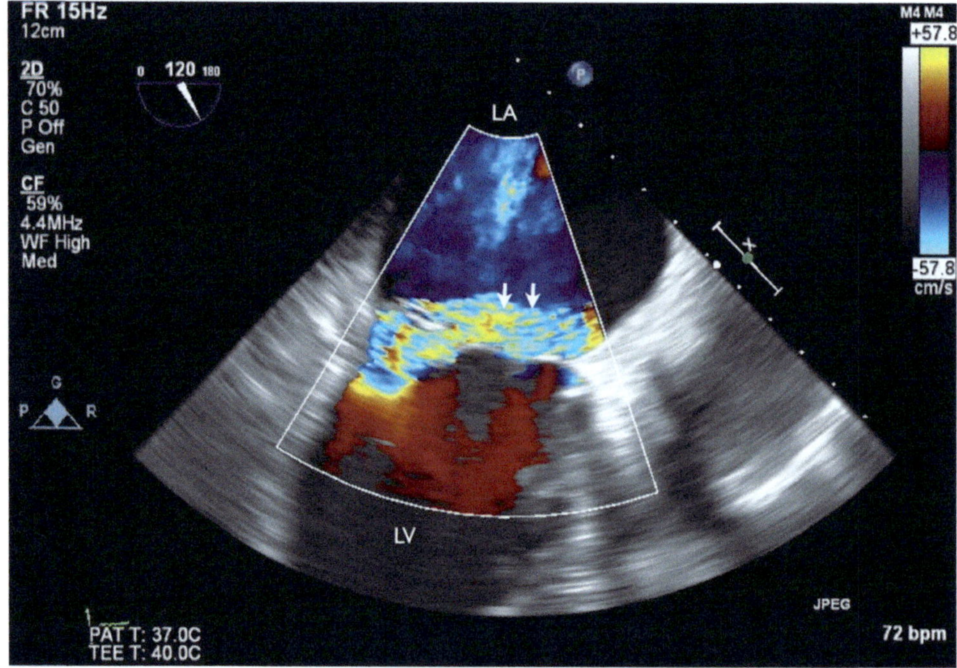

Fig. 10.6 TEE at 120° with color flow Doppler imaging demonstrated anteriorly directed mitral regurgitation jet (*arrows*). *LA* left atrium, *LV* left ventricle

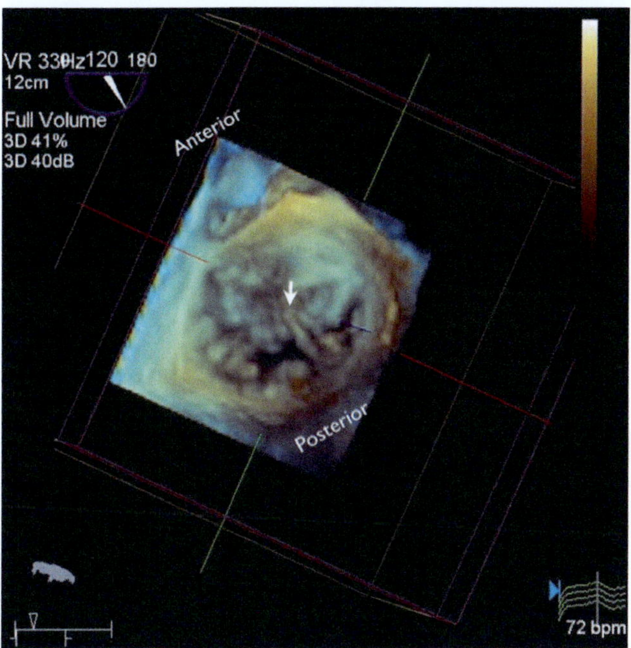

Fig. 10.7 Three-dimensional (3D) reconstruction imaging of the mitral valve (surgical view) showed a flail P3 segment of the mitral valve with ruptured papillary muscle (*arrow*)

10.1.1 Learning Points

Papillary muscle rupture (PMR) is a catastrophic mechanical complication of acute myocardial infarction (AMI). Patients with PMR typically present 2–7 days after AMI with acute pulmonary edema and are often in cardiogenic shock. The absence of new heart murmur after AMI does not exclude the diagnosis. PMR is far more common in patients with inferior wall infarction because the posteromedial papillary muscle has a single blood supply via the posterior descending coronary artery, whereas the anterolateral papillary muscle has a dual blood supply from both the left anterior descending and the left circumflex coronary arteries. The ruptured head or heads are seen to be attached to the leaflets by the mitral chordae. These can mimic vegetations, but the clinical presentation, the chordal attachment to the leaflets, and the usual attachment to both leaflets help to distinguish them from vegetations.

10.2 Case 2. Chronic Ischemic Mitral Regurgitation

A 75-year-old man with a remote history of AMI presented with shortness of breath. His primary care physician heard systolic murmur, so echocardiography was performed. Transthoracic echocardiography (TTE) revealed mitral regurgitation with impaired left ventricular systolic function. The patient was referred for further management (Figs. 10.8, 10.9, 10.10, and 10.11).

Video 10.8 Transthoracic echocardiography (TTE) apical long-axis view showed anteroseptal wall hypokinesia. The zona coapta of the mitral valve was apically displaced (AVI 6579 kb)

Video 10.9 TTE apical long-axis view with color Doppler flow imaging showed a posteriorly directed mitral regurgitation jet (AVI 4392 kb)

Video 10.10 TTE apical four-chamber view showed anterolateral and apical hypokinesia. The posterior mitral leaflet has restricted motion throughout the cardiac cycle (AVI 6328 kb)

Video 10.11 TTE apical four-chamber view with color Doppler flow imaging showed posteriorly directed mitral regurgitation (AVI 4777 kb)

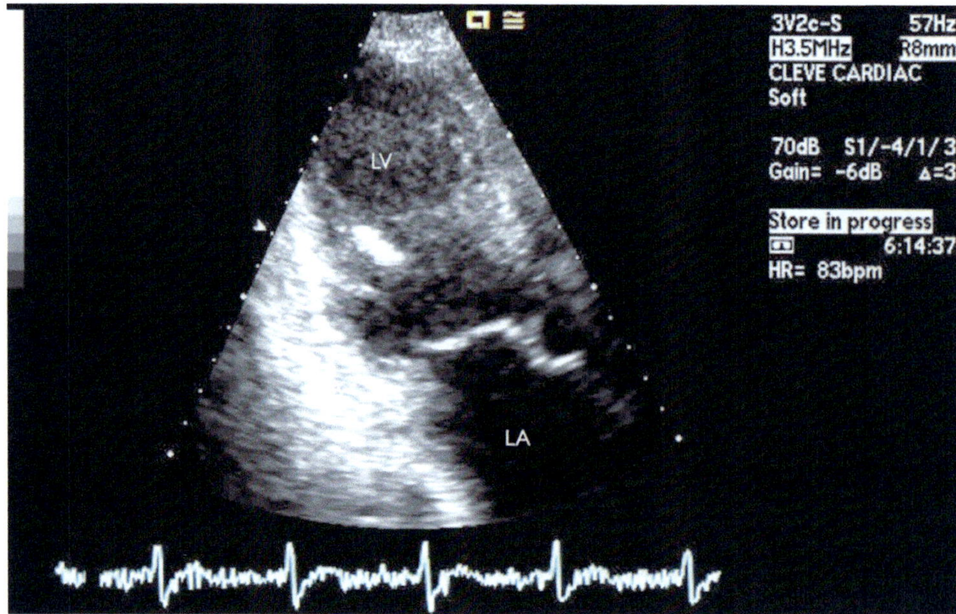

Fig. 10.8 Transthoracic echocardiography (TTE) apical long-axis view showed anteroseptal wall hypokinesia. The zona coapta of the mitral valve was apically displaced. *LA* left atrium, *LV* left ventricle

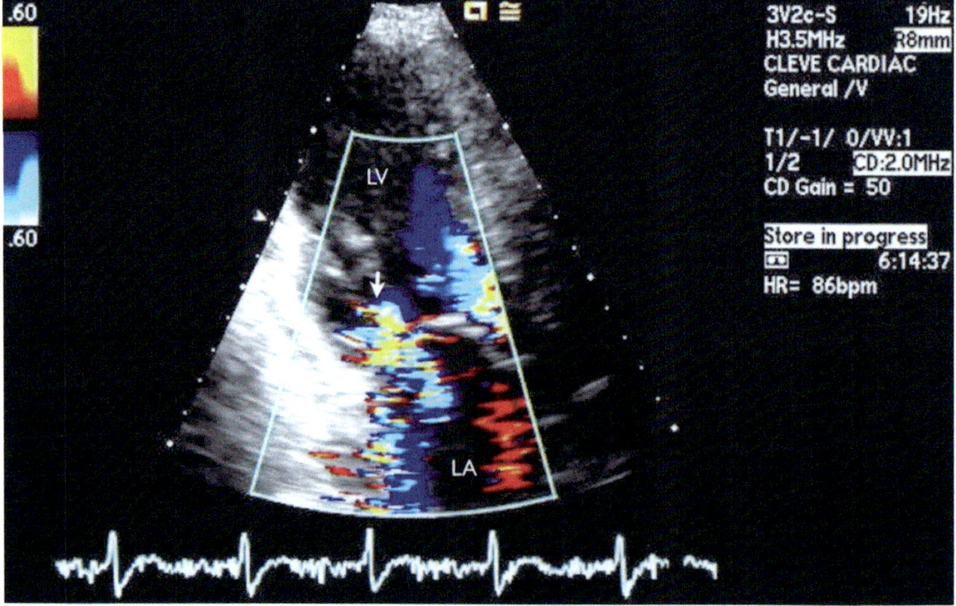

Fig. 10.9 TTE apical long-axis view with color Doppler flow imaging showed posteriorly directed mitral regurgitation jet (*arrow*). *LA* left atrium, *LV* left ventricle

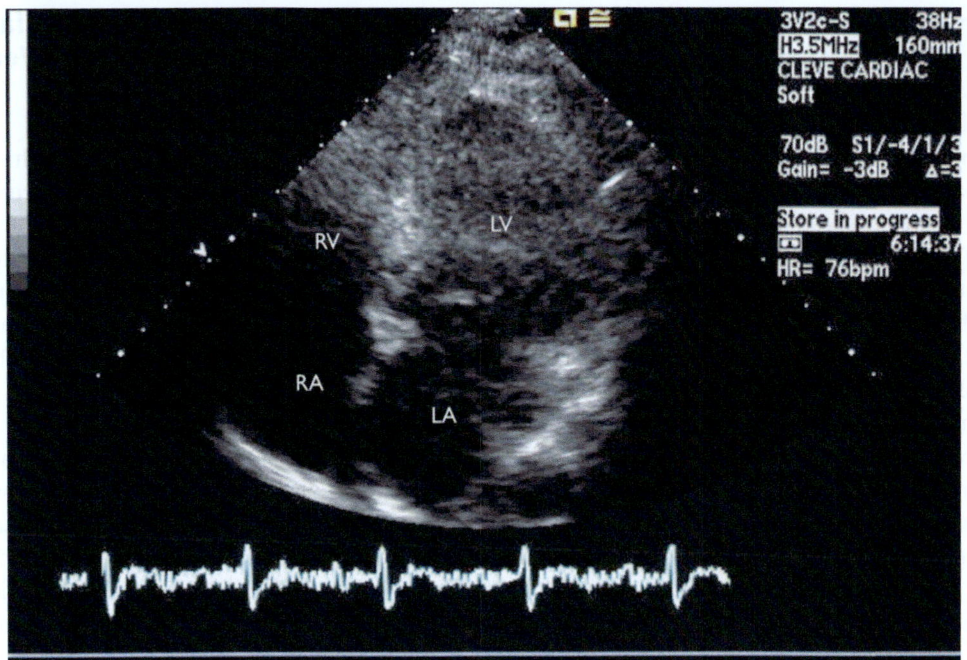

Fig. 10.10 TTE apical four-chamber view showed anterolateral and apical hypokinesia. The posterior mitral leaflet has restricted motion throughout the cardiac cycle. *RA* right atrium, *RV* right ventricle, *LA* left atrium, *LV* left ventricle

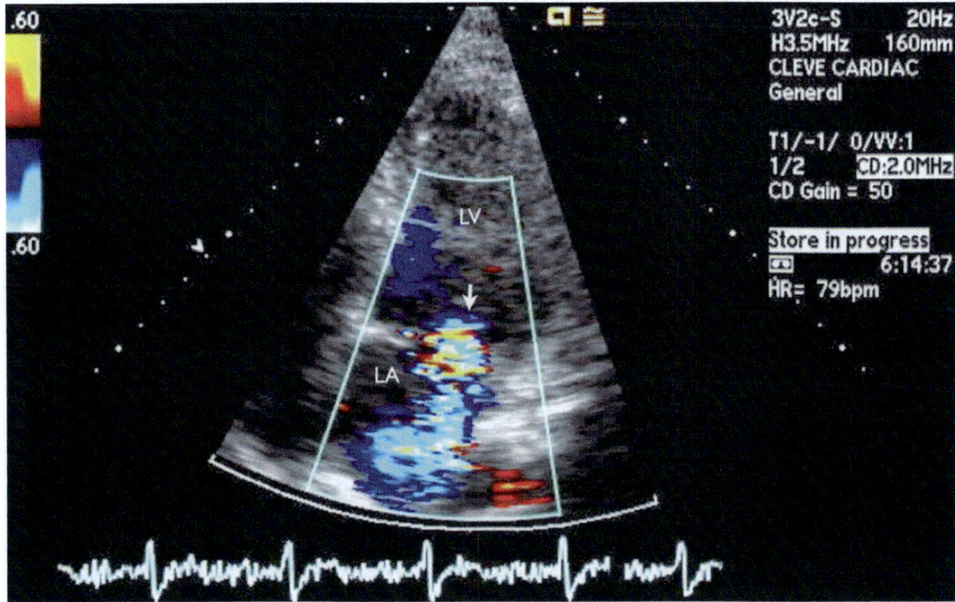

Fig. 10.11 TTE apical four-chamber view with color Doppler flow imaging showed posteriorly directed mitral regurgitation (*arrow*). *LA* left atrium, *LV* left ventricle

10.2.1 Learning Points

Mitral regurgitation (MR) after AMI is a multifactorial process involving both local and global left ventricular remodeling. The presence of significant MR in this setting portends a bad prognosis and increased risk of death and heart failure independently of previously known indicators of risk after myocardial infarction. MR is often clinically silent, so it should be systematically evaluated by echocardiography. Wall motion abnormalities are a common cause of chronic secondary MR, and their presence worsens the condition. Coronary revascularization and cardiac resynchronization therapy may improve the symptoms and outcome in appropriately selected patients. The new 2014 ACC/AHA guidelines for management of valvular heart diseases [1] considered that an effective regurgitant orifice (ERO) of 0.20 cm^2 or larger and regurgitant volume of 30 mL or more are markers of severe MR. These changes are based on the fact that the measurement of the proximal isovelocity surface area by two-dimensional TTE in patients with secondary MR underestimates the true ERO because of the crescentic shape of the proximal convergence. Furthermore, a smaller calculated ERO is associated with adverse outcomes in patients with secondary MR than in patients with primary MR. The MR will also likely progress because of the associated progressive left ventricular systolic dysfunction and adverse remodeling [1]. Current medical options rely chiefly on standard anti–heart failure medications; surgical approaches or mitral valve intervention offer future promise.

10.3 Case 3. Post-myocardial Infarction Mitral Regurgitation and Ventricular Septal Rupture

A 75-year-old man with a past medical history of AMI 2 months ago presented to our institute with cardiogenic shock. Physical examination revealed blood pressure of 80/60 mmHg, jugular venous distension up to the mandible, and systolic thrill palpable at the left lower parasternal border. A 3/6 pansystolic murmur was heard at the left lower parasternal border and radiated to the axilla (Figs. 10.12, 10.13, 10.14, and 10.15).

Video 10.12 TTE apical four-chamber view, zoomed at LV and RV, showed severely impaired left ventricular systolic function with regional wall motion abnormalities in the left anterior descending coronary artery territory. An echo dropout is seen at the distal septum (AVI 562 kb)

Video 10.13 TTE apical four-chamber view with color Doppler flow imaging, zoomed at LV and RV, showed left-to-right shunt during systole at the distal septum and significant mitral regurgitation (AVI 522 kb)

Video 10.14 TTE apical four-chamber view showed apical displacement of the mitral valve zona coapta (AVI 951 kb)

Video 10.15 TTE apical four-chamber view with color Doppler flow imaging showed significant mitral regurgitation (AVI 460 kb)

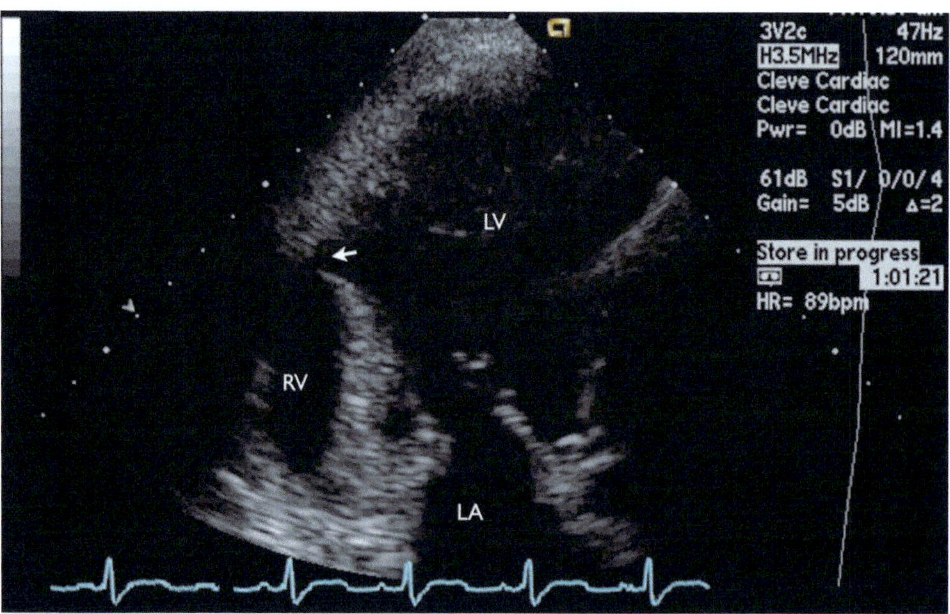

Fig. 10.12 TTE apical four-chamber view, zoomed at LV and RV, showed severely impaired left ventricular systolic function with regional wall motion abnormalities in the left anterior descending coronary artery territory. An echo dropout is seen at the distal septum (*arrow*). *LA* left atrium, *LV* left ventricle, *RV* right ventricle

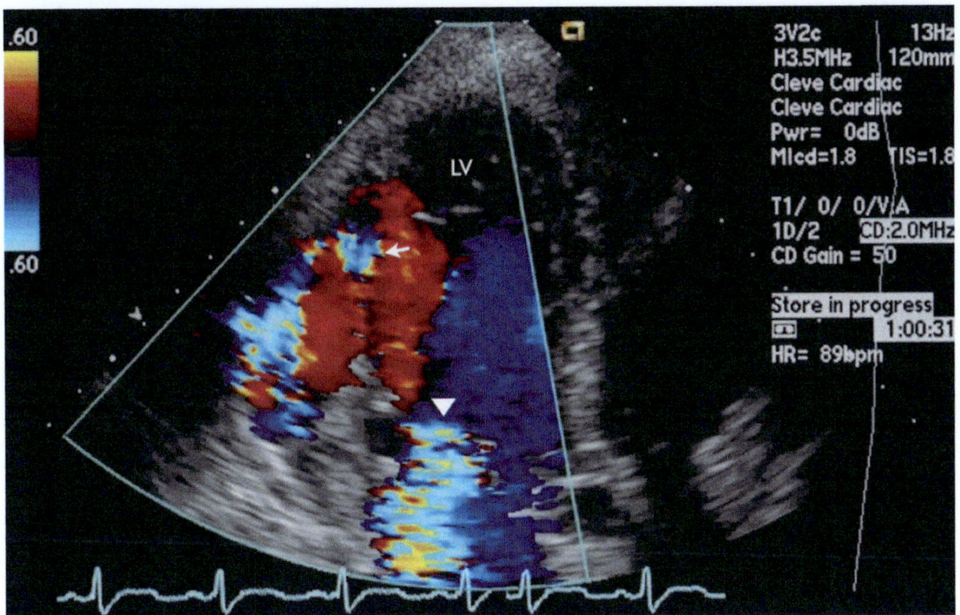

Fig. 10.13 TTE apical four-chamber view with color Doppler flow imaging, zoomed at LV and RV, showed left-to-right shunt during systole at the distal septum (*arrow*) and significant mitral regurgitation (*arrowhead*). *LV* left ventricle

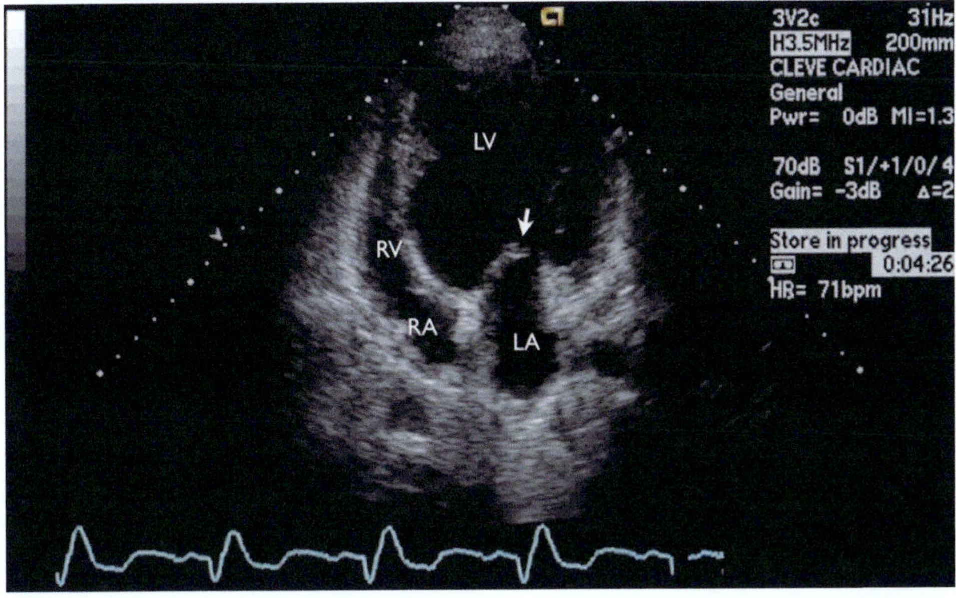

Fig. 10.14 TTE apical four-chamber view showed apical displacement of the mitral valve zona coapta (*arrow*). *LA* left atrium, *LV* left ventricle, *RA* right atrium, *RV* right ventricle

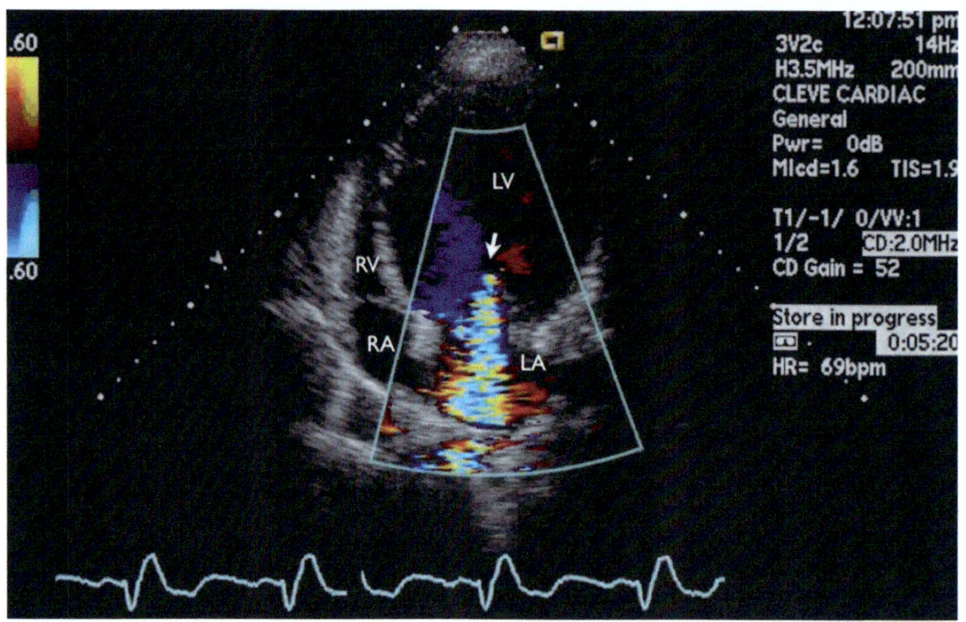

Fig. 10.15 TTE apical four-chamber view with color Doppler flow imaging showed significant mitral regurgitation (*arrow*). *LA* left atrium, *LV* left ventricle, *RA* right atrium, *RV* right ventricle

10.3.1 Learning Points

The differential diagnoses of a systolic murmur following AMI include papillary muscle dysfunction or rupture, ventricular septal rupture (VSR), and left ventricular dilatation with resultant MR. The combination of post-MI VSR and MR is rare and devastating. The mechanical lesions of VSR and MR are amenable to surgical intervention if a sufficient amount of residual functional muscle can be preserved in the left ventricle. Intraaortic balloon counterpulsation allows a period of time to stabilize the condition of patients with these lesions, to reduce myocardial ischemia, and to carry out studies to determine the extent of coronary artery disease [2].

References

1. Nishimura RA, Otto CM, Bonow RO, Carabello BA, Erwin 3rd JP, Guyton RA, et al. 2014 AHA/ACC guideline for the management of patients with valvular heart disease: a report of the American College of Cardiology/American Heart Association Task Force on Practice Guidelines. J Am Coll Cardiol. 2014;63:e57–185.
2. Buckley MJ, Mundth ED, Daggett WM, Gold HK, Leinbach RC, Austen WG. Surgical management of ventricular septal defects and mitral regurgitation complicating acute myocardial infarction. Ann Thorac Surg. 1973;16:598–609.

Mitral Valve Prostheses

11

Christine Jellis

Mitral valve surgery is one of the most technically demanding aspects of cardiac surgery, owing both to the valve's location and to its complicated structure. Overall cardiac surgical performance is gauged by the rate of successful mitral valve repair. Typically, the best short-term and long-term outcomes are achieved by surgeons who have a subspecialized interest in mitral valve surgery and perform large numbers of repairs in high-volume centers. A repair is usually preferred over a replacement, owing to both longevity and the avoidance of anticoagulation, but repair is not always technically feasible if the valve is stenotic, calcified, significantly thickened, or morphologically unsuitable. A good replacement is always better than a poor repair, which may lead to premature redo surgery. Mitral valve repairs typically involve plication of the posterior leaflet and insertion of an annuloplasty ring. An Alfieri stitch is sometimes included to optimize leaflet coaptation. Mitral valve replacements can be both bioprosthetic and mechanical. Individualized factors including the patient's age, suitability for anticoagulation, and plans for future pregnancies are all important to consider when deciding on the best approach. Robotic mitral valve surgery with femoral cannulation via a mini-thoracotomy is now providing an alternative to traditional approaches via a median sternotomy. Percutaneous valve replacement or repair using various clip devices is now a viable alternative for some patients [*see* Chap. 6]. Valvuloplasty may be adjunctively performed as a temporizing bridge to surgery or a more palliative procedure in the setting of significant mitral stenosis, although factors such as valve and subvalvular thickening and calcification will ultimately govern suitability for this procedure.

Like all surgery, mitral valve surgery can be associated with complications. Echocardiography plays an important role in the perioperative and long-term monitoring of valve function. Transesophageal echocardiography is often useful to overcome issues with poor leaflet visualization and valve shadowing on transthoracic echo. 3D/4D imaging of the mitral valve has revolutionized prosthetic valve assessment by providing better temporal and spatial resolution than traditional 2D imaging (Fig. 11.1). Small paravalvular leaks can be readily identified and localized, thereby allowing better preoperative surgical planning or consideration of percutaneous options. In additional to prosthetic valve degeneration with associated regurgitation or stenosis, other complications include paravalvular leaks due to valve dehiscence and valvular dysfunction due to pannus, inflammatory response, thrombus, or endocarditis.

Video 11.1 A 3D image of a normally functioning, trileaflet, Biocor bioprosthetic mitral valve replacement viewed from the left atrium. High image resolution enables the leaflets, annulus, and even sutures to be clearly demonstrated. The 3D image is conventionally orientated with the aortic valve at the 12 o'clock position, thereby allowing consistency of image description and better ease of interpretation (AVI 1528 kb)

Electronic supplementary material The online version of this chapter (doi:10.1007/978-1-4471-6672-6_11) contains supplementary material, which is available to authorized users.

C. Jellis
Department of Cardiovascular Medicine, Cleveland Clinic, 9500 Euclid Avenue, Cleveland, OH 44195, USA
e-mail: jellisc@ccf.org

M. Desai et al. (eds.), *An Atlas of Mitral Valve Imaging*, DOI 10.1007/978-1-4471-6672-6_11, © Springer-Verlag London 2015

Fig. 11.1 A 3D image of a normally functioning, trileaflet, Biocor bioprosthetic mitral valve replacement viewed from the left atrium. High image resolution enables the leaflets, annulus, and even sutures to be clearly demonstrated. The 3D image is conventionally orientated with the aortic valve at the 12 o'clock position, thereby allowing consistency of image description and better ease of interpretation

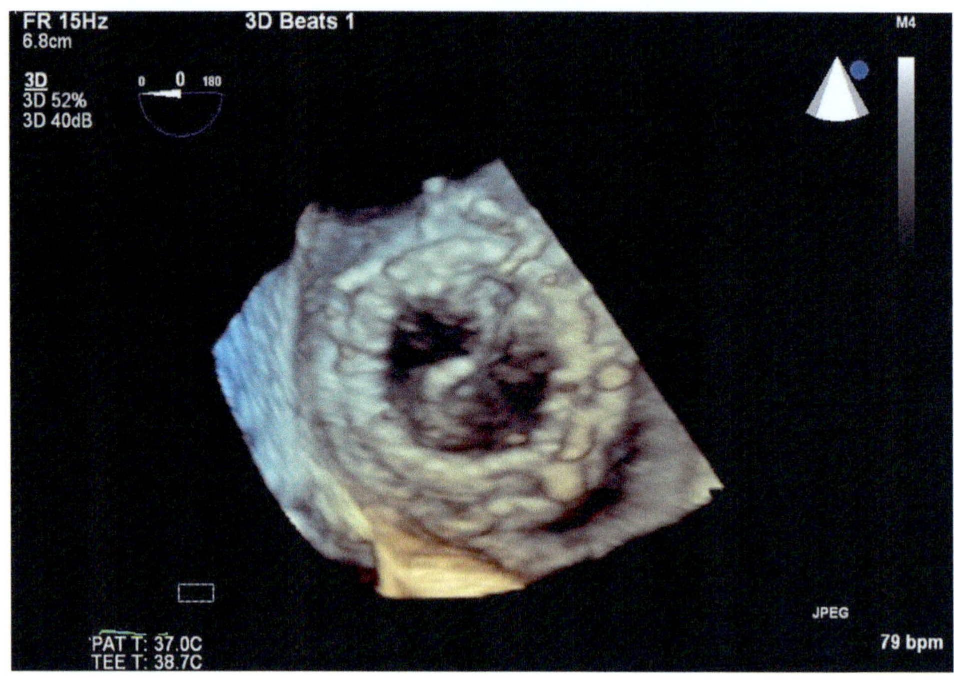

11.1   Case 1. Alfieri Stitch

A 70-year-old woman presented with long-standing mitral regurgitation, aortic regurgitation, and paroxysmal atrial fibrillation. She demonstrated increasing left atrial and left ventricular enlargement, which prompted surgical referral. Despite prominent mitral annular calcification, the surgeon was able to successfully repair her mitral valve, using plication of the middle scallop of the posterior leaflet, an Alfieri stitch, and placement of a 35-mm annuloplasty ring. She also underwent replacement of the aortic valve with a #23 Carpentier-Edwards bovine pericardial heterograft, isolation of the pulmonary veins, and ligation of the left atrial appendage (Figs. 11.2, 11.3, 11.4, and 11.5).

Video 11.2 A parasternal long-axis view demonstrates the repaired mitral valve, with the aortic valve replacement in situ (AVI 2992 kb)

Video 11.3 Slight angulation of the probe demonstrates a parasternal long-axis view of the mitral valve at the position of the Alfieri stitch. This appearance may be mistaken for mitral stenosis. The annuloplasty ring in short axis can be best appreciated at the posterior aspect of the annulus (AVI 2244 kb)

Video 11.4 A parasternal short-axis view at the left ventricular base demonstrates the double-orifice mitral valve with the Alfieri stitch joining the middle aspects of both mitral valve leaflets and improving overall leaflet coaptation (AVI 3100 kb)

Video 11.5 The mitral valve is viewed from an apical four-chamber view. The Alfieri stitch can be seen joining the leaflet tips centrally. The annuloplasty ring is appreciated laterally. The posterior leaflet appears small and somewhat restricted, consistent with the known repair and plication of the middle posterior scallop (AVI 2712 kb)

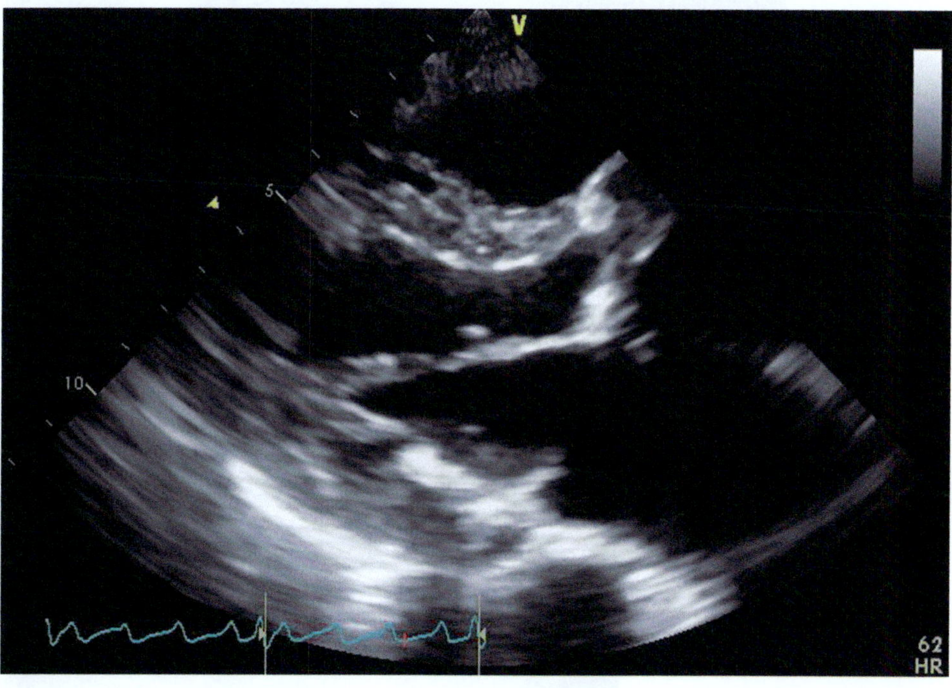

Fig. 11.2 A parasternal long-axis view demonstrates the repaired mitral valve, with the aortic valve replacement in situ

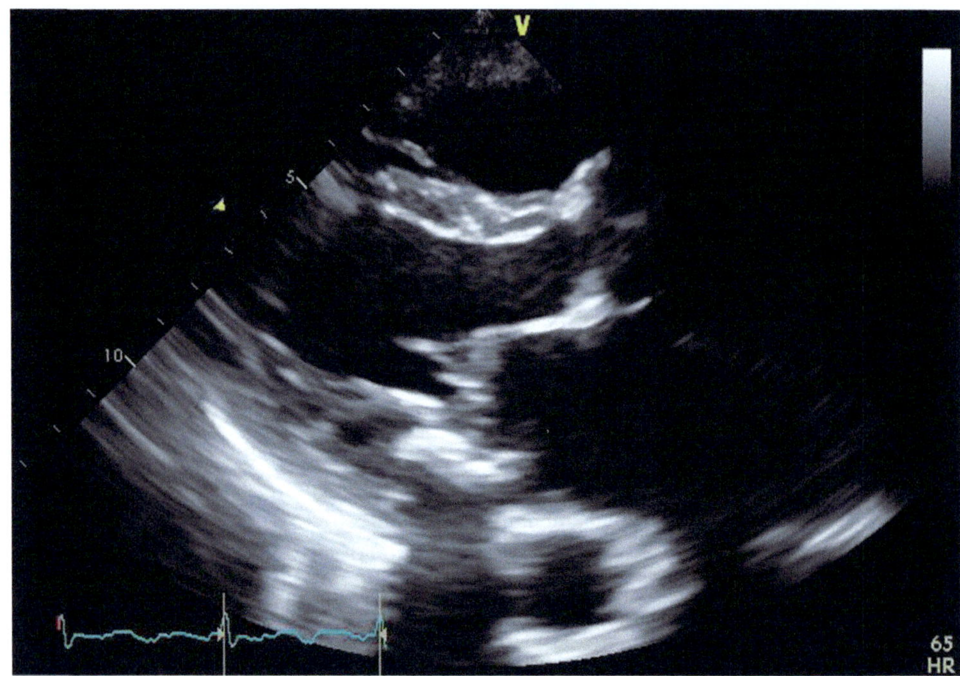

Fig. 11.3 Slight angulation of the probe demonstrates a parasternal long-axis view of the mitral valve at the position of the Alfieri stitch. This appearance may be mistaken for mitral stenosis. The annuloplasty ring in short axis can be best appreciated at the posterior aspect of the annulus

Fig. 11.4 A parasternal short-axis view at the left ventricular base demonstrates the double-orifice mitral valve with the Alfieri stitch joining the middle aspects of both mitral valve leaflets and improving overall leaflet coaptation

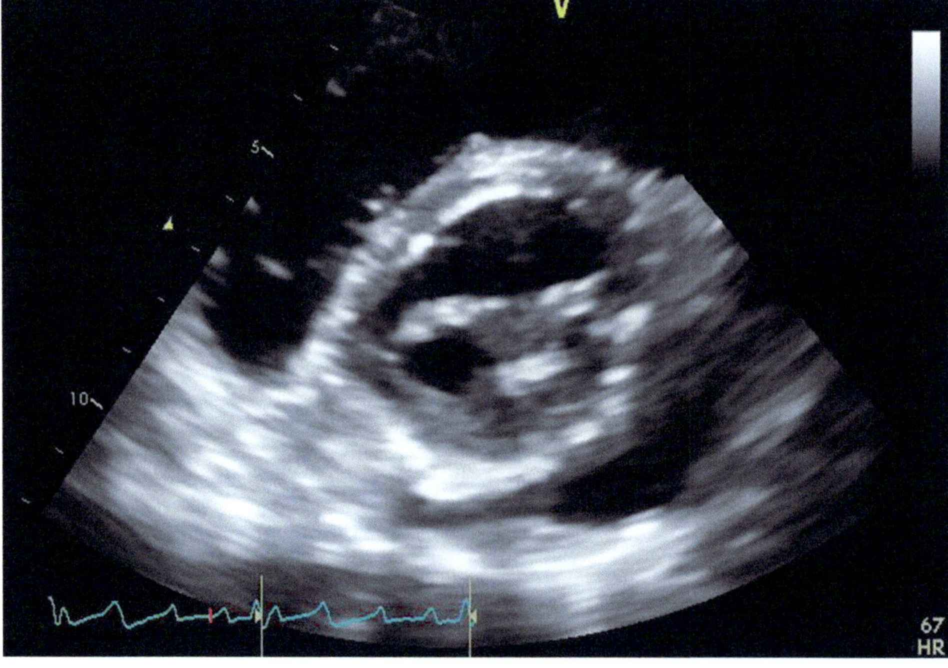

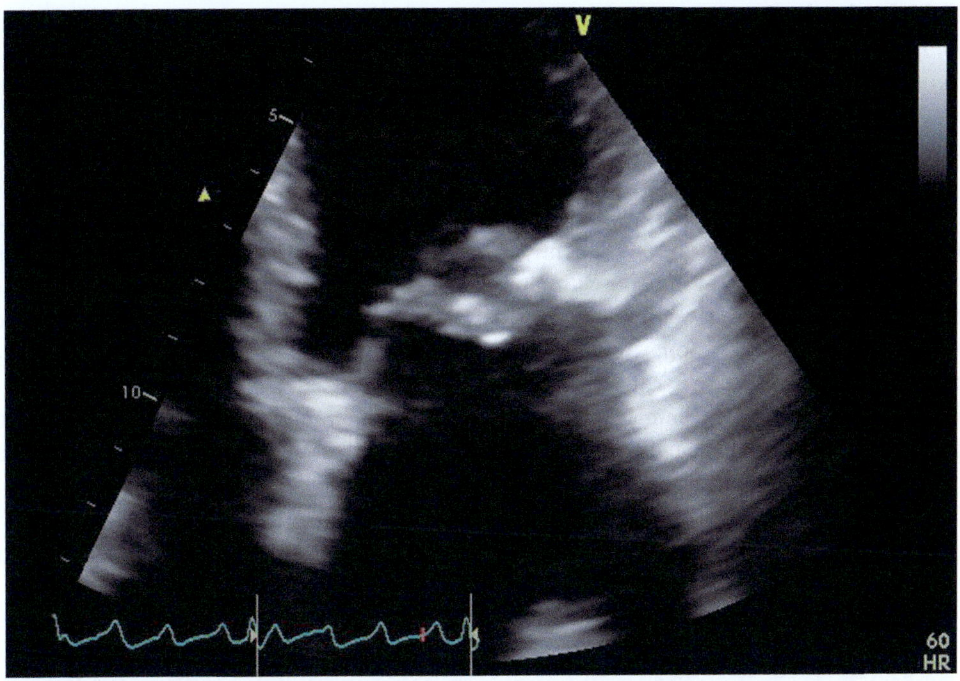

Fig. 11.5 The mitral valve is viewed from an apical four-chamber view. The Alfieri stitch can be seen joining the leaflet tips centrally. The annuloplasty ring is appreciated laterally. The posterior leaflet appears small and somewhat restricted, consistent with the known repair and plication of the middle posterior scallop

11.2 Case 2. Valvuloplasty

A 43-year-old woman in previously excellent health presented with a cerebrovascular accident due to middle cerebral artery occlusion. She was emergently treated with fibrinolysis and achieved full recovery. She subsequently was found to have severe mitral stenosis, despite an absence of previous symptoms. The transvalvular peak gradient was 23 mmHg and the mean gradient was 14 mmHg, with moderate (2–3+) mitral regurgitation. She was anticoagulated and then referred for mitral balloon valvuloplasty, which was performed via a trans-septal puncture. After the procedure, the gradients were reduced to 16 and 9 mmHg, with only mild (1+) residual mitral regurgitation, and the estimated mitral valve area (by pressure half time) was 1.9 cm^2 (Figs. 11.6, 11.7, 11.8, 11.9, 11.10, 11.11, 11.12, and 11.13).

Video 11.6 Transesophageal echocardiogram (TEE) at 0°, demonstrating severe thickening and tethering of both mitral valve leaflets (predominantly involving the leaflet tips). This appearance is typical for rheumatic heart disease (AVI 4855 kb)

Video 11.7 TEE at 0° demonstrating moderate (2–3+) regurgitation at baseline. A septostomy has been performed in preparation for the valvuloplasty, and the catheter can be seen traversing the interatrial septum (AVI 1992 kb)

Video 11.8 A 3D image of the mitral valve viewed from the left atrium. The leaflets are thickened, with commissural fusion and a resultant reduced valve area (AVI 1077 kb)

Video 11.9 Balloon inflation within the mitral valve at the time of valvuloplasty (AVI 6410 kb)

Video 11.10 After valvuloplasty, biplane color Doppler imaging through the mitral valve demonstrates no significant increase in severity of mitral regurgitation from baseline (AVI 1806 kb)

Video 11.11 A 3D image of the mitral valve (viewed from the left atrium) after valvuloplasty shows that leaflet mobility has improved, with a reduction in commissural fusion and an increased valve area (AVI 1272 kb)

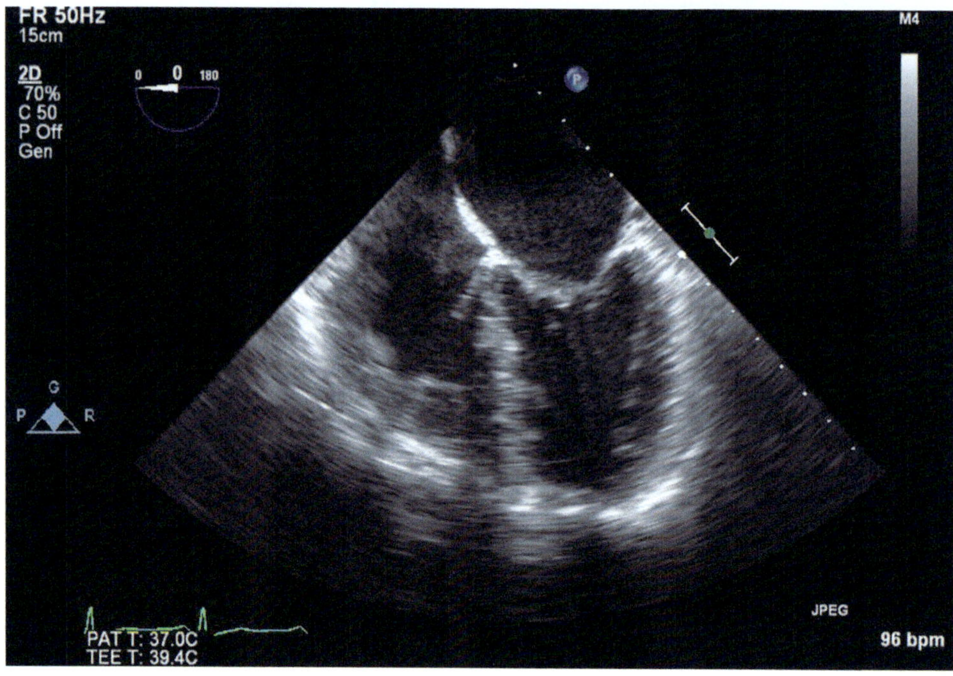

Fig. 11.6 Transesophageal echocardiogram (TEE) at 0°, demonstrating severe thickening and tethering of both mitral valve leaflets (predominantly involving the leaflet tips). This appearance is typical for rheumatic heart disease

Fig. 11.7 TEE at 0° demonstrating moderate (2–3+) regurgitation at baseline. A septostomy has been performed in preparation for the valvuloplasty, and the catheter can be seen traversing the interatrial septum

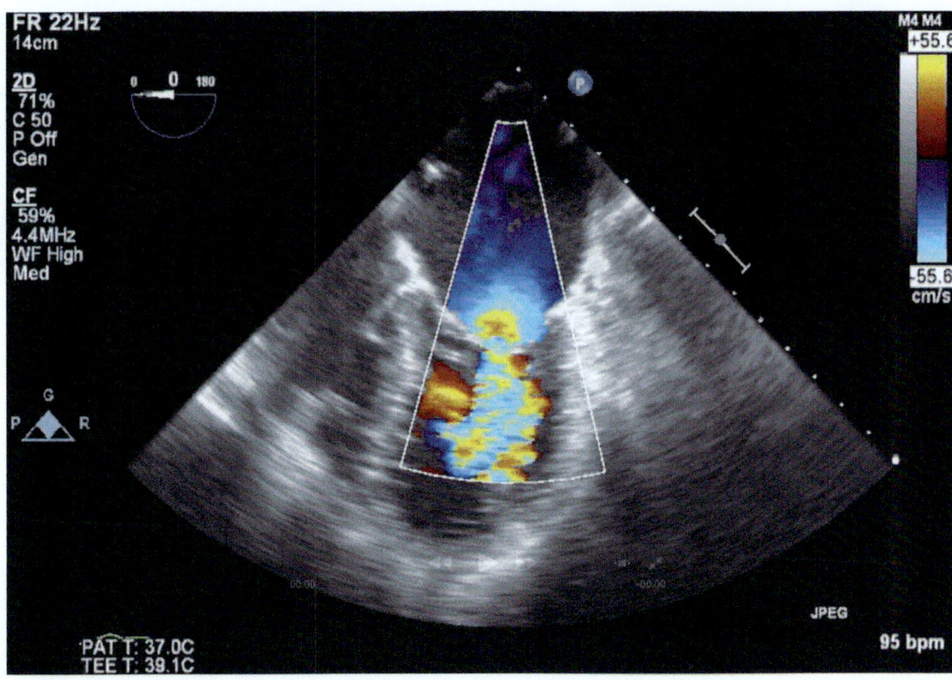

Fig. 11.8 3D image of the mitral valve viewed from the left atrium. The leaflets are thickened, with commissural fusion and a resultant reduced valve area

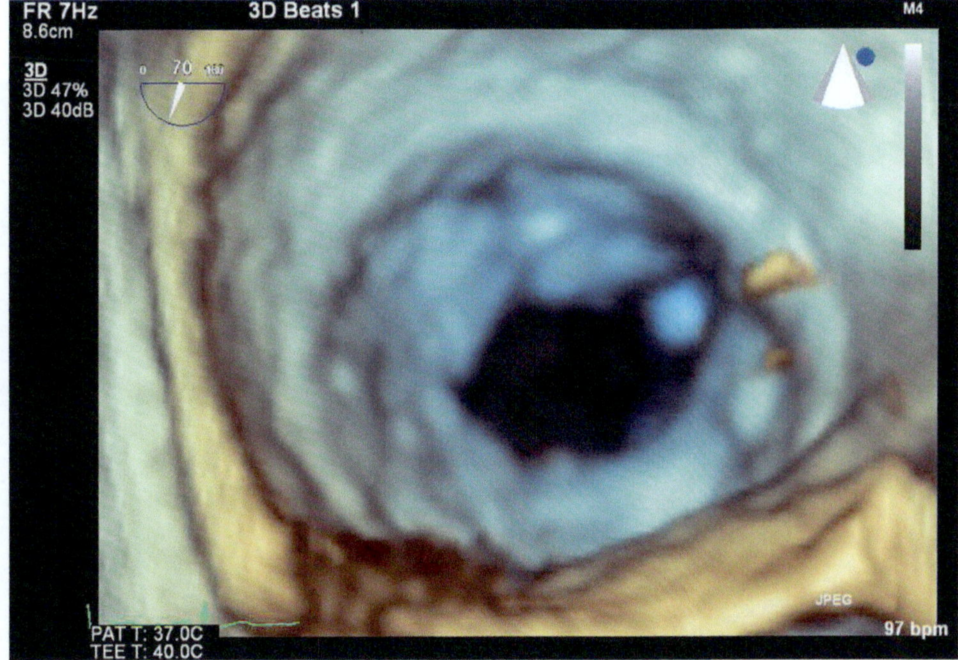

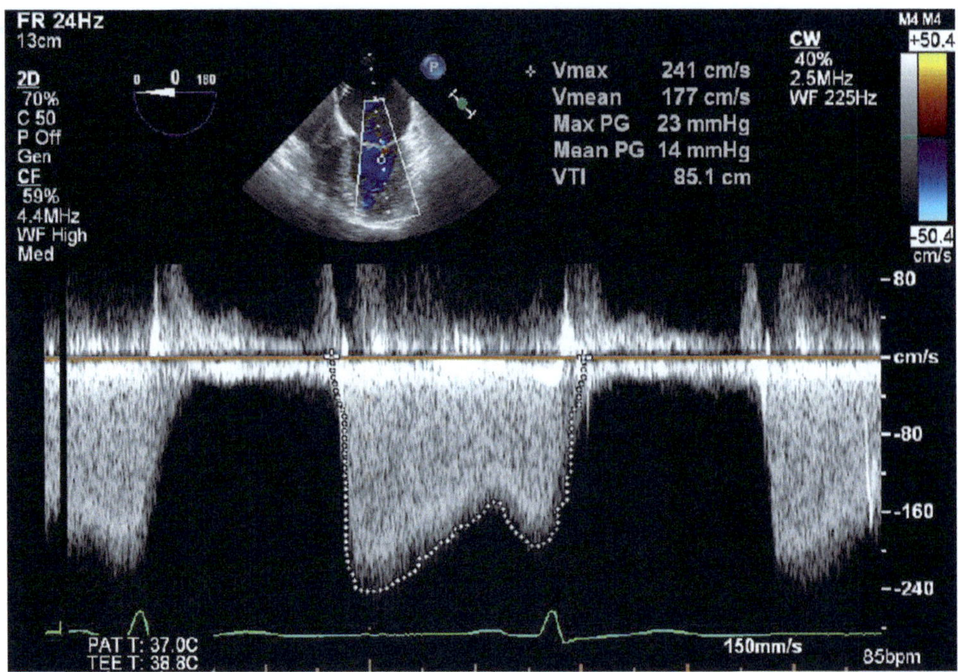

Fig. 11.9 Continuous wave Doppler through the mitral valve demonstrates severe stenosis with a peak gradient of 23 mmHg and a mean gradient of 14 mmHg

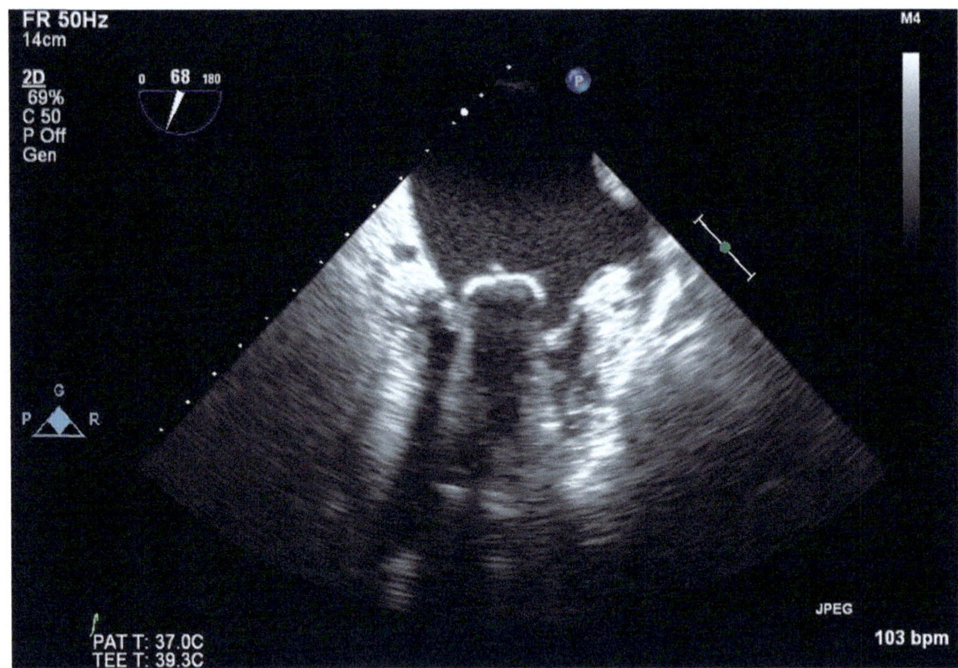

Fig. 11.10 Balloon inflation within the mitral valve at the time of valvuloplasty

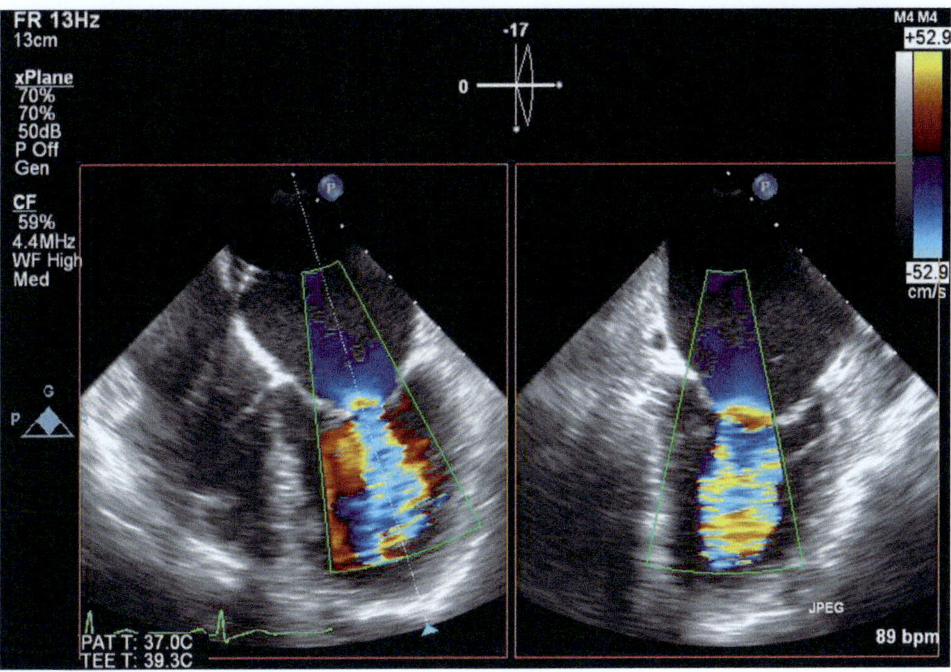

Fig. 11.11   After valvuloplasty, biplane color Doppler imaging through the mitral valve demonstrates no significant increase in severity of mitral regurgitation from baseline

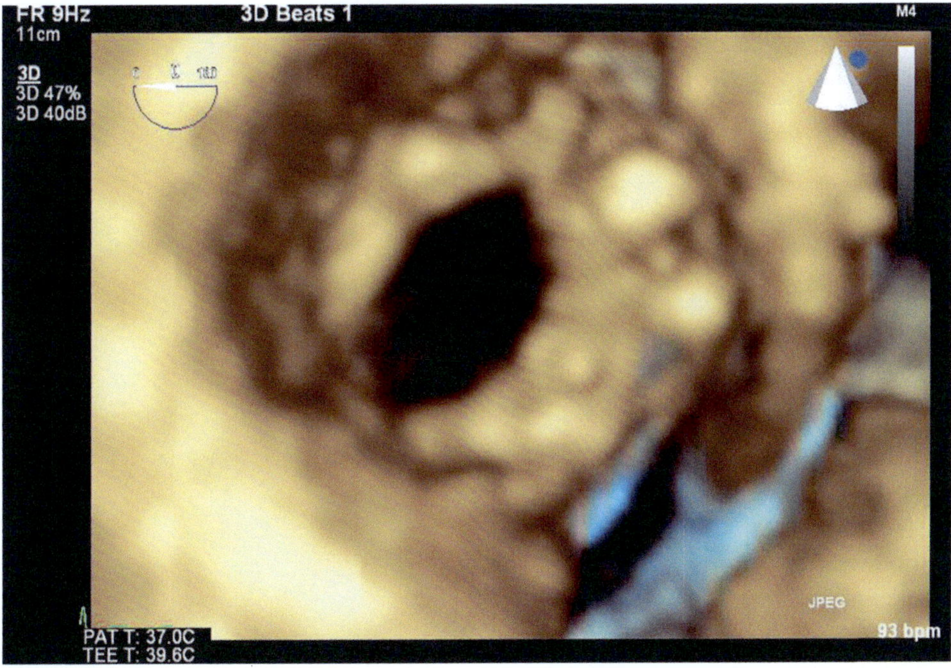

Fig. 11.12   A 3D image of the mitral valve (viewed from the left atrium) after valvuloplasty shows that leaflet mobility has improved, with a reduction in commissural fusion and an increased valve area

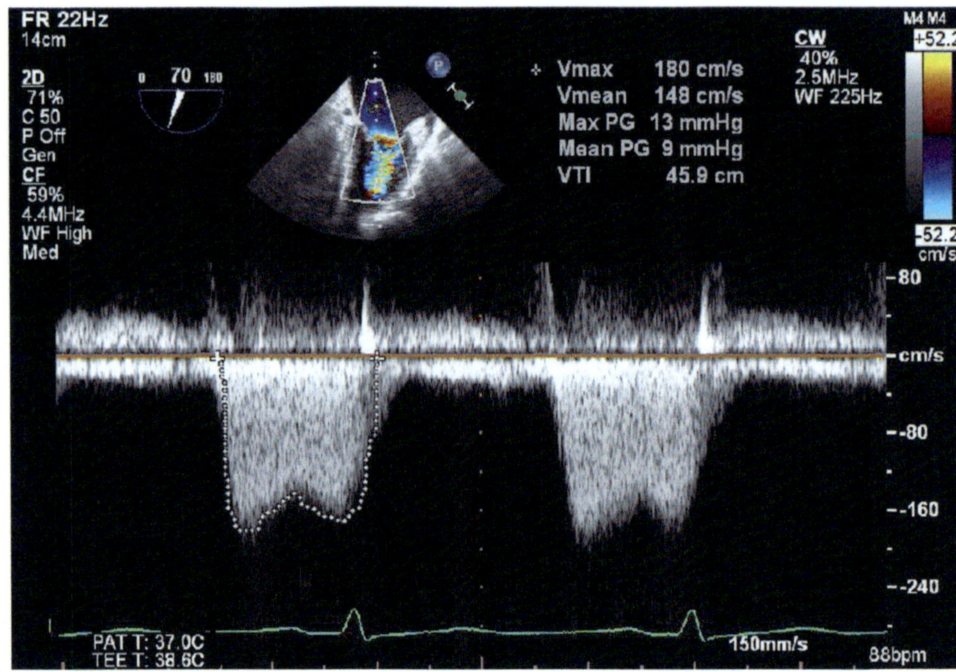

Fig. 11.13 Continuous wave Doppler through the mitral valve after valvuloplasty demonstrates an improvement in transmitral gradients to a peak of 13 mmHg and a mean of 9 mmHg

11.3   Case 3. Paravalvular Leak 1

A 62-year-old woman with end-stage renal failure on hemodialysis presented with a severe paravalvular mitral valve leak, severe tricuspid regurgitation, and moderate aortic stenosis on a background history of previous bioprosthetic mitral valve replacement and coronary artery bypass graft surgery 3 years earlier. She underwent a mitral valve replacement with an On-X mechanical valve (#33), a tricuspid valve repair with a Carpentier ring (#30), an aortic valve replacement with a Trifecta bioprosthesis (#23), and coronary artery bypass graft surgery.

Preoperative echocardiography demonstrated a paravalvular leak originating at the anterolateral aspect of the mitral annulus. The eccentric, regurgitant jet hugged the wall of the left atrium and was difficult to quantitate, but visually it appeared severe. Transvalvular peak and mean gradients of 17 and 9 mmHg were noted (Figs. 11.14, 11.15, and 11.16).

Video 11.12 TEE at 50° demonstrates an eccentric paravalvular leak originating at the anterolateral aspect of the mitral annulus (AVI 1485 kb)

Video 11.13 With 3D reconstruction of the mitral valve, orientated with the aortic valve at the top of the image, the small paravalvular defect can be seen adjacent to the valve annulus at the 6 o'clock position (AVI 845 kb)

Video 11.14 Color 3D imaging clearly demonstrates the small paravalvular leak (AVI 953 kb)

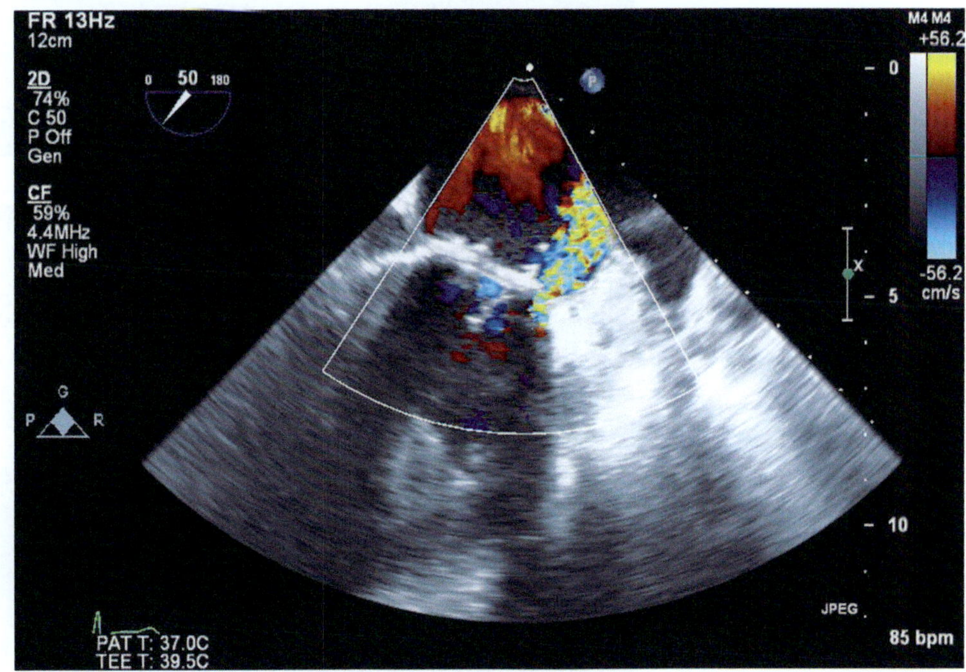

Fig. 11.14 TEE at 50° demonstrates an eccentric paravalvular leak originating at the anterolateral aspect of the mitral annulus

Fig. 11.15 With 3D reconstruction of the mitral valve, orientated with the aortic valve at the top of the image, the small paravalvular defect can be seen adjacent to the valve annulus at the 6 o'clock position

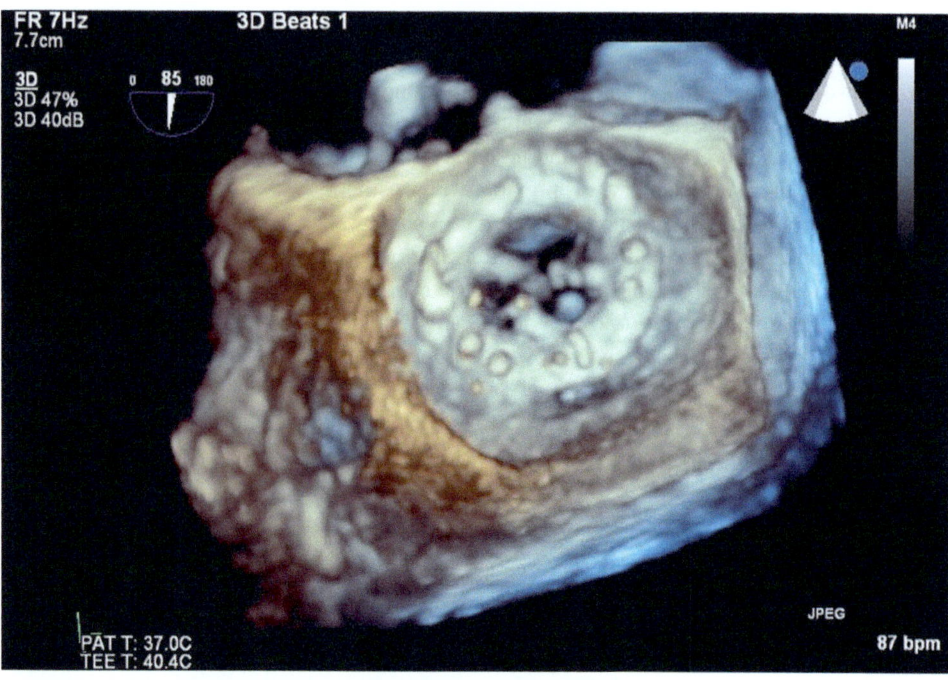

Fig. 11.16 3D color Doppler imaging clearly demonstrates the small paravalvular leak

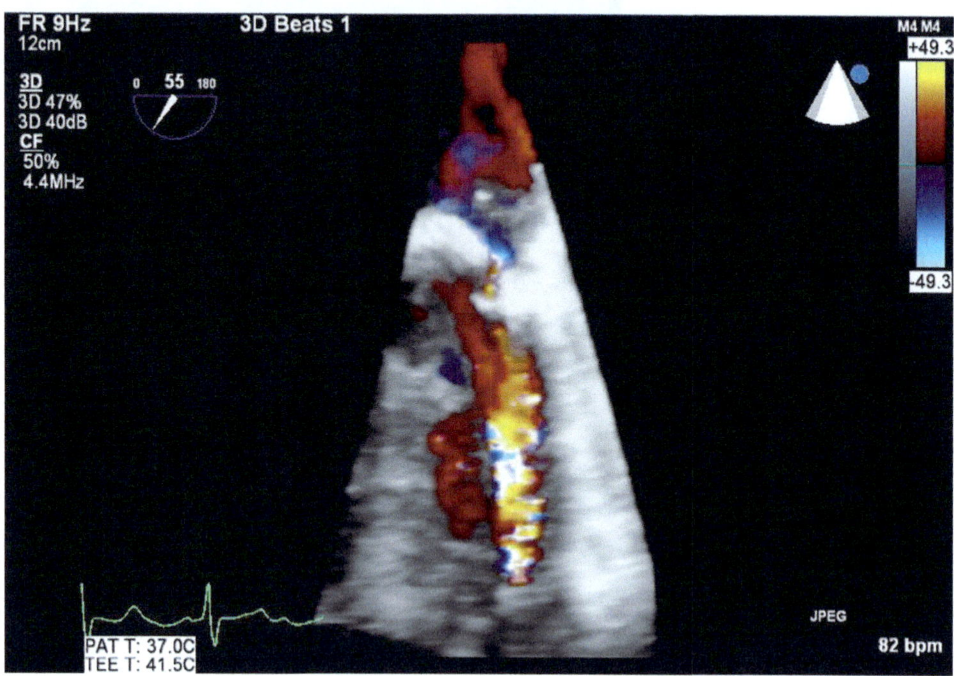

11.4 Case 4. Paravalvular Leak 2

A 51-year-old woman with a past history of mitral valve replacements 20 and 27 years previously now presents with hemolytic anemia, atrial fibrillation, and a small (5 mm) mitral paravalvular leak with severe tricuspid regurgitation. She has symptoms of right heart failure with evidence of fluid overload. She has known biventricular dysfunction, with implantation of an implantable cardiac defibrillator.

Echocardiography demonstrated biventricular enlargement. The St. Jude mechanical prosthetic mitral valve replacement was associated with a moderate (2–3+), posterolaterally directed paravalvular leak, which originated adjacent to the lateral aspect of the valve near the left atrial appendage ostium, although the valve itself remained well seated. There was severe (4+) tricuspid regurgitation related to annular dilatation.

She successfully underwent her third cardiac surgery involving mitral valve replacement with an On-X mechanical valve (#33) and a tricuspid valve repair with a Carpentier classic annuloplasty ring (#30) (Figs. 11.17, 11.18, 11.19, and 11.20).

Video 11.15 TEE at 60° demonstrating the mechanical mitral valve with normally functioning leaflets. A small paravalvular region of defect can be seen adjacent to the lateral aspect of the valve (AVI 8981 kb)

Video 11.16 The same 60° TEE view demonstrates a small jet of flow through the paravalvular defect on color Doppler imaging (AVI 1539 kb)

Video 11.17 Rotating the TEE probe to 90° demonstrates the paravalvular leak adjacent to the lateral aspect of the valve, perpendicular to the orifice of the left atrial appendage (AVI 1689 kb)

Video 11.18 3D imaging of the mechanical mitral valve demonstrates a normally functioning, well-seated bileaflet prosthesis (AVI 1277 kb)

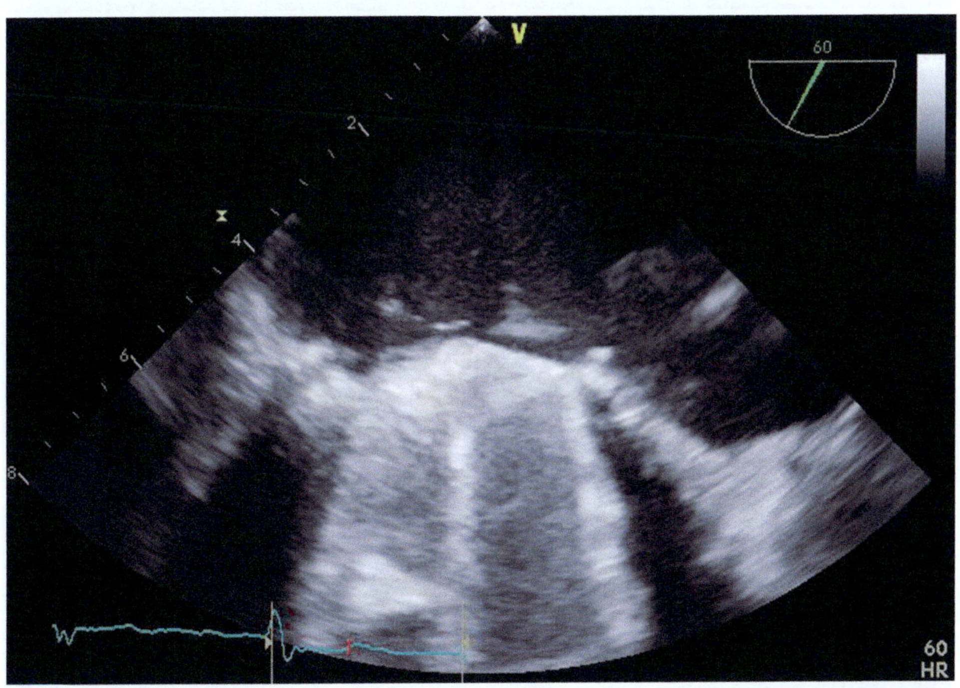

Fig. 11.17 TEE at 60° demonstrating the mechanical mitral valve with normally functioning leaflets. A small paravalvular region of defect can be seen adjacent to the lateral aspect of the valve

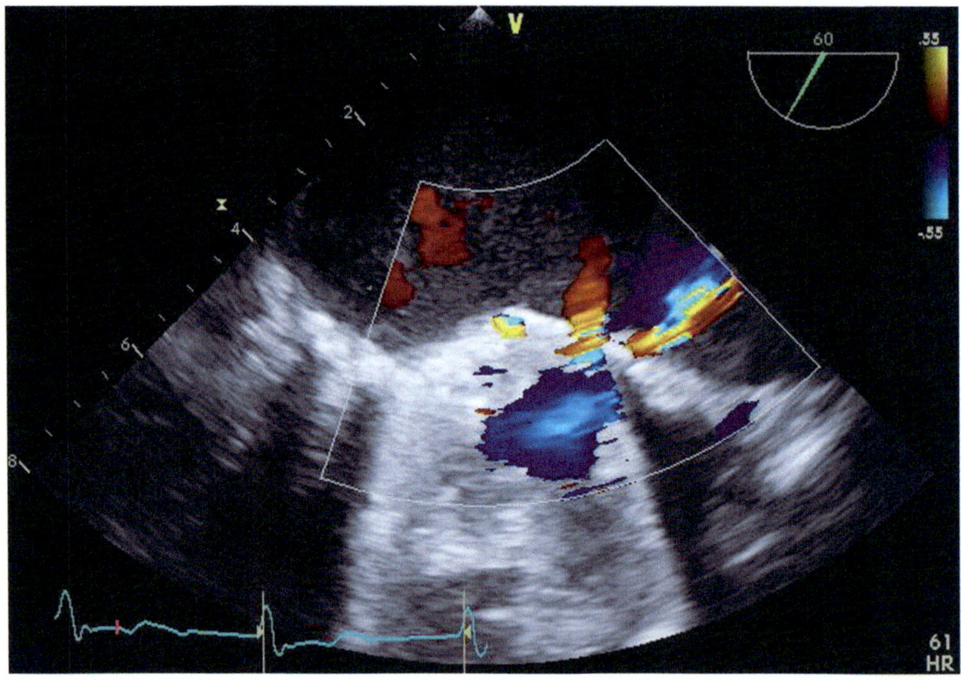

Fig. 11.18 The same 60° transesophageal view demonstrates a small jet of flow through the paravalvular defect on color Doppler imaging

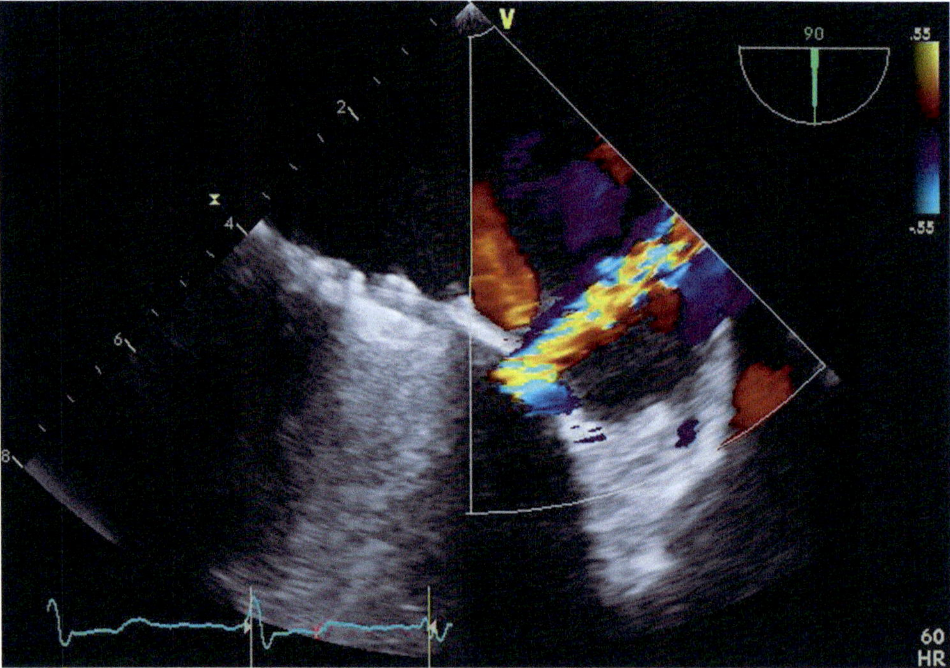

Fig. 11.19 Rotating the transesophageal probe to 90° demonstrates the paravalvular leak adjacent to the lateral aspect of the valve, perpendicular to the orifice of the left atrial appendage

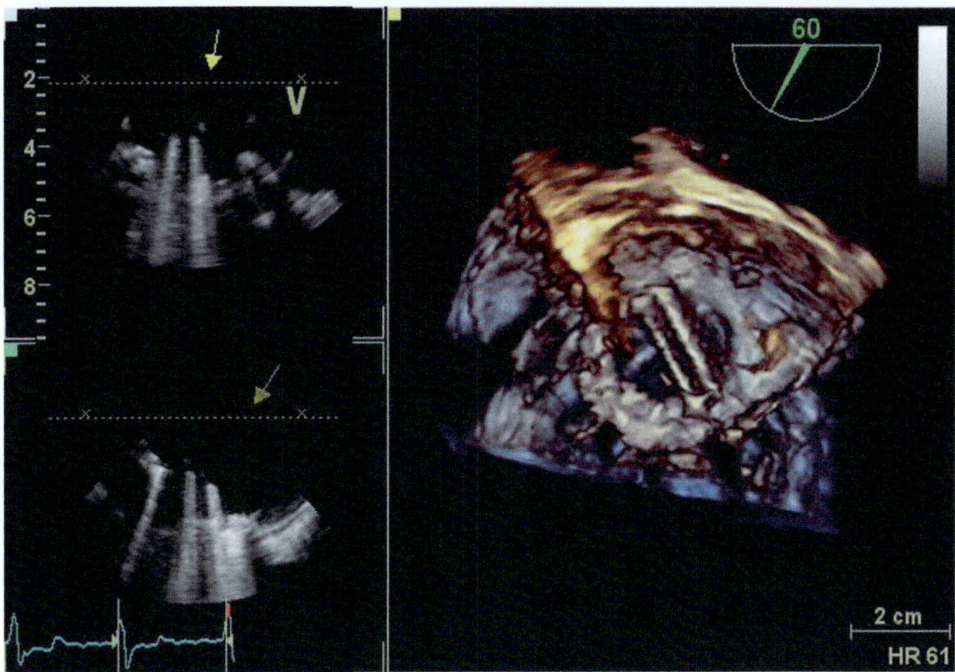

Fig. 11.20   3D imaging (*right-hand panel*) of the mechanical mitral valve demonstrates a normally functioning, well-seated bileaflet prosthesis

11.5 Case 5. Paravalvular Leaks 3

A 67-year-old woman presented with mild exertional dyspnea and mild hemolytic anemia. Her background history included myxomatous mitral valve disease, for which she underwent mitral valve replacement over 10 years ago, followed by replacement with a porcine valve and tricuspid repair 3 years ago.

Transthoracic and transesophageal echocardiograms were remarkable for a moderate (2+), anterolateral mitral paravalvular leak, although the mitral valve prosthesis appeared otherwise well-seated. The vena contracta measured 0.1 cm². Otherwise, there was only trivial valvular regurgitation, with no restriction of leaflet excursion. The peak and mean gradients were 22 and 6 mmHg. The tricuspid valve repair appeared intact, with only trivial regurgitation and a mean gradient of 4 mmHg (Figs. 11.21, 11.22, 11.23, and 11.24).

Given her lack of symptoms and only mild anemia, she will have ongoing follow-up with serial echocardiography every 6–12 months, or sooner if her symptoms worsen.

Video 11.19 Transesophageal long-axis view demonstrating a normally functioning bioprosthetic mitral valve replacement (AVI 4234 kb)

Video 11.20 Transesophageal long-axis view with a moderate (2+) paravalvular leak anteriorly on color Doppler imaging (AVI 2679 kb)

Video 11.21 3D left atrial view of the mitral valve, atypically orientated with the aortic valve at 3 o'clock and the anterior paravalvular defect at the 9 o'clock position (AVI 745 kb)

Video 11.22 3D left ventricular view of the mitral valve, with the anterior paravalvular defect now visible at the 3 o'clock position (AVI 755 kb)

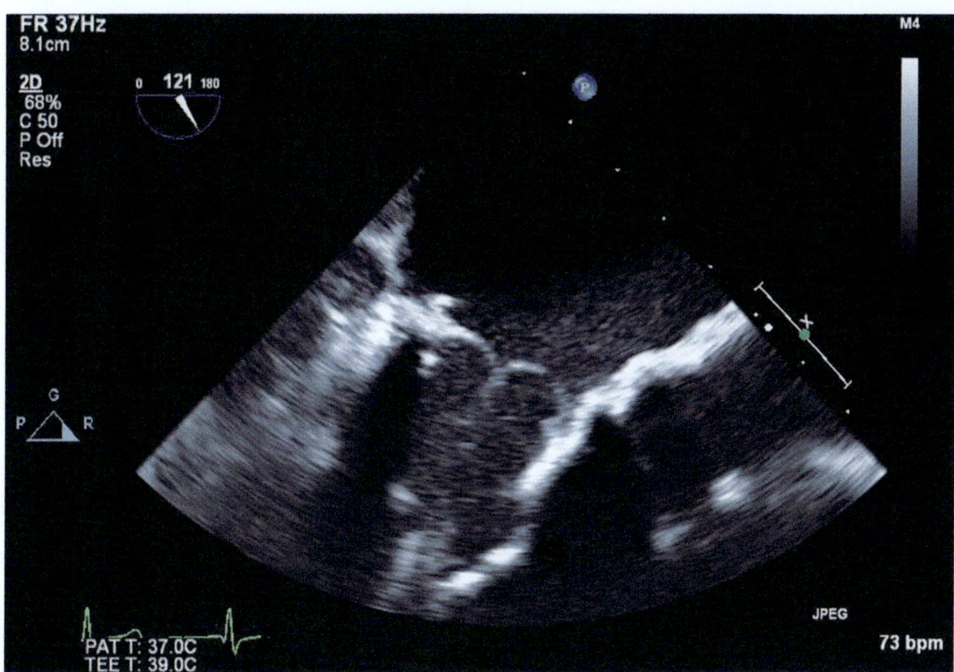

Fig. 11.21 TEE long-axis view demonstrating a normally functioning bioprosthetic mitral valve replacement

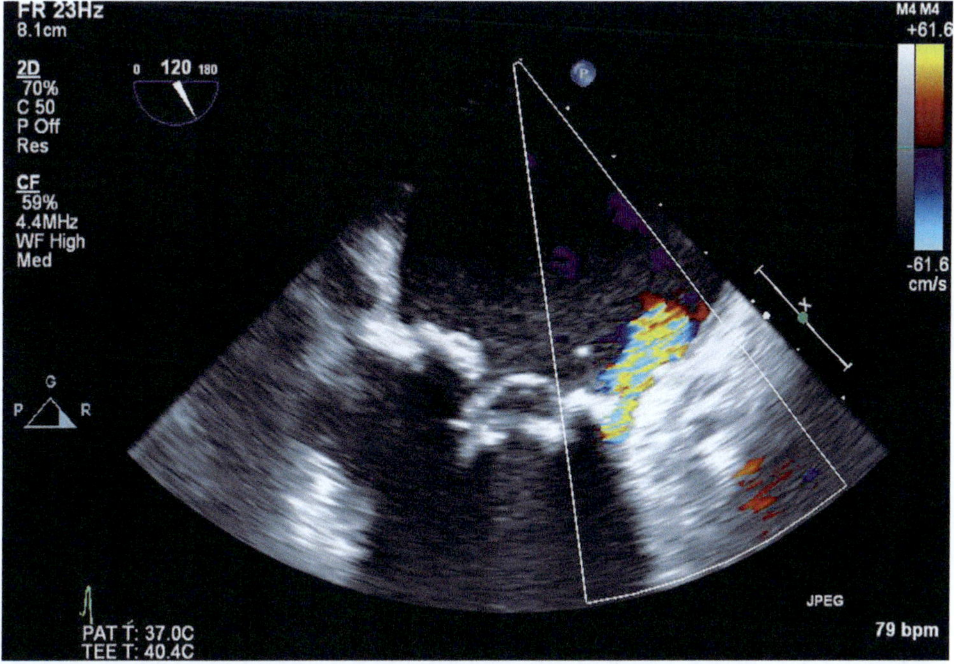

Fig. 11.22 TEE long-axis view with a moderate (2+) paravalvular leak anteriorly on color Doppler imaging

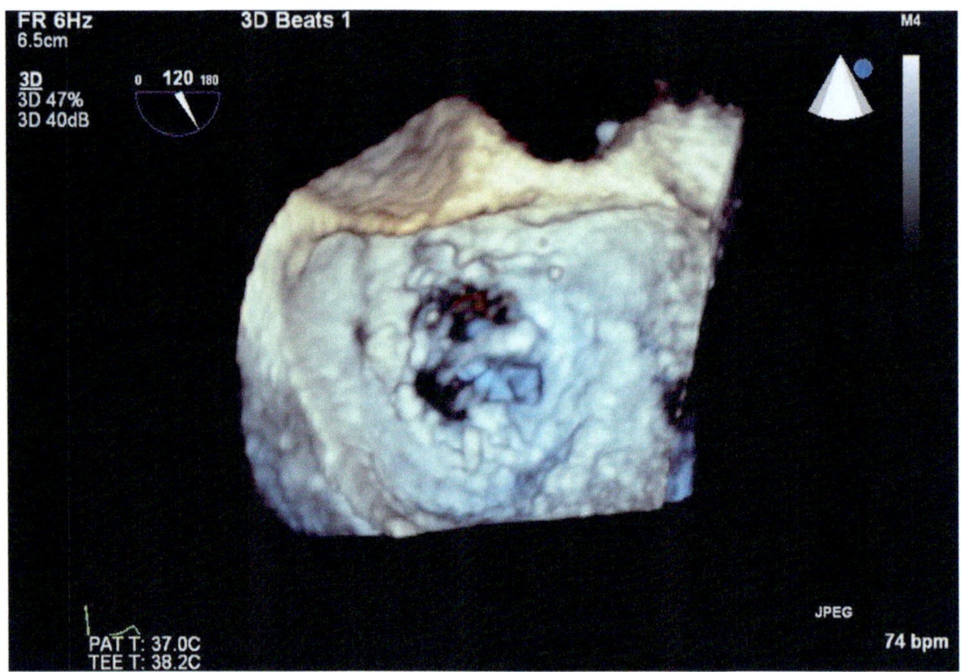

Fig. 11.23 3D left atrial view of the mitral valve, atypically orientated with the aortic valve at 3 o'clock and the anterior paravalvular defect at the 9 o'clock position

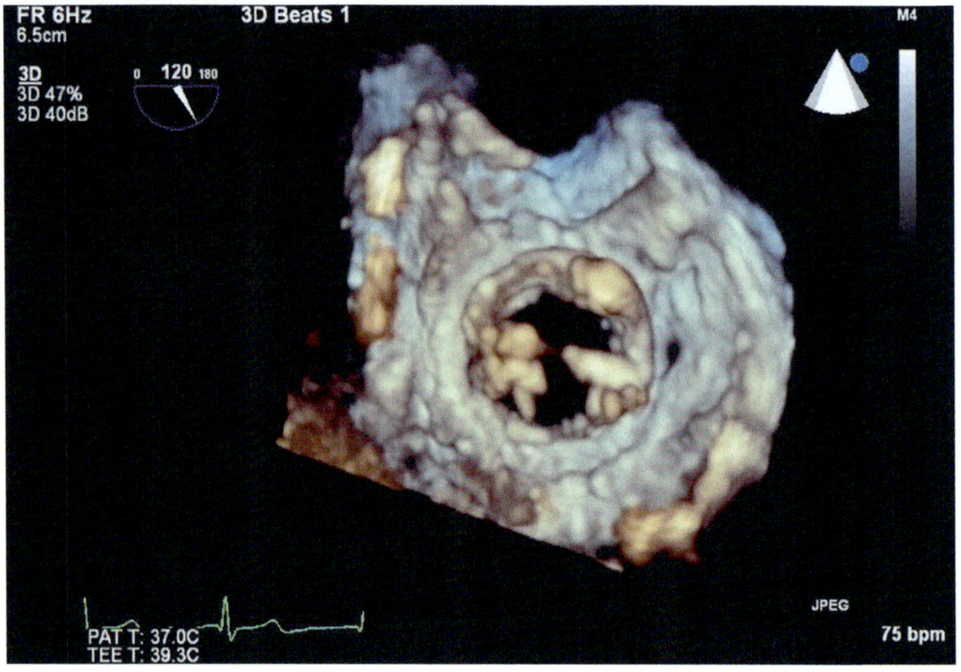

Fig. 11.24 3D left ventricular view of the mitral valve, with the anterior paravalvular defect now visible at the 3 o'clock position

11.6   Case 6. Bioprosthetic Mitral Valve Replacement and Pseudoaneurysm

A 77-year-old woman was referred with a history of coronary artery bypass graft surgery and bioprosthetic aortic (#21) and mitral (#25) valve replacements for aortic stenosis and mitral regurgitation 2 months earlier. The surgery had been complicated by severe mitral annular calcification and bleeding from the AV groove and posterior ventricle, which required a pericardial patch. She now reported worsening symptoms of heart failure, and echocardiography demonstrated partial dehiscence of the mitral valve with a resultant severe, posterior paravalvular leak (measuring 1.0 cm in maximal diameter), which was in direct communication with a large (5.0×4.1 cm) pseudoaneurysm adjacent to the left atrium, which obstructed pulmonary venous drainage (Figs. 11.25, 11.26, 11.27, and 11.28). The aortic valve replacement was well seated, with only trivial regurgitation. Reoperation was performed involving removal of the old prosthesis, unroofing and repair of the pseudoaneurysm, and replacement of the mitral valve with a Biocor #29 prosthesis.

Video 11.23 TEE imaging of the bioprosthetic mitral valve replacement at 38°, demonstrating the large pseudoaneurysm adjacent to the valve annulus and left atrium laterally (AVI 4606 kb)

Video 11.24 The addition of color Doppler imaging demonstrates regurgitant flow directly from the left ventricle into the pseudoaneurysm via a communication located just below the level of the valve annulus laterally (AVI 2413 kb)

Video 11.25 Transesophageal biplane view of the bioprosthetic mitral valve replacement at 0 and 90°, demonstrating the large lateral pseudoaneurysm, which expands during systole, when there is retrograde flow into the cavity (AVI 3898 kb)

Video 11.26 3D reconstruction of the mitral valve viewed from the left atrium. The large pseudoaneurysm can be seen adjacent to the lateral aspect of the valve and left atrium (AVI 1886 kb)

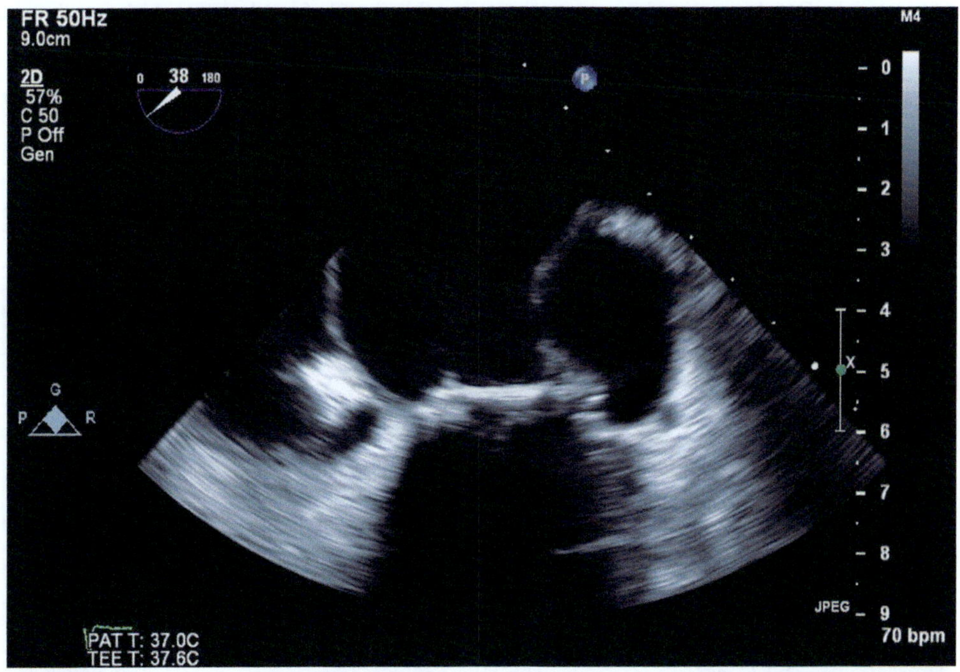

Fig. 11.25 TEE imaging of the bioprosthetic mitral valve replacement at 38°, demonstrating the large pseudoaneurysm adjacent to the valve annulus and left atrium laterally

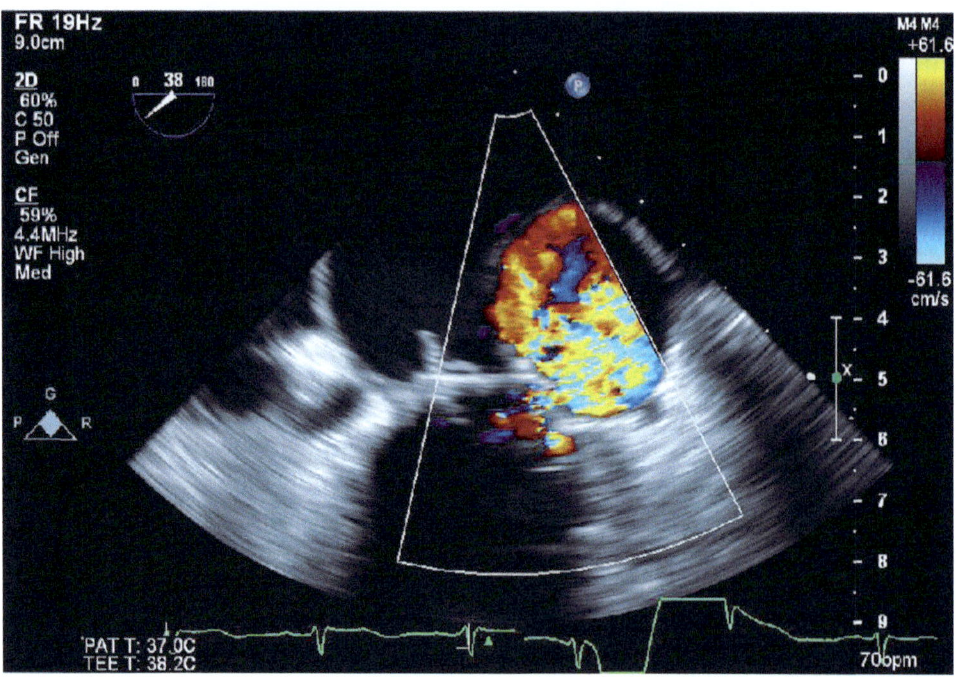

Fig. 11.26 The addition of color Doppler imaging demonstrates regurgitant flow directly from the left ventricle into the pseudoaneurysm via a communication located just below the level of the valve annulus laterally

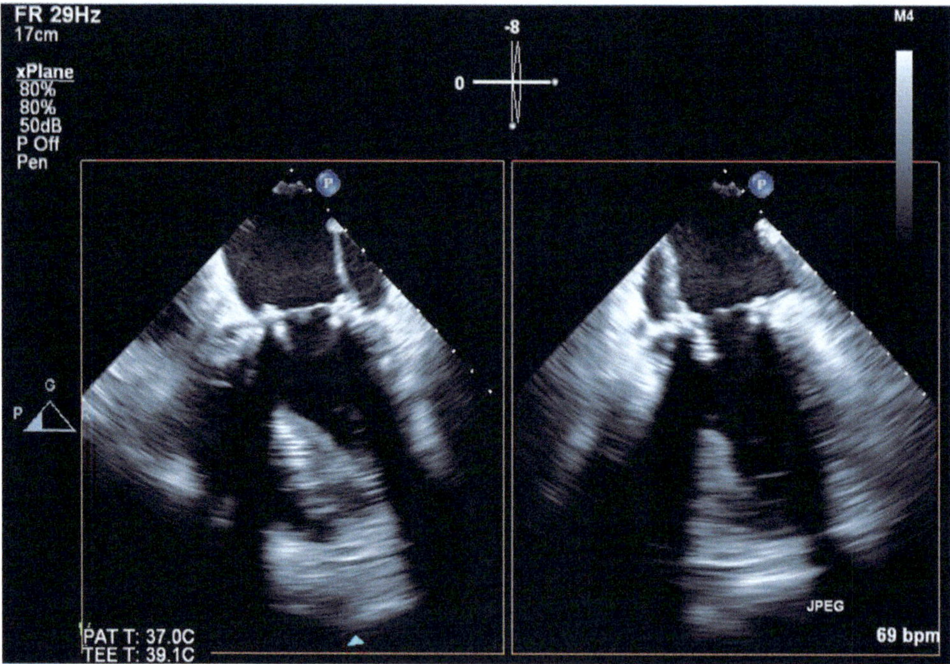

Fig. 11.27 Transesophageal biplane view of the bioprosthetic mitral valve replacement at 0 and 90°, demonstrating the large lateral pseudoaneurysm, which expands during systole, when there is retrograde flow into the cavity

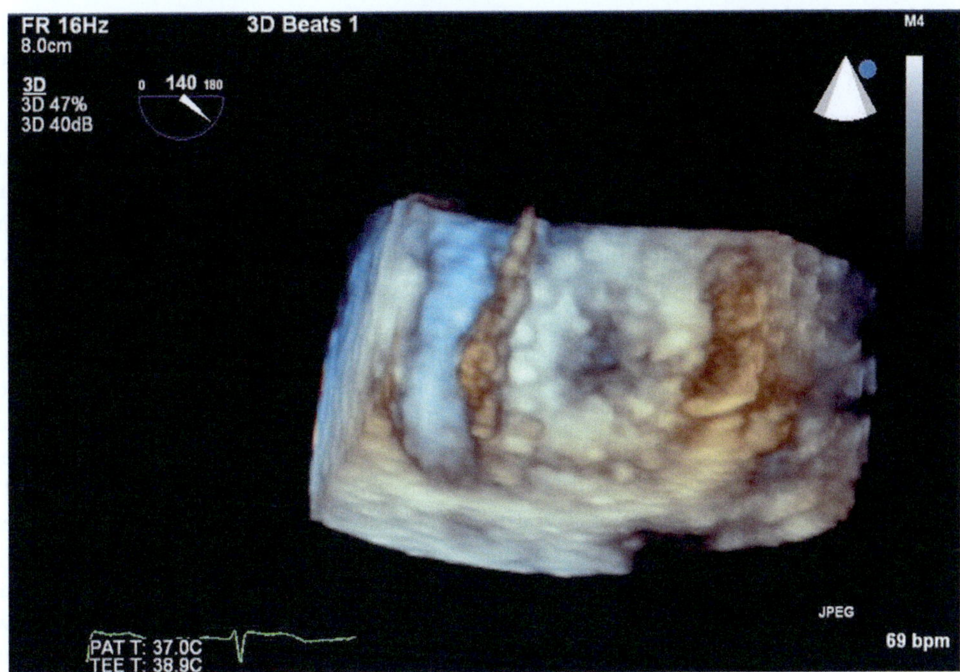

Fig. 11.28 3D reconstruction of the mitral valve viewed from the left atrium. The large pseudoaneurysm can be seen adjacent to the lateral aspect of the valve and left atrium

11.7 Case 7. Mechanical Valve Replacement and Pseudoaneurysm

A 33-year-old man presents with increasing dyspnea and fatigue. His past history was remarkable for bileaflet mechanical mitral valve replacement 5 years earlier, as a result of mitral valve infection endocarditis secondary to intravenous drug use. He has abstained from drug use since this time and remained compliant with oral anticoagulation, but he has not had an echocardiogram for several years.

Echocardiography was performed and demonstrated a mechanical mitral valve replacement with moderate (2+) valvular regurgitation, a moderate (2+) paravalvular jet with flow directed into the left atrial appendage, and a further small paravalvular leak communicating with a small lateral pseudoaneurysm located between the valve annulus and the left atrial appendage (Figs. 11.29, 11.30, and 11.31). Given his lack of constitutional symptoms and negative blood cultures, it was suspected that the pseudoaneurysm was related to an old abscess cavity rather than active infection.

He was taken to the operating room, where the echocardiographic findings were confirmed. The mitral valve prosthesis was left alone, as it appeared normal and was well seated, with preserved function. The pseudoaneurysm was resected, and a patch repair of remaining paravalvular defects was performed. There was no evidence of infective endocarditis or abscess formation visually or on microbiology of the resected tissue.

Video 11.27 TEE imaging of the bileaflet mechanical mitral valve prosthesis at 58°. The valve appears well seated, with normal leaflet opening. A large left atrial appendage can be seen laterally to the right of the image. Between the appendage and the valve is a small cavity demonstrating expansion during systole. This dynamic appearance is suggestive of a pseudoaneurysm (AVI 4572 kb)

Video 11.28 Color Doppler imaging, in the same 58° TEE plane, demonstrates three separate jets of systole flow. There is a moderate (2+) valvular regurgitant jet, a moderate (2+) paravalvular jet originating laterally with flow directed into the left atrial appendage, and a small amount of systolic flow going directly from the left ventricle into the pseudoaneurysm (AVI 1335 kb)

Video 11.29 A 3D reconstruction of the mitral valve prosthesis from the left atrial aspect. The valve appears well seated, with normal motion of both leaflets. The large left atrial appendage can be seen adjacent to the valve laterally to the left of the image. Between the appendage and the valve ring is a small slit-like annular defect (9 o'clock position), which represents the cause of the paravalvular leak (AVI 927 kb)

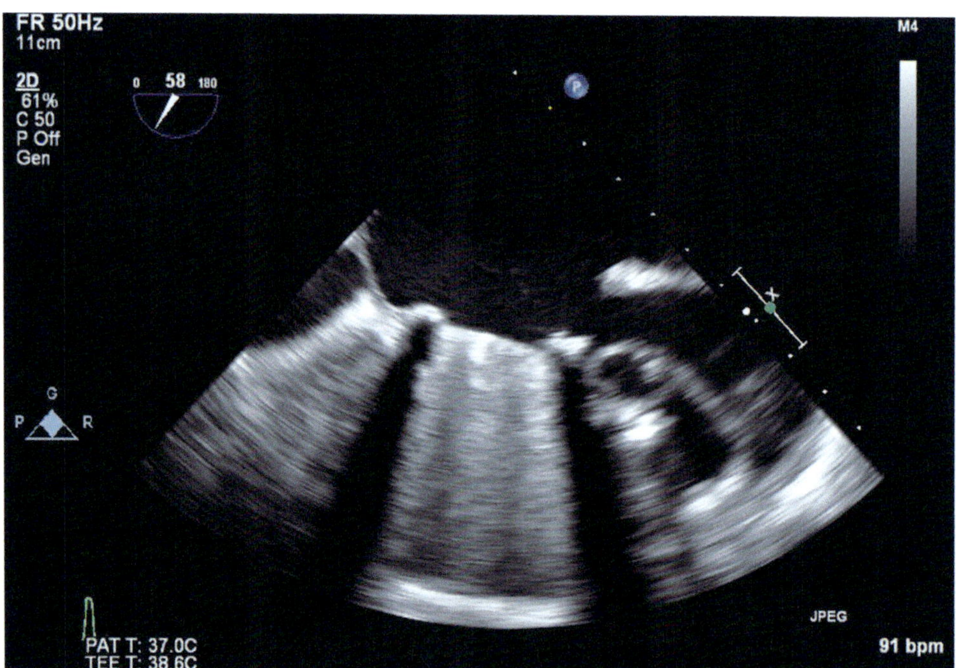

Fig. 11.29 TEE imaging of the bileaflet mechanical mitral valve prosthesis at 58°. The valve appears well seated, with normal leaflet opening. A large left atrial appendage can be seen laterally to the right of the image. Between the appendage and the valve is a small cavity demonstrating expansion during systole. This dynamic appearance is suggestive of a pseudoaneurysm

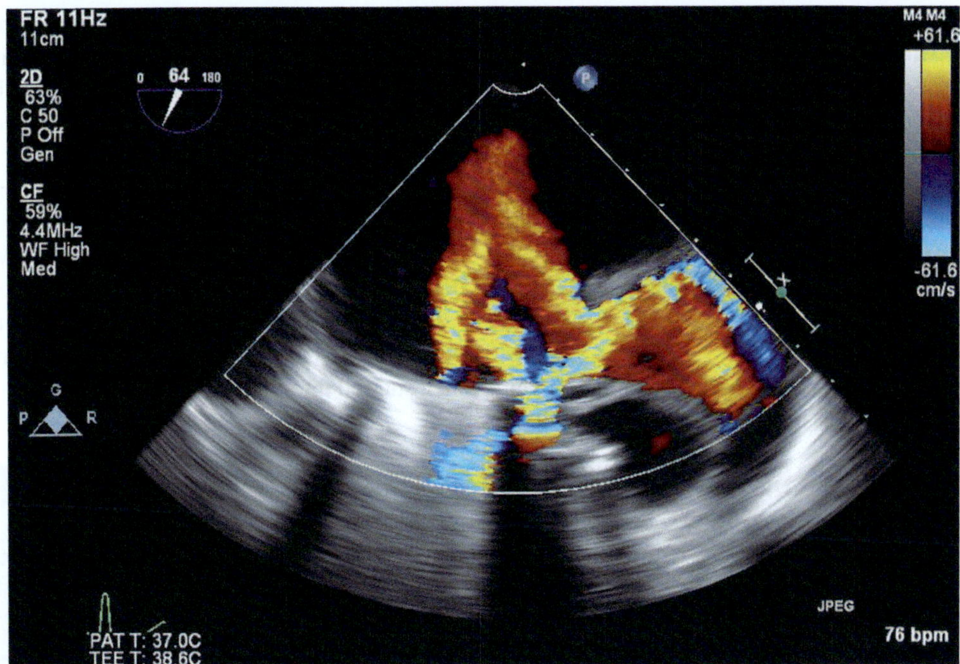

Fig. 11.30 Color Doppler imaging, in the same 58° TEE plane, demonstrates three separate jets of systole flow. There is a moderate (2+) valvular regurgitant jet, a moderate (2+) paravalvular jet originating laterally with flow directed into the left atrial appendage, and a small amount of systolic flow going directly from the left ventricle into the pseudoaneurysm

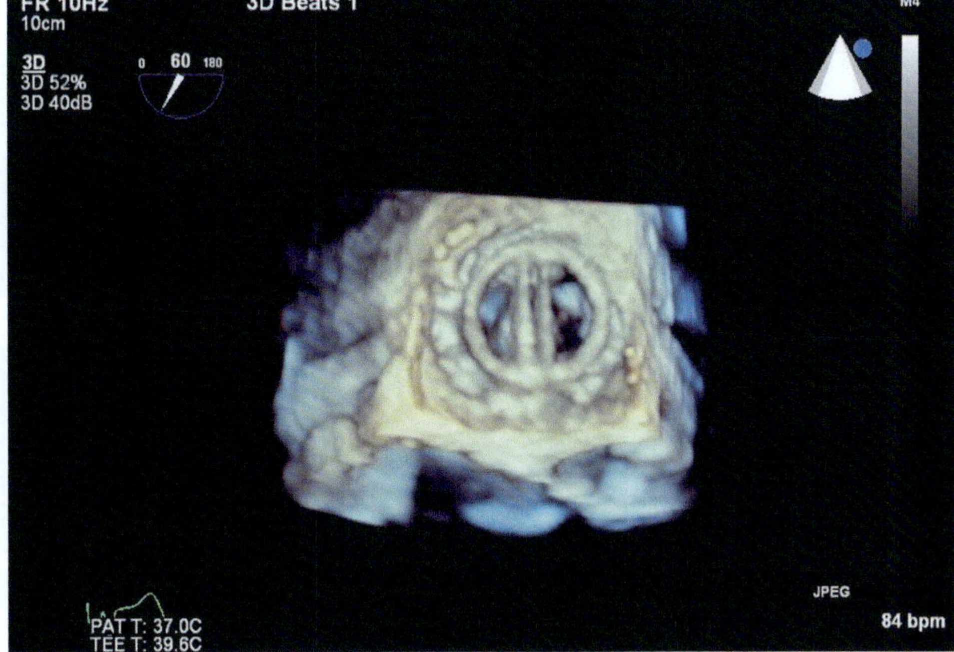

Fig. 11.31 A 3D reconstruction of the mitral valve prosthesis from the left atrial aspect. The valve appears well seated, with normal motion of both leaflets. The large left atrial appendage can be seen adjacent to the valve laterally to the left of the image. Between the appendage and the valve ring is a small slit-like annular defect (9 o'clock position), which represents the cause of the paravalvular leak

11.8 Case 8. Bioprosthetic Valve Dehiscence

A 74-year-old woman presented in congestive heart failure. She was known to have a history of mitral valve replacement (St. Jude Biocor #29) 1 year earlier at another hospital for *Streptococcus viridans* infective endocarditis. Her other comorbidities involved atrial fibrillation with sick sinus syndrome (necessitating pacemaker implantation), hypertension, hyperlipidemia, chronic renal insufficiency, and moderate to severe chronic lung disease.

Transthoracic echocardiography revealed mild left ventricular dysfunction and a moderate (3+) posterolateral paravalvular mitral leak in addition to severe (3–4+) tricuspid regurgitation. Blood cultures were negative on this occasion, although there was clinical concern that an infective cause of valve dehiscence was masked by recent oral antibiotic use (Figs. 11.32, 11.33, and 11.34).

She underwent redo mitral valve surgery. The surgeon noted that there was clear dehiscence of the prosthesis from the posterolateral annulus of the mitral valve, with no evidence of any active infection. As a precaution, however, the valve's original prosthesis was removed and the annulus was débrided. A 31-mm St. Jude Biocor porcine mitral valve was then sutured into place.

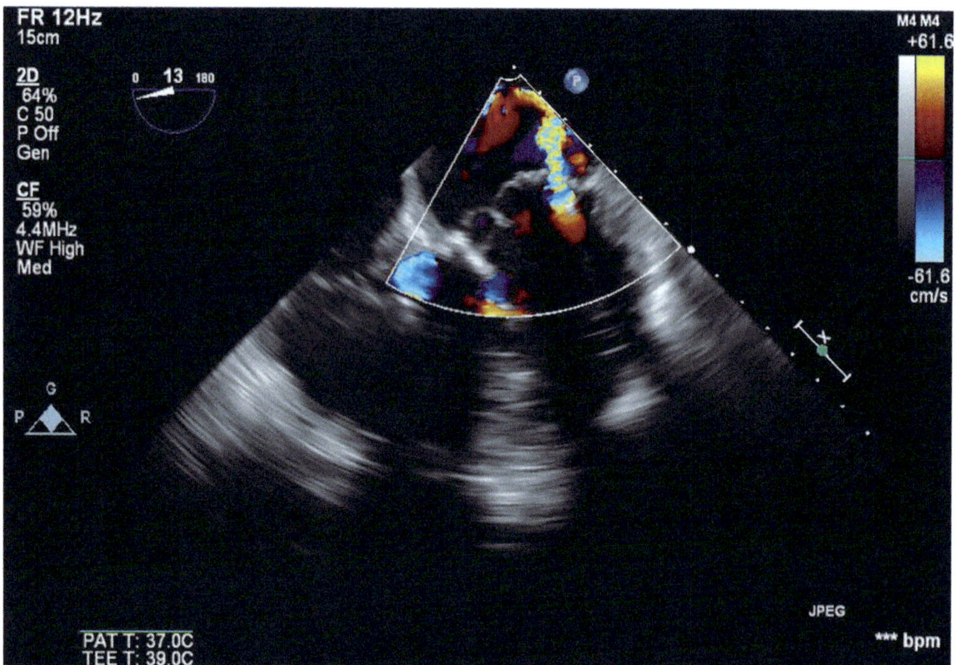

Fig. 11.32 TEE four-chamber view (13°) demonstrating a moderately severe lateral paravalvular leak on color Doppler imaging

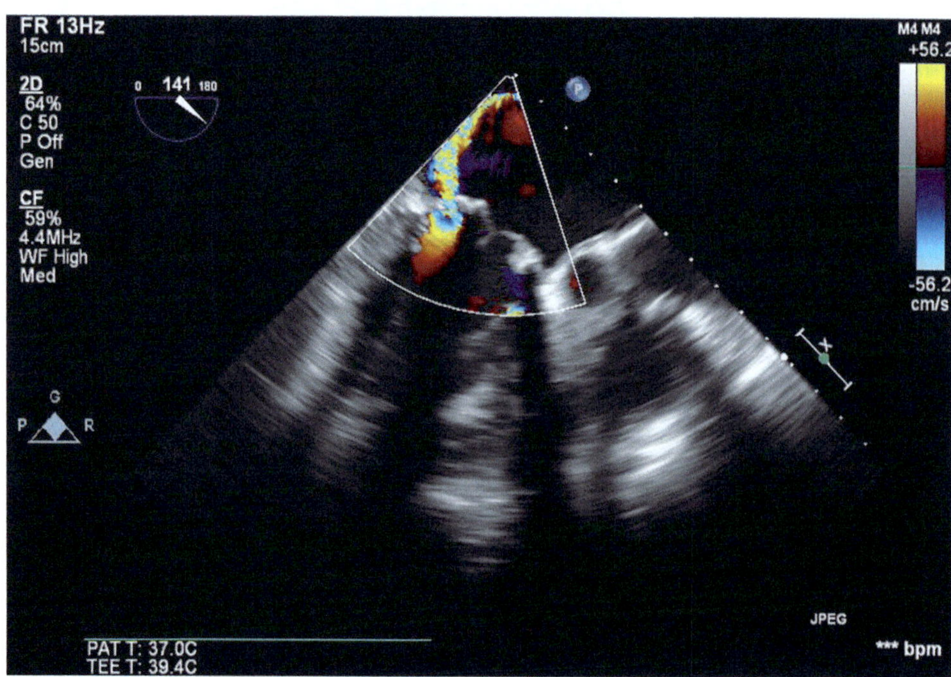

Fig. 11.33 TEE long-axis view (141°) demonstrating the same moderately severe paravalvular leak viewed more posteriorly

Fig. 11.34 3D reconstruction of the mitral valve viewed from the left atrium (**a**) and left ventricle (**b**). Significant dehiscence of the valve bioprosthesis is evident

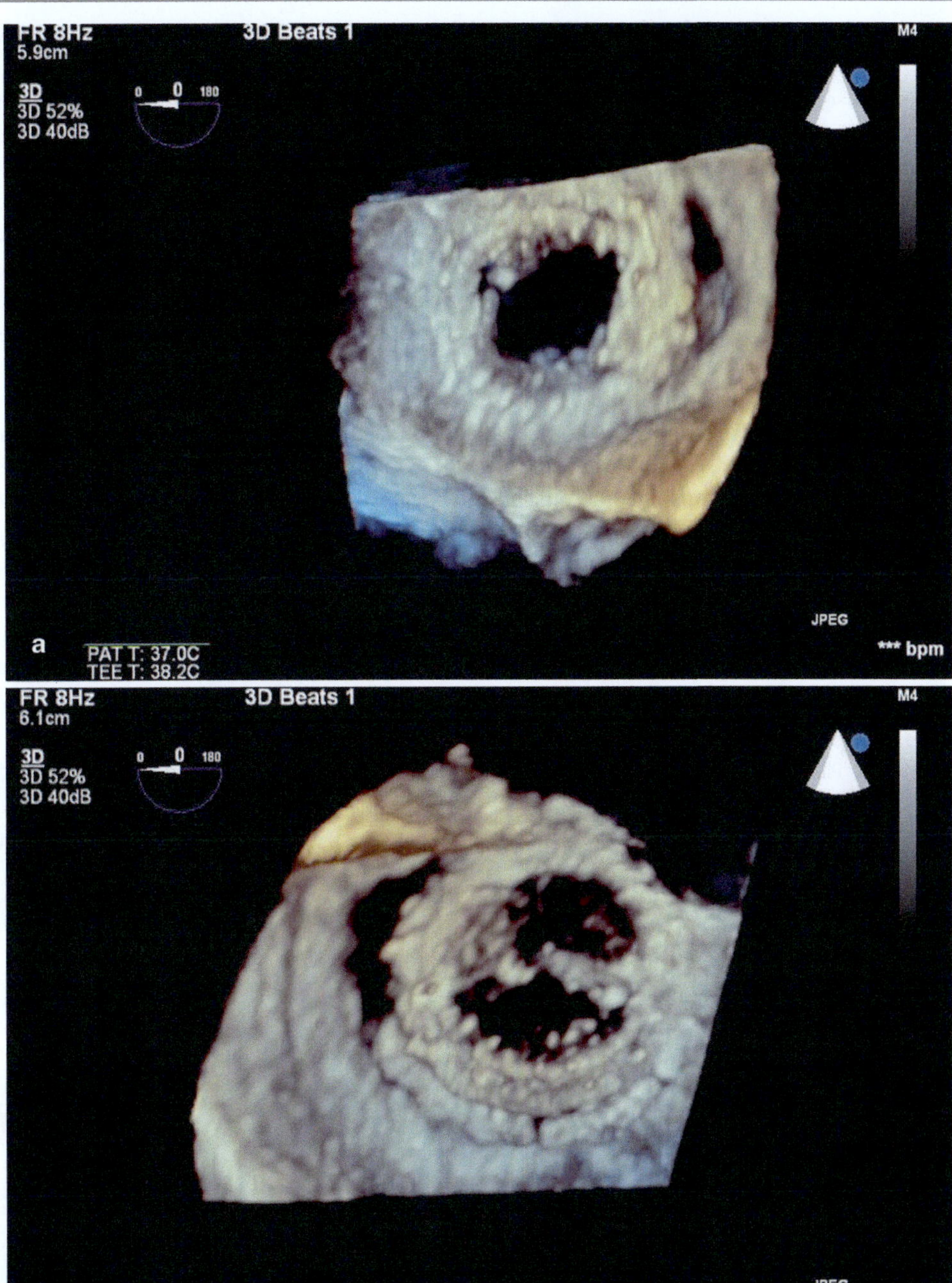

11.9   Case 9. Annuloplasty Ring Dehiscence

A 58-year-old man with a history of myocardial infarction presented with symptoms of heart failure. Transthoracic echocardiography revealed severe functional ischemic mitral regurgitation, and coronary angiography revealed multivessel coronary artery disease. After extensive discussion of the risks, benefits, and alternatives, he elected to proceed with surgery. He understood that the risk of surgery was somewhat increased because of his ischemic mitral regurgitation.

He underwent coronary artery bypass grafting and insertion of a 30-mm Carpentier-McCarthy-Adams ischemic annuloplasty ring. Unfortunately, 2 years later he again started developing symptoms of heart failure. Echocardiography demonstrated significant left ventricular enlargement and dysfunction, with pulmonary hypertension and severe mitral insufficiency due to partial ring dehiscence (Figs. 11.35, 11.36, 11.37, 11.38, 11.39, 11.40, and 11.41).

Video 11.30 Parasternal long-axis view on transthoracic echocardiography (TTE), demonstrating dehiscence of the mitral annuloplasty ring, which can be seen partially hanging below the native valve within the left atrium (AVI 4432 kb)

Video 11.31 The same parasternal long-axis view with color Doppler imaging shows a severe paravalvular regurgitant jet (AVI 1942 kb)

Video 11.32 An apical four-chamber transthoracic view also shows the partially dehisced annuloplasty ring hanging below the native valve annulus in the left atrium (AVI 9310 kb)

Video 11.33 Color Doppler imaging of the same four-chamber view confirms a severe paravalvular jet laterally (AVI 2219 kb)

Video 11.34 Biplane imaging of the mitral valve at 40 and 130° on TEE also demonstrates a moderate central jet of valvular regurgitation (AVI 896 kb)

Video 11.35 3D transesophageal imaging of the mitral valve demonstrates severe dehiscence of the annuloplasty ring, involving nearly 50 % of its circumference (AVI 1046 kb)

Video 11.36 3D transesophageal imaging with color Doppler demonstrates the severe paravalvular regurgitation associated with the annuloplasty ring dehiscence (AVI 1533 kb)

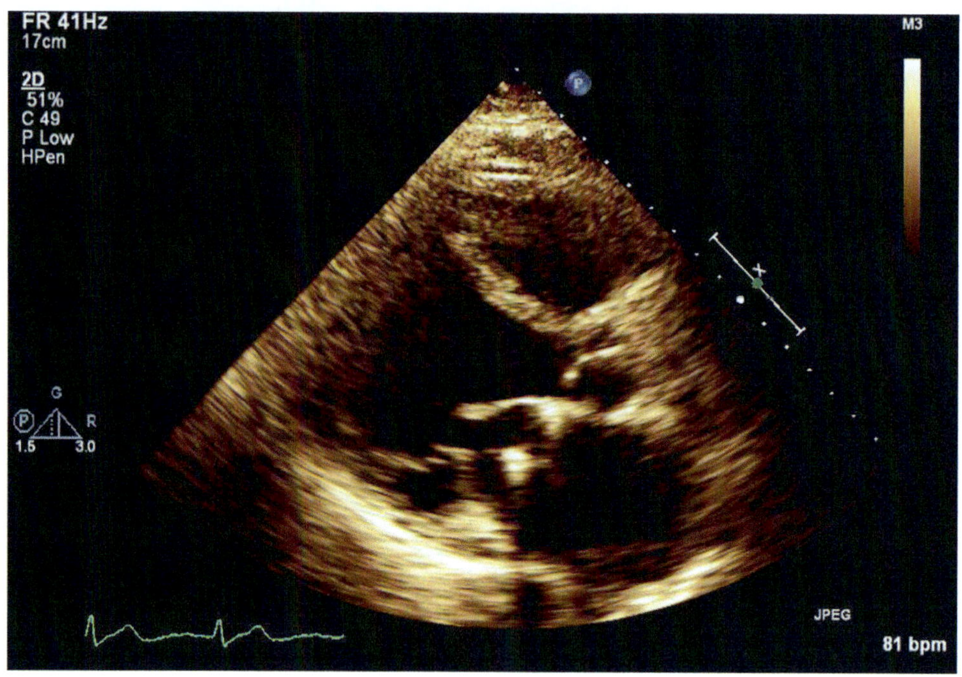

Fig. 11.35 Parasternal long-axis view on transthoracic echocardiography (TTE), demonstrating dehiscence of the mitral annuloplasty ring, which can be seen partially hanging below the native valve within the left atrium

Fig. 11.36 The same parasternal long-axis view with color Doppler imaging shows a severe paravalvular regurgitant jet

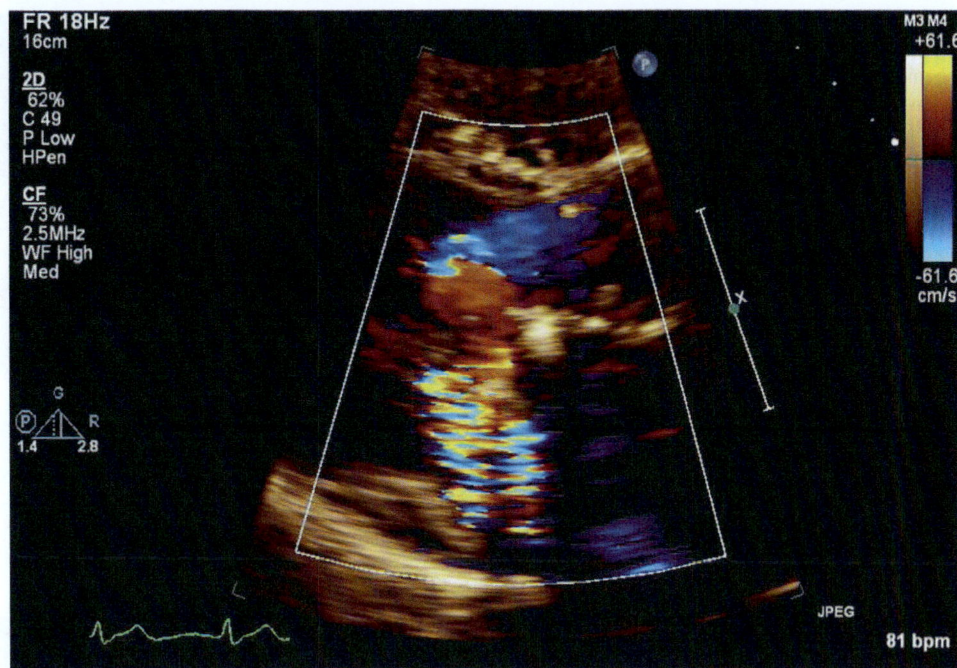

Fig. 11.37 An apical four-chamber transthoracic view also shows the partially dehisced annuloplasty ring hanging below the native valve annulus in the left atrium

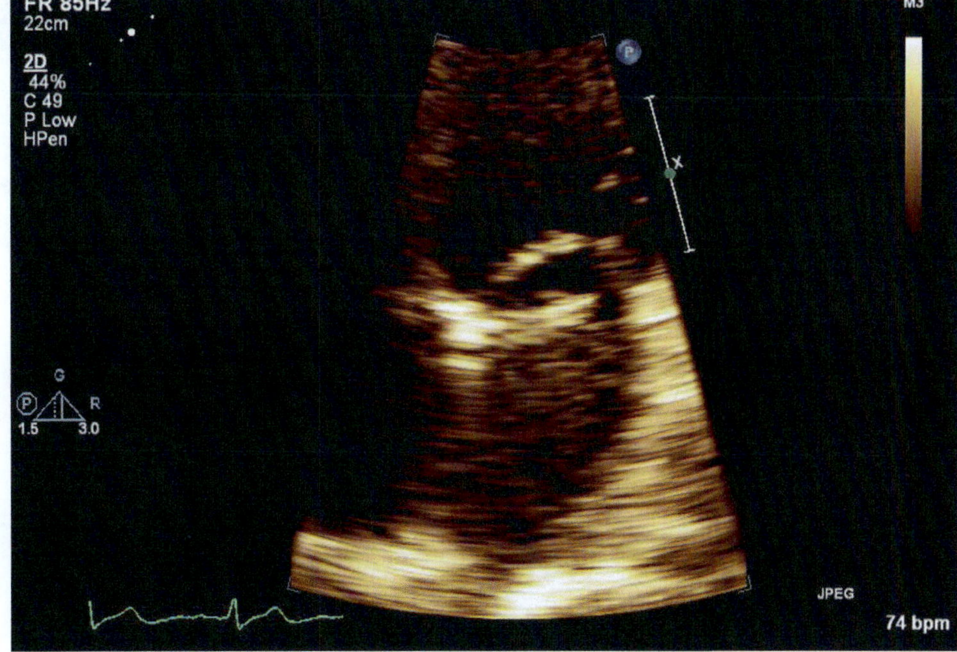

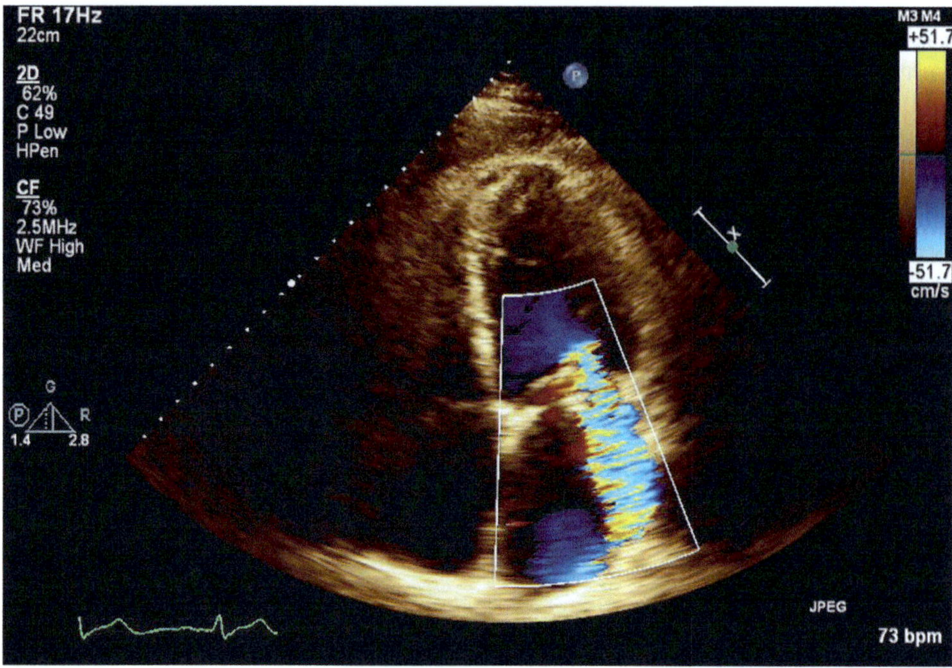

Fig. 11.38 Color Doppler imaging of the same four-chamber view confirms a severe paravalvular jet laterally

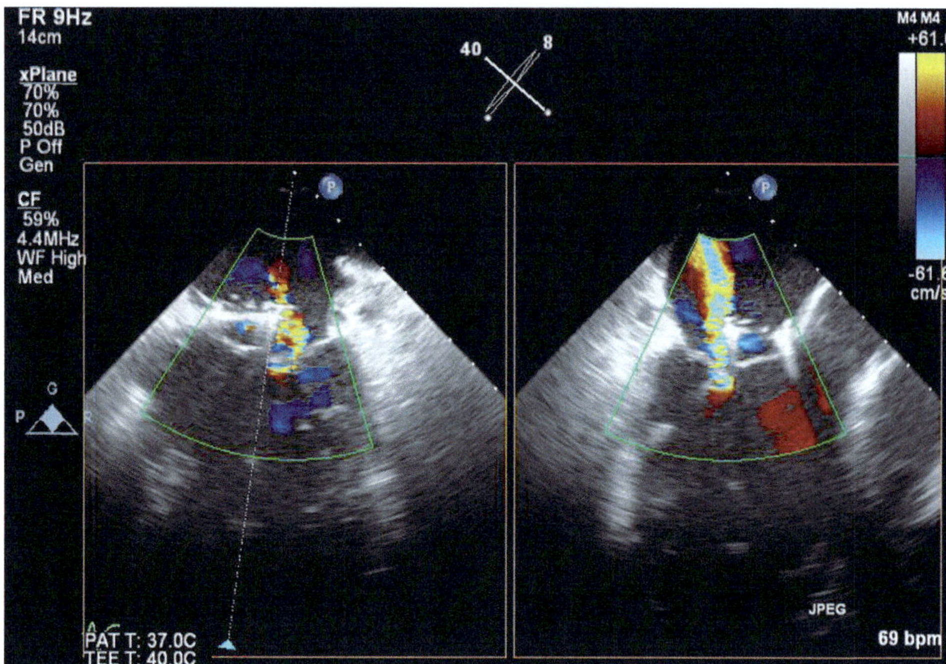

Fig. 11.39 Biplane imaging of the mitral valve at 40 and 130° on TEE also demonstrates a moderate central jet of valvular regurgitation

Fig. 11.40 3D transesophageal imaging of the mitral valve demonstrates severe dehiscence of the annuloplasty ring, involving nearly 50 % of its circumference

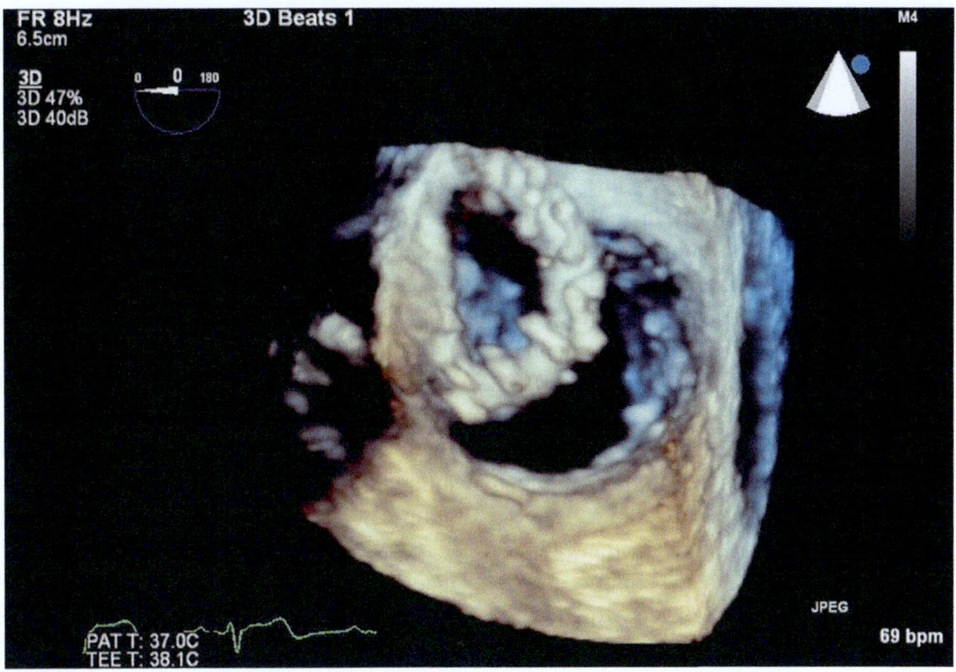

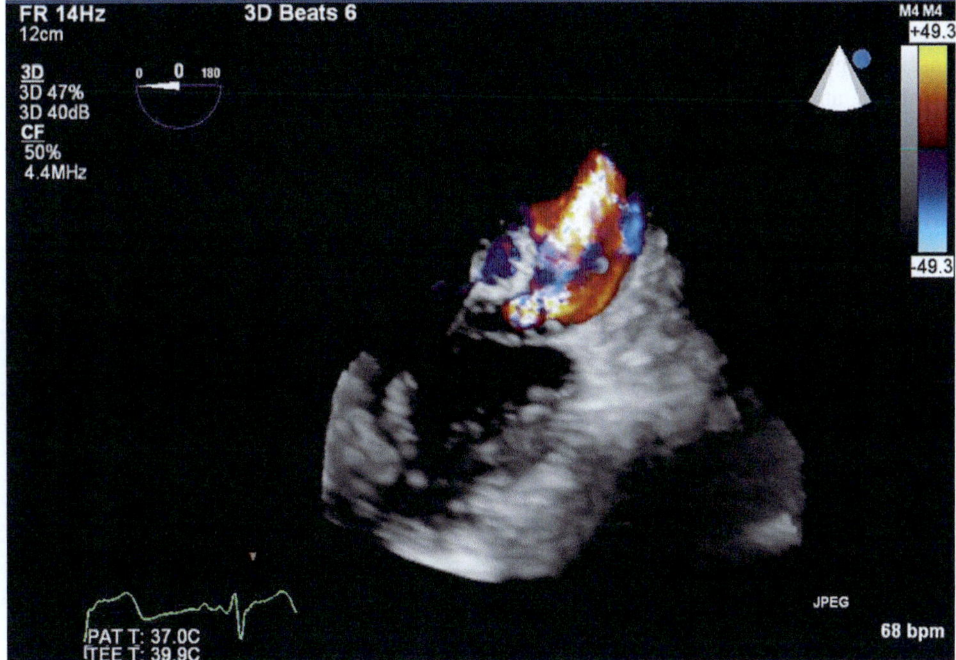

Fig. 11.41 3D transesophageal imaging with color Doppler demonstrates the severe paravalvular regurgitation associated with the annuloplasty ring dehiscence

11.10 Case 10. Inflammatory Response

A 51-year-old man with a history of mitral valve repair (35-mm Duran annuloplasty ring) for mitral valve prolapse 2 years earlier (Figs. 11.42, 11.43, 11.44, 11.45, and 11.46) presented with a transient ischemic attack and severe mitral stenosis. The peak and mean transvalvular gradients measured 23 mmHg and 14 mmHg respectively. Transesophageal echocardiography demonstrated the mitral annulus to be severely thickened globally (0.6 cm), with laminated echogenic material extending from the annulus onto both leaflet bodies (Figs. 11.47, 11.48, 11.49, 11.50, 11.51, and 11.52). This thickening severely restricted the valve orifice and leaflet opening. The appearance was felt to be suspicious for infective endocarditis or laminar thrombus, although he denied any constitutional symptoms suggestive of infection. Multiple blood cultures remained negative.

He was commenced on empiric antibiotic therapy and therapeutically anticoagulated with heparin prior to redo mitral valve surgery. The ring and adjacent tissue was resected and a mechanical mitral valve was sutured in place. Histology revealed extensive inflammatory response with no evidence of thrombus or infection.

Video 11.37 Transesophageal view (at 91°) of the repaired mitral valve with an annuloplasty ring in situ, taken immediately after the original valve surgery. There is good leaflet coaptation without restriction of leaflet movement (AVI 4700 kb)

Video 11.38 Another transesophageal view (at 139°) taken immediately after the original valve surgery, showing good leaflet coaptation without restriction of leaflet movement (AVI 4752 kb)

Video 11.39 Color Doppler imaging at the same transesophageal 139° view immediately after the original valve repair confirms that there was no residual regurgitation (AVI 1148 kb)

Video 11.40 A TEE image (0°) obtained 2 years later showed that the mitral annulus was severely thickened circumferentially, with laminated echogenic material extending from the annulus onto both leaflet bodies. This thickening restricted leaflet opening and resulted in a small, stenotic valve orifice (AVI 3941 kb)

Video 11.41 TEE view at 60°, also obtained 2 years later, showing thickening of the mitral annulus (AVI 5445 kb)

Video 11.42 TEE view at 90°, also obtained 2 years later, showing thickening of the mitral annulus (AVI 5005 kb)

Video 11.43 TEE view at 120°, also obtained 2 years later, showing thickening of the mitral annulus (AVI 3815 kb)

Video 11.44 3D imaging of the mitral valve demonstrated a significant reduction in valve orifice area related to the smooth, laminated echogenic material overlying the annuloplasty ring and extending onto the leaflet bases. Severe associated valve leaflet thickening was also evident (AVI 681 kb)

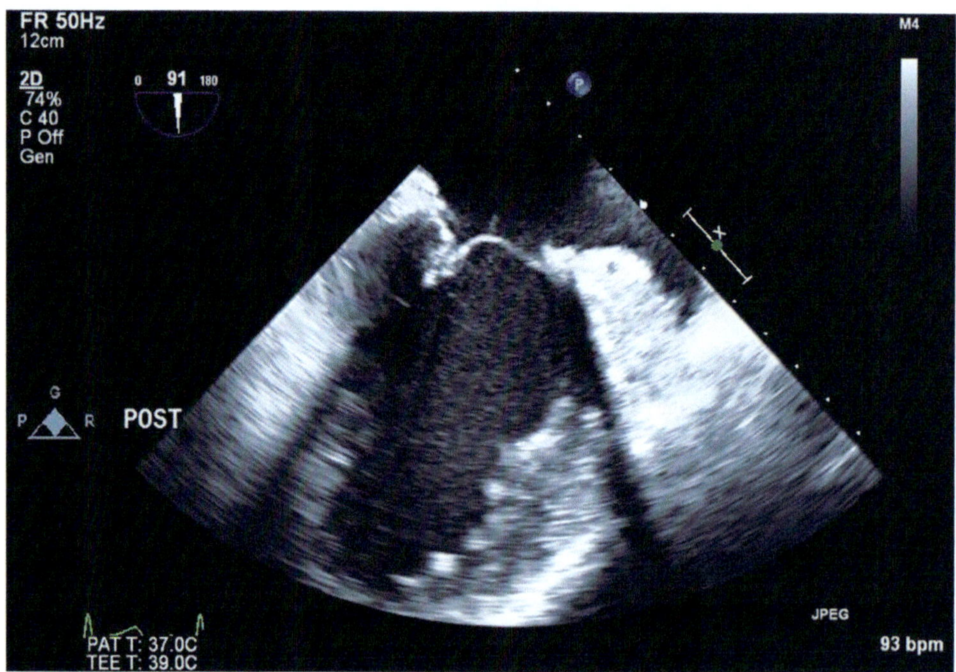

Fig. 11.42 Transesophageal view (91°) of the repaired mitral valve with an annuloplasty ring in situ, taken immediately after the original valve surgery. There is good leaflet coaptation without restriction of leaflet movement

Fig. 11.43 Another transesophageal view (139°) taken immediately after the original valve surgery. There is good leaflet coaptation without restriction of leaflet movement

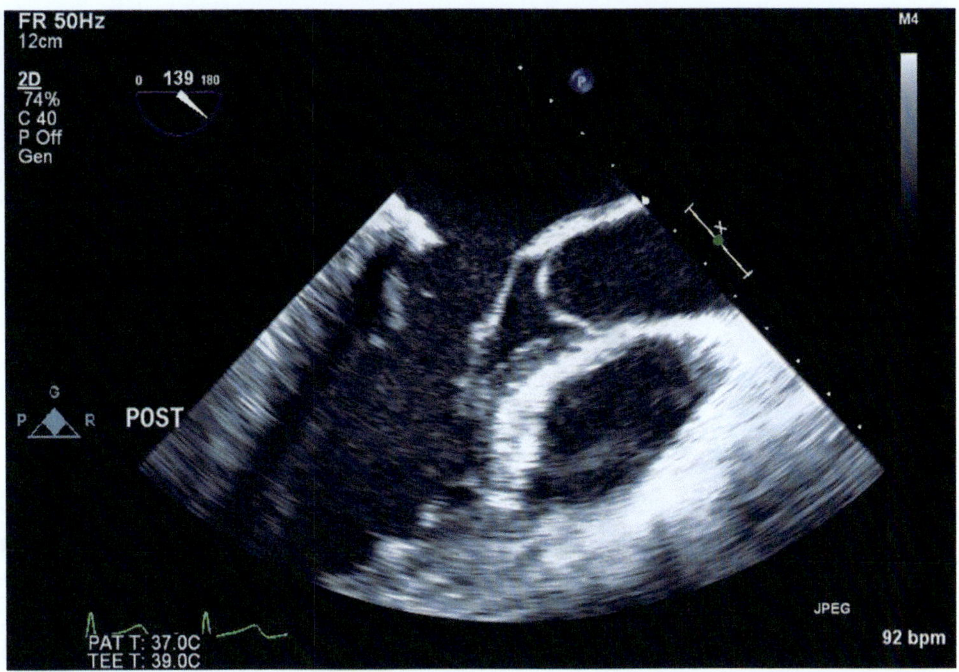

Fig. 11.44 Color Doppler imaging at the same transesophageal 139° view immediately after the original valve repair confirms that there was no residual regurgitation

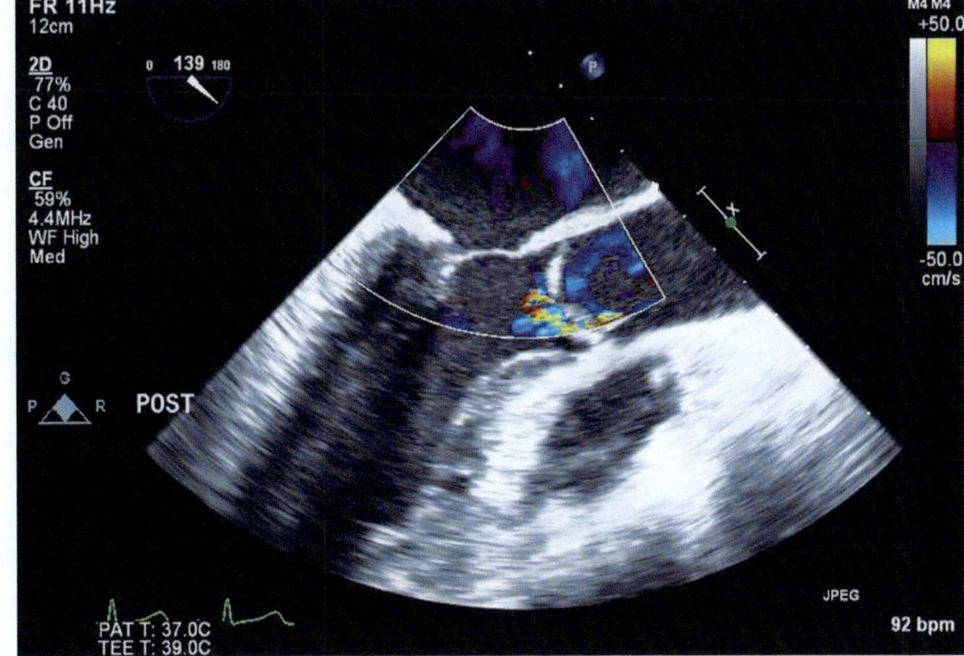

Fig. 11.45 3D imaging immediately after the original valve repair confirms good leaflet excursion with a normal-sized valve orifice area during diastole

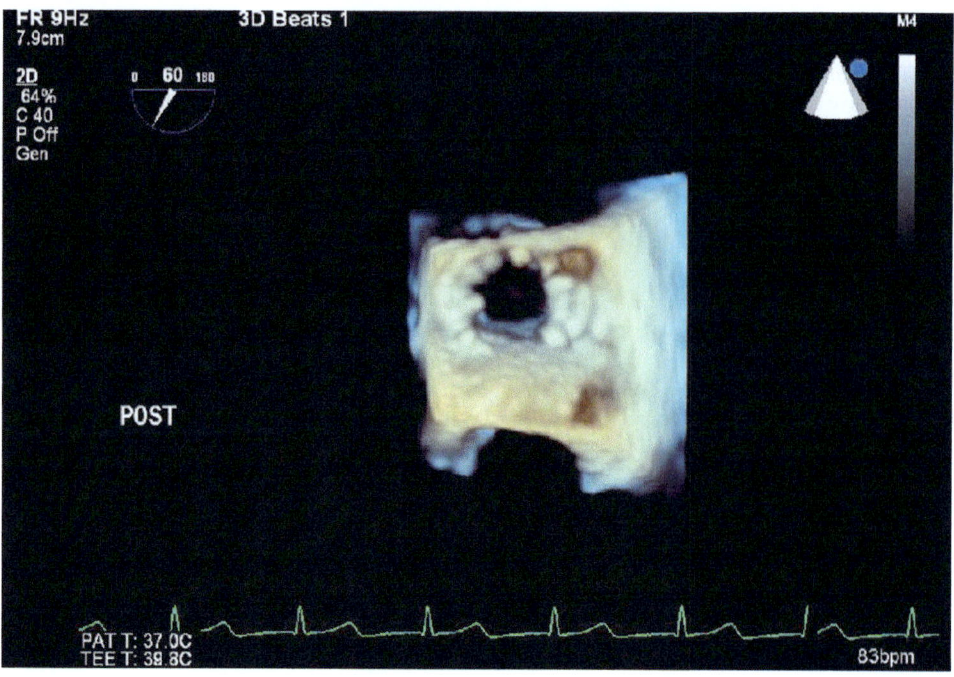

Fig. 11.46 Transvalvular gradients immediately after the original valve repair were within acceptable limits, with a peak gradient of 9 mmHg and a mean gradient of 5 mmHg

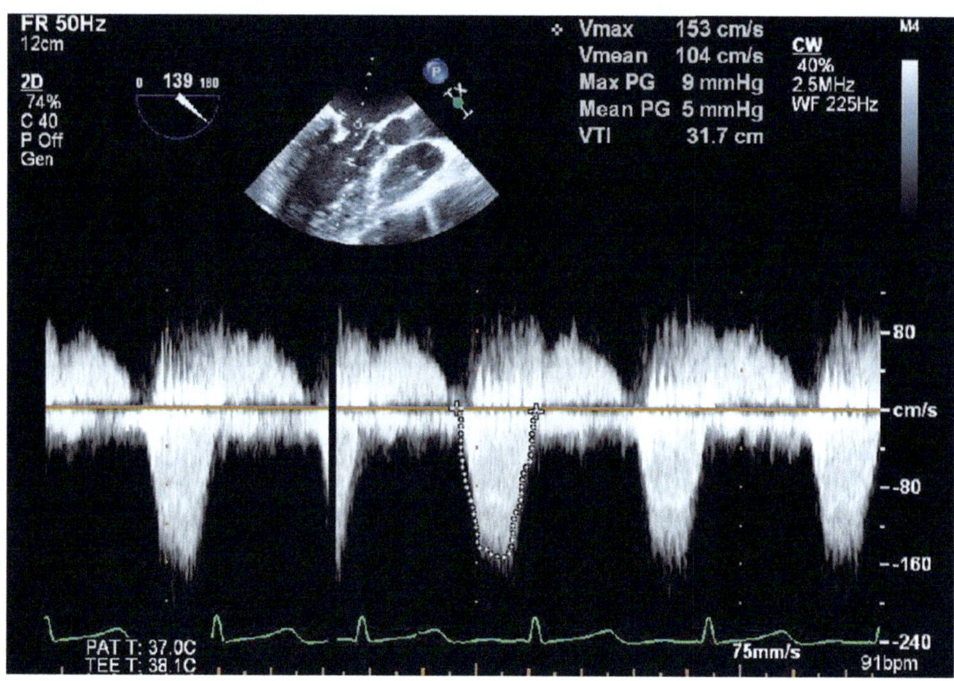

Fig. 11.47 A TEE image (0°) obtained 2 years later showed that the mitral annulus was severely thickened circumferentially, with laminated echogenic material extending from the annulus onto both leaflet bodies. This thickening restricted leaflet opening and resulted in a small, stenotic valve orifice

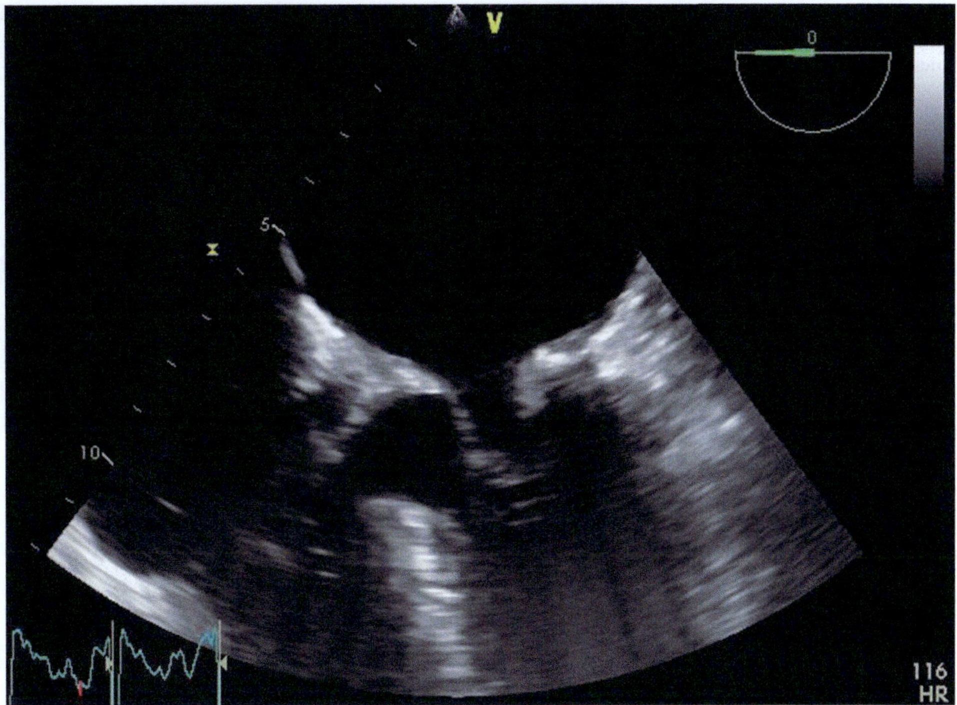

Fig. 11.48 TEE view at 60° also obtained 2 years later, showing thickening of the mitral annulus

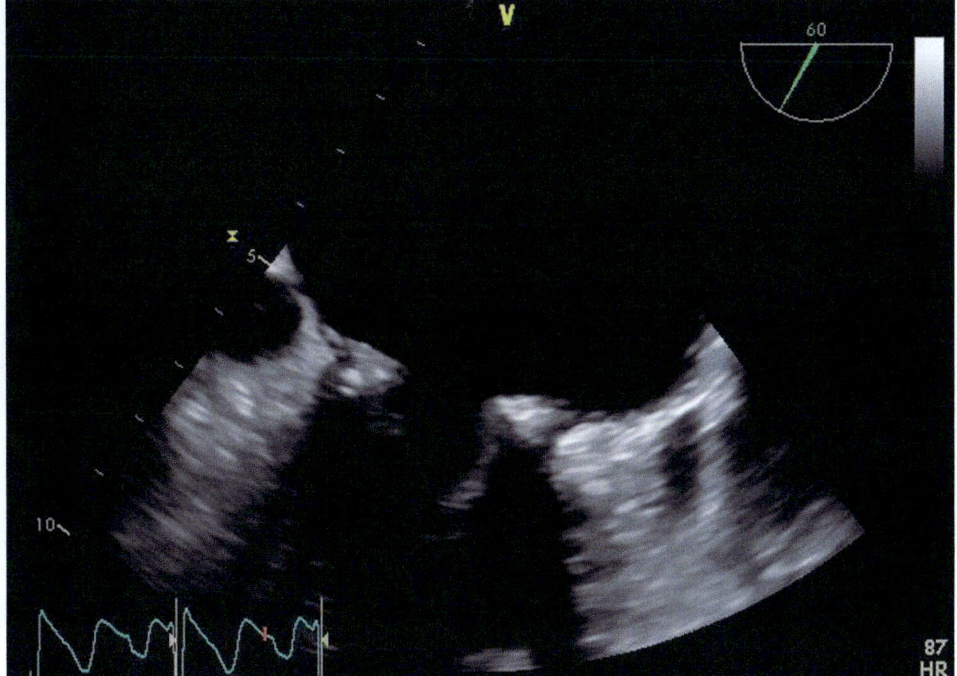

Fig. 11.49 TEE view at 90° also obtained 2 years later, showing thickening of the mitral annulus

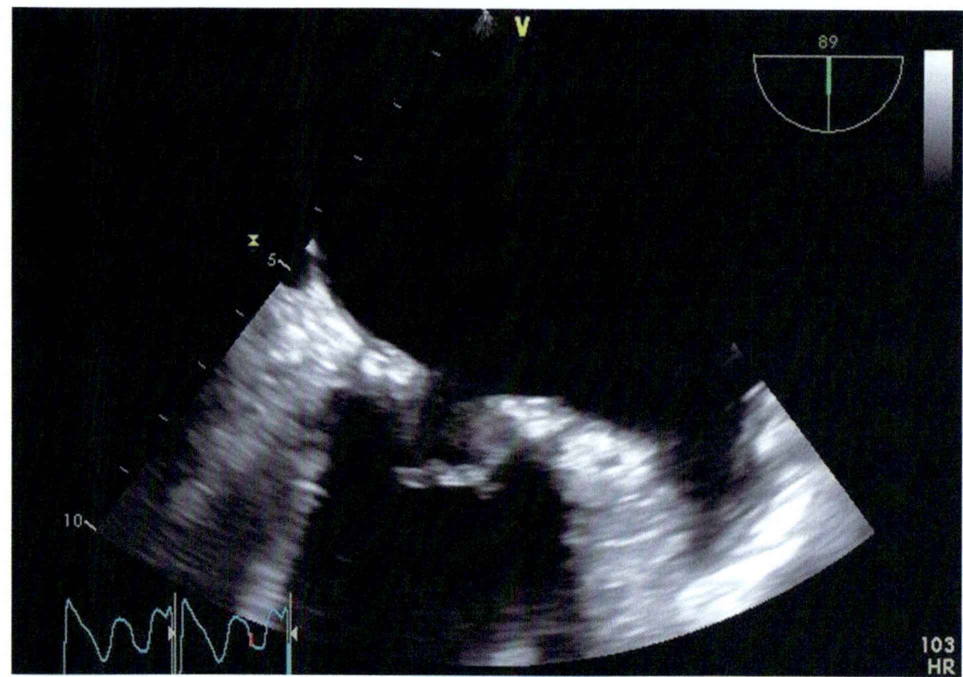

Fig. 11.50 TEE view at 120° also obtained 2 years later, showing thickening of the mitral annulus

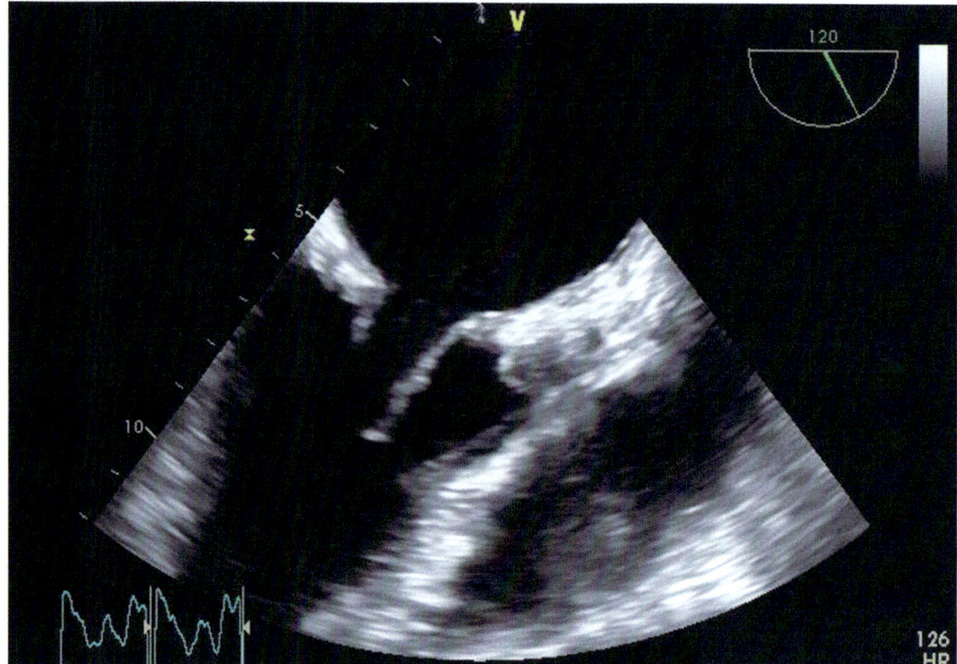

Fig. 11.51 A significant interval increase in transvalvular gradients was noted, to peak and mean gradients of 23 and 14 mmHg respectively

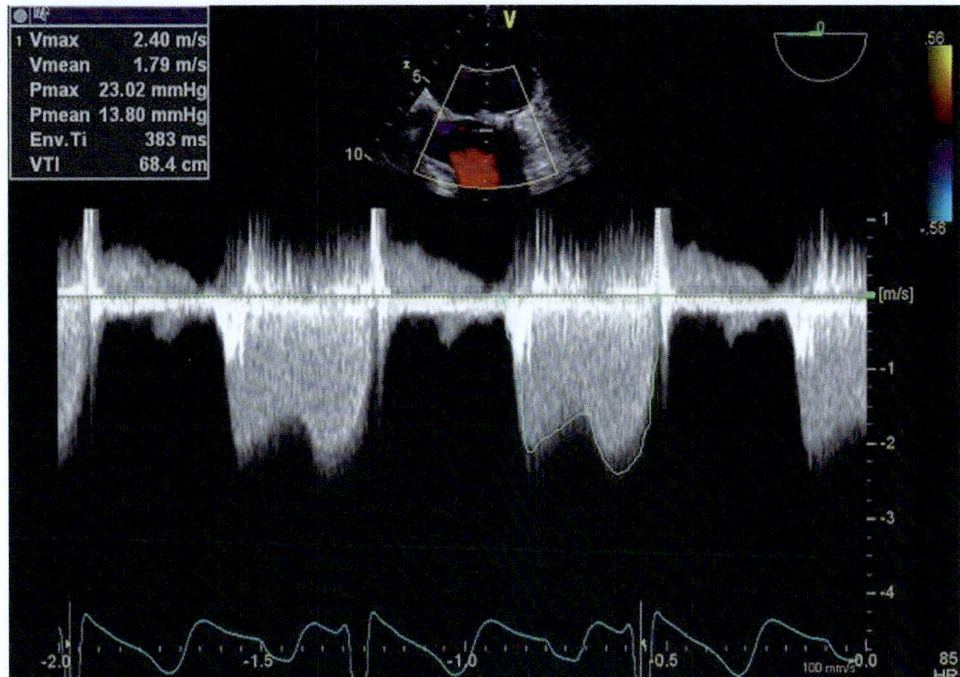

Fig. 11.52 3D imaging of the mitral valve demonstrated a significant reduction in valve orifice area related to the smooth, laminated echogenic material overlying the annuloplasty ring and extending onto the leaflet bases. Severe associated valve leaflet thickening was also evident

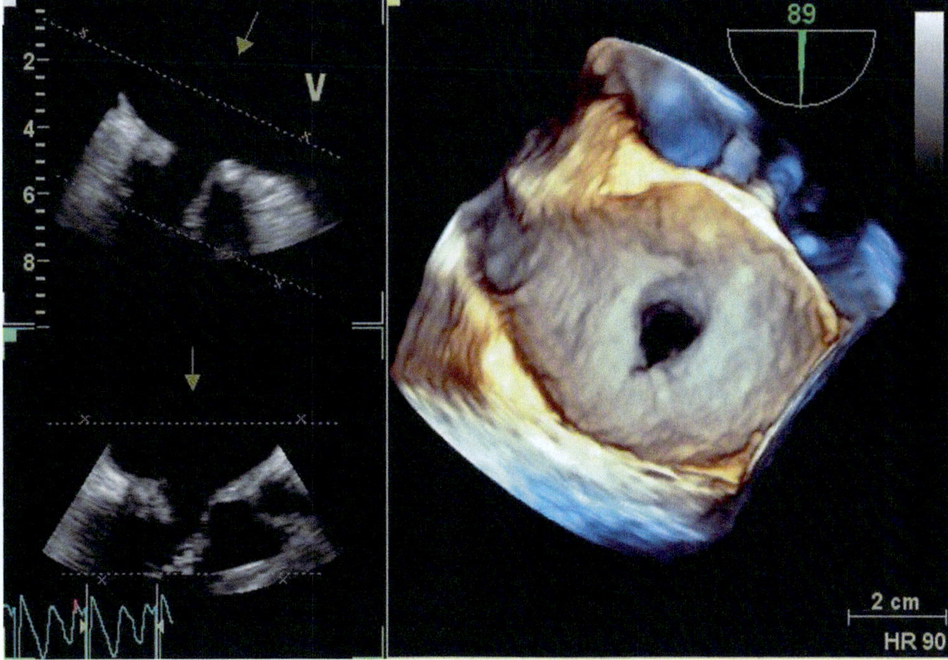

11.11 Case 11. Inflammatory Response

A 60-year-old woman was noted to have a new murmur, shortness of breath, and fatigue when presenting for routine cardiology review. She denied any constitutional symptoms, including fever, diaphoresis, or change in weight. Three months earlier she had undergone a mitral valve repair for severe symptomatic mitral regurgitation secondary to prolapse (Fig. 11.53).

She underwent a transesophageal echocardiogram, which demonstrated multiple mobile echodensities attached to the left atrial aspect of the mitral valve annuloplasty prosthesis, with suggestion of abscess formation along the intervalvular fibrosa and a small (0.6 cm, Qp:Qs 1.1) Gerbode-type defect (left ventricle to right atrial shunt) without evidence of right ventricular volume overload (Figs. 11.54, 11.55, 11.56, 11.57, and 11.58).

The appearance was felt to be concerning for vegetations or thrombi. She underwent cardiac surgery with resection of the previous annuloplasty ring, insertion of a bioprosthetic mitral valve replacement, and closure of the Gerbode defect. Histological assessment of the resected tissue revealed extensive chronic inflammation with a small amount of acute fibrinous exudate. No microorganisms or organized thrombi were identified.

On routine review 6 months later, she remained well, with no symptoms of heart failure or constitutional symptoms including fever, but repeat echocardiography again demonstrated multiple echodensities attached to the new valve prosthesis (Figs. 11.59 and 11.60). In view of her stable clinical status, it was felt that these new abnormalities represented a further inflammatory response to another valve prosthesis. She was managed conservatively with ongoing discussion regarding the need for therapeutic anticoagulation.

Video 11.45 Normal TEE (119° long-axis view) of the first bioprosthetic valve immediately after replacement (AVI 7356 kb)

Video 11.46 Standard TEE (0° view) demonstrating extensive multiple mobile echodensities attached to the left atrial aspect of the valve leaflets and annulus (AVI 8015 kb)

Video 11.47 Standard TEE (61° view) demonstrating extensive multiple mobile echodensities attached to the left atrial aspect of the valve leaflets and annulus (AVI 6522 kb)

Video 11.48 Standard TEE (94° view) demonstrating extensive multiple mobile echodensities attached to the left atrial aspect of the valve leaflets and annulus (AVI 6563 kb)

Video 11.49 Biplane 0/90° view demonstrating orthogonal views of the mitral valve prosthesis with multiple mobile echodensities attached (AVI 4399 kb)

Video 11.50 3D reconstruction of the mitral valve prosthesis with multiple mobile echodensities attached to the valve annulus and leaflets (AVI 1340 kb)

Video 11.51 Repeat TEE after the redo bioprosthetic mitral valve replacement also demonstrated small, mobile echodensities adherent to the left atrial aspect of the prosthetic valve annulus (AVI 7291 kb)

Video 11.52 Repeat TEE after the redo bioprosthetic mitral valve replacement also demonstrated small, mobile echodensities adherent to the left atrial aspect of the prosthetic valve annulus (AVI 3147 kb)

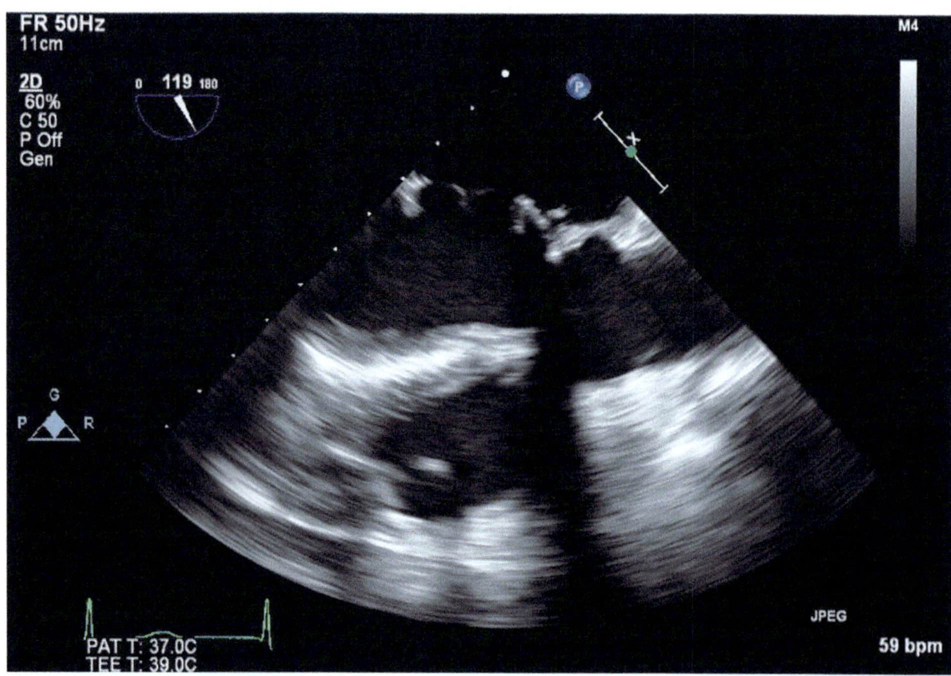

Fig. 11.53 Normal TEE (119° long-axis view) of the first bioprosthetic valve immediately after replacement

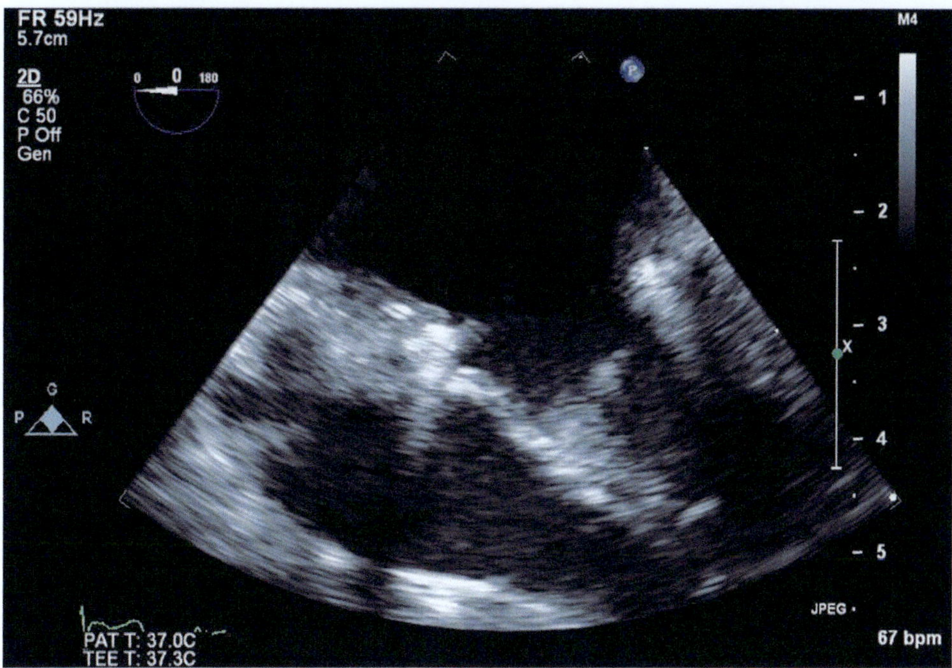

Fig. 11.54 Standard TEE (0° view) demonstrating extensive multiple mobile echodensities attached to the left atrial aspect of the valve leaflets and annulus

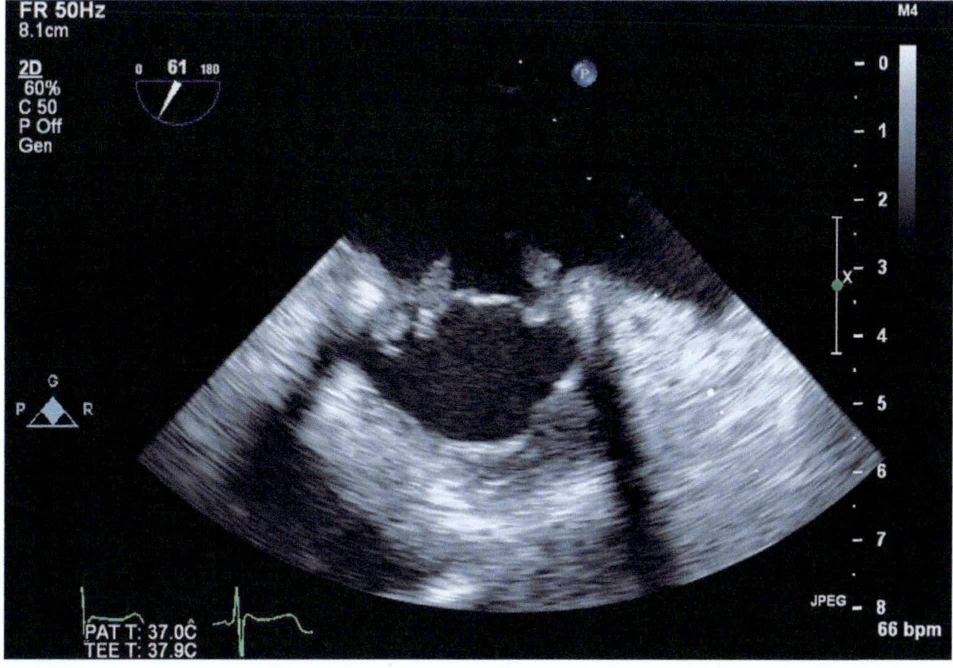

Fig. 11.55 Standard TEE (61° view) demonstrating extensive multiple mobile echodensities attached to the left atrial aspect of the valve leaflets and annulus

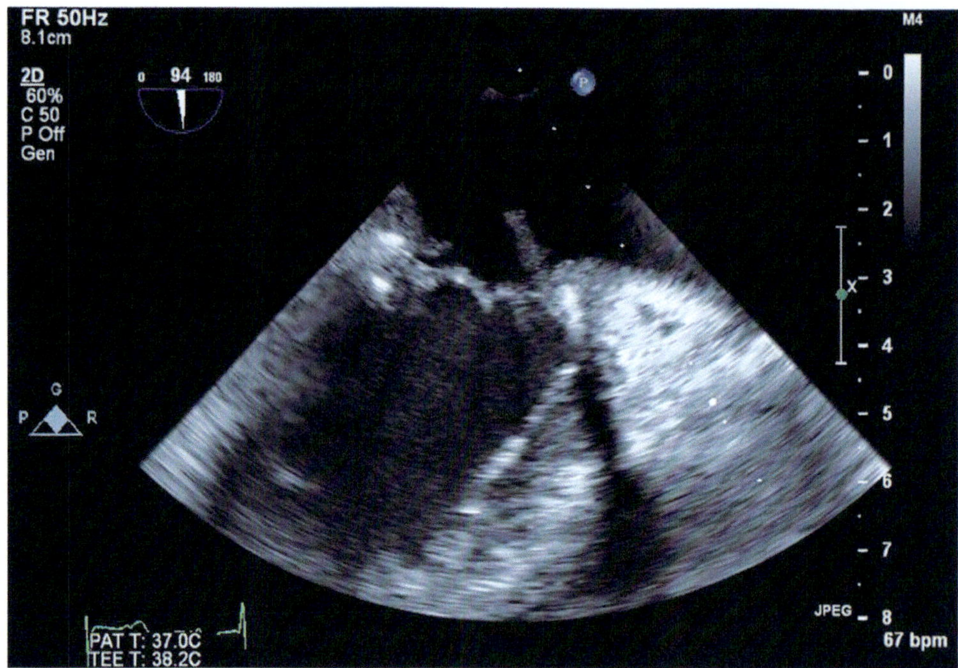

Fig. 11.56 Standard TEE (94° view) demonstrating extensive multiple mobile echodensities attached to the left atrial aspect of the valve leaflets and annulus

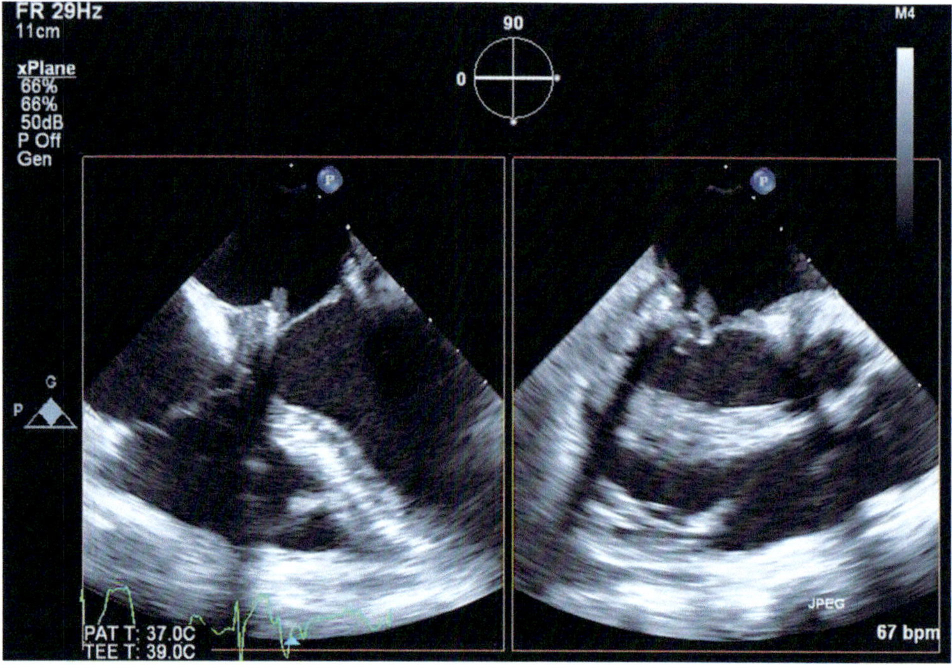

Fig. 11.57 Biplane 0/90° view demonstrating orthogonal views of the mitral valve prosthesis with multiple mobile echodensities attached

Fig. 11.58 3D reconstruction of the mitral valve prosthesis with multiple mobile echodensities attached to the valve annulus and leaflets

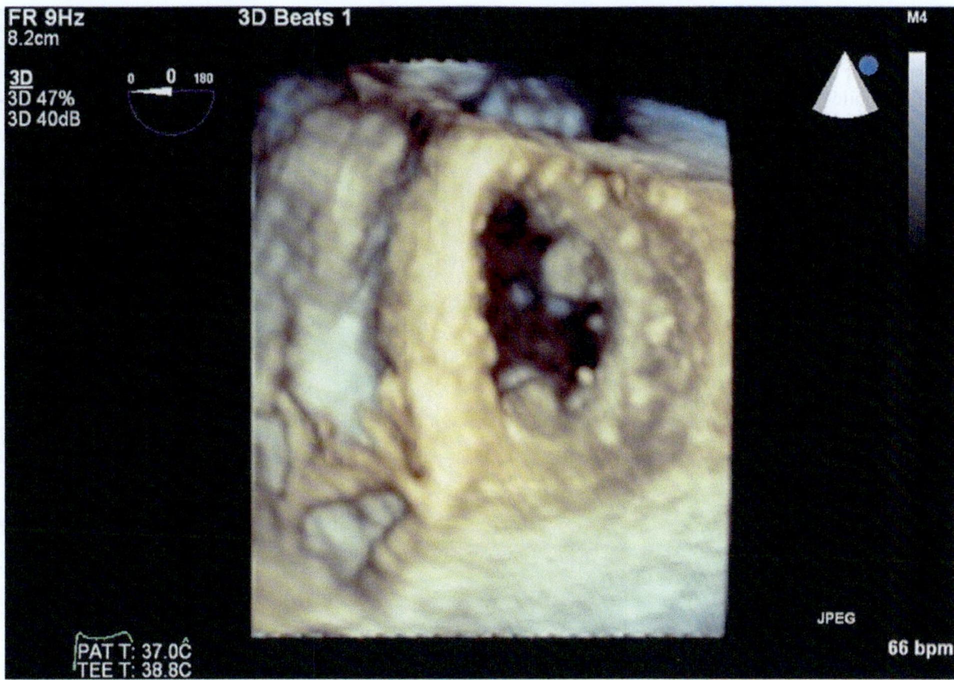

Fig. 11.59 Repeat TEE after the redo bioprosthetic mitral valve replacement also demonstrated small, mobile echodensities adherent to the left atrial aspect of the prosthetic valve annulus

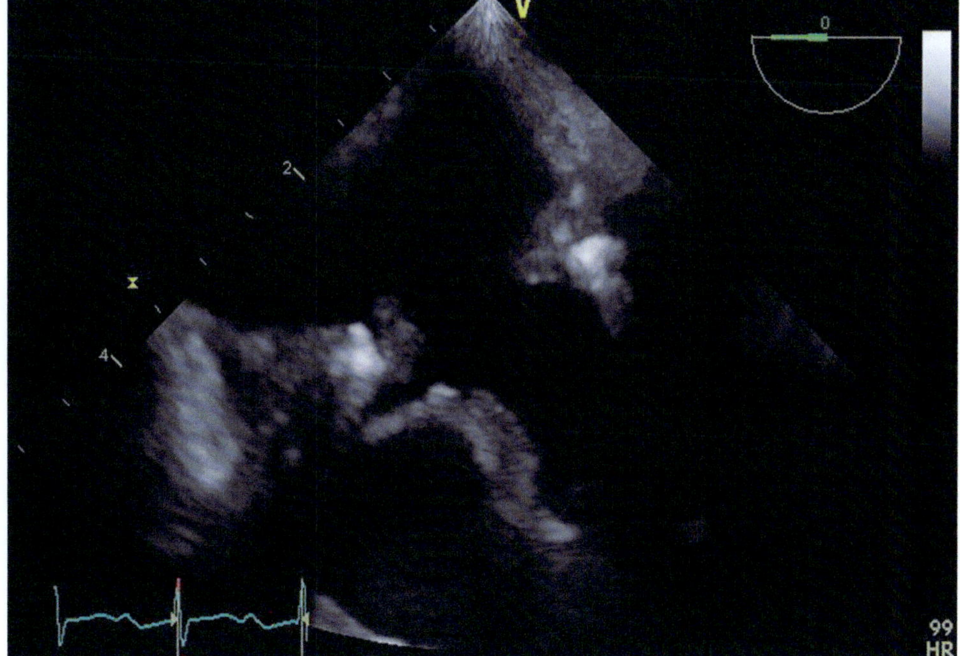

Fig. 11.60 Repeat TEE after the redo bioprosthetic mitral valve replacement also demonstrated small, mobile echodensities adherent to the left atrial aspect of the prosthetic valve annulus

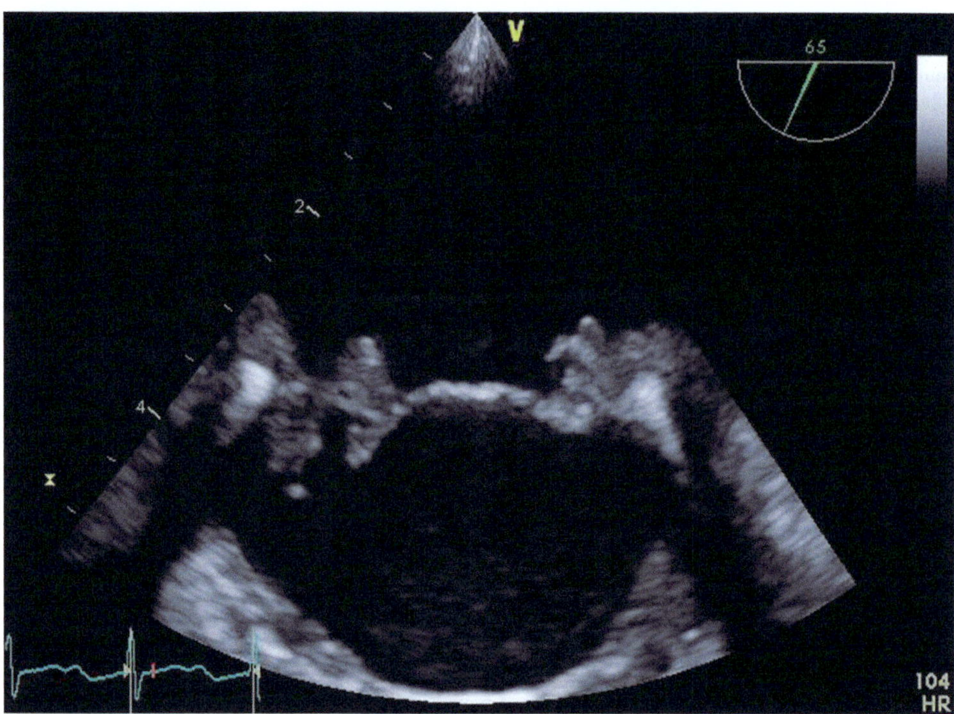

11.12 Case 12. Mitral Valve Prosthesis Thrombus

A 72-year-old woman with a history of rheumatic heart disease, obstructive lung disease, hypertension, and chronic kidney disease underwent a third-time redo double valve replacement involving a mitral valve replacement (27-mm Biocor bioprosthesis), aortic root replacement with reimplantation of the coronary arteries, an aortic valve replacement (25-mm Freestyle bioprosthesis), and ascending aorta graft repair. The redo mitral valve replacement had required extensive annular débridement and reconstruction of the fibrous skeleton of the heart with pericardial patches because of heavy calcification. The postoperative period was complicated by shock requiring arteriovenous extracorporeal membrane oxygenation support. Thrombus formation within the left atrium involved the mitral valve prosthesis, and she was returned to surgery for urgent thrombectomy of the mitral valve. Layered thrombus was found within the left atrium, which extended across the mitral valve and impeded its opening (Figs. 11.61, 11.62, 11.63, 11.64, 11.65, 11.66, 11.67, 11.68, and 11.69).

Video 11.53 3D reconstruction of the mitral valve immediately after initial implantation, demonstrating a normal, functioning valve (AVI 996 kb)

Video 11.54 Two days after surgery, while the patient was on arteriovenous extracorporeal membrane oxygenation support, TEE (0° view) demonstrated severe biventricular dysfunction and severe mitral valve dysfunction. Both leaflets demonstrated very poor mobility and were severely restricted by overlying thrombus, which extended into the left atrium. Swirling sludge could be seen throughout the left atrium. The left atrial appendage had been ligated at the time of the original surgery (AVI 7260 kb)

Video 11.55 TEE (138° view) performed at the same time as Video 11.54 also demonstrated severe biventricular dysfunction and severe mitral valve dysfunction. Both leaflets demonstrated very poor mobility and were severely restricted by overlying thrombus, which extended into the left atrium. Swirling sludge could be seen throughout the left atrium (AVI 7232 kb)

Video 11.56 Color Doppler imaging demonstrated only a small jet of turbulent forwards flow across the severely stenotic mitral valve (AVI 2125 kb)

Video 11.57 3D reconstruction of the mitral valve showed a severely stenotic valve with only a slit-like valve orifice remaining (AVI 1136 kb)

Video 11.58 After the thrombectomy, leaflet mobility improved, but a degree of restricted leaflet excursion persisted because of residual thrombus on the valve leaflets and annulus. Biventricular function remained severely impaired (AVI 3627 kb)

Video 11.59 Zoomed view of Video 11.58 (AVI 5439 kb)

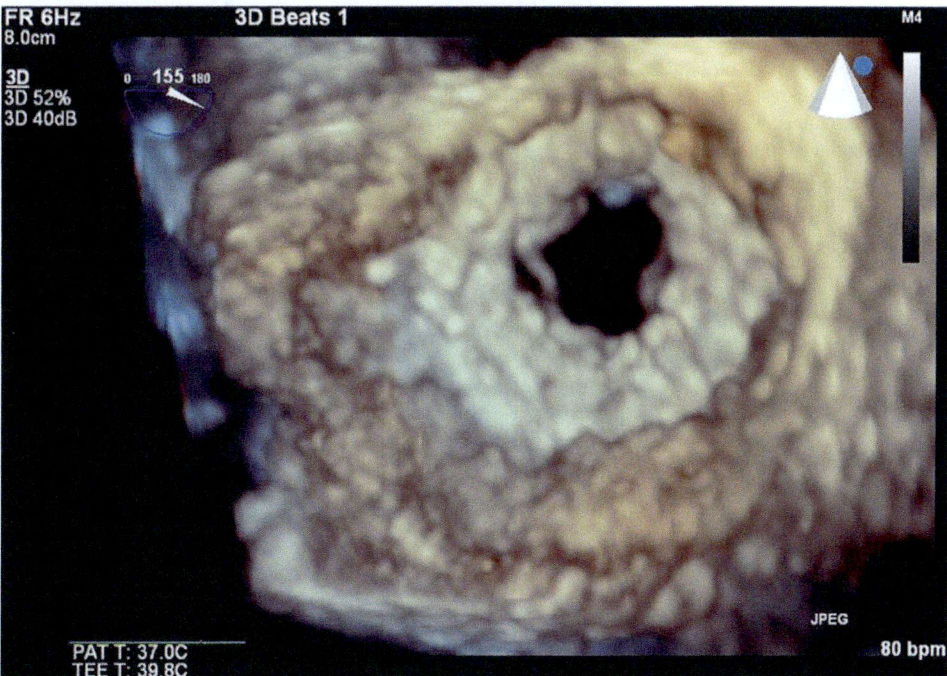

Fig. 11.61 3D reconstruction of the mitral valve immediately after initial implantation, demonstrating a normal, functioning valve

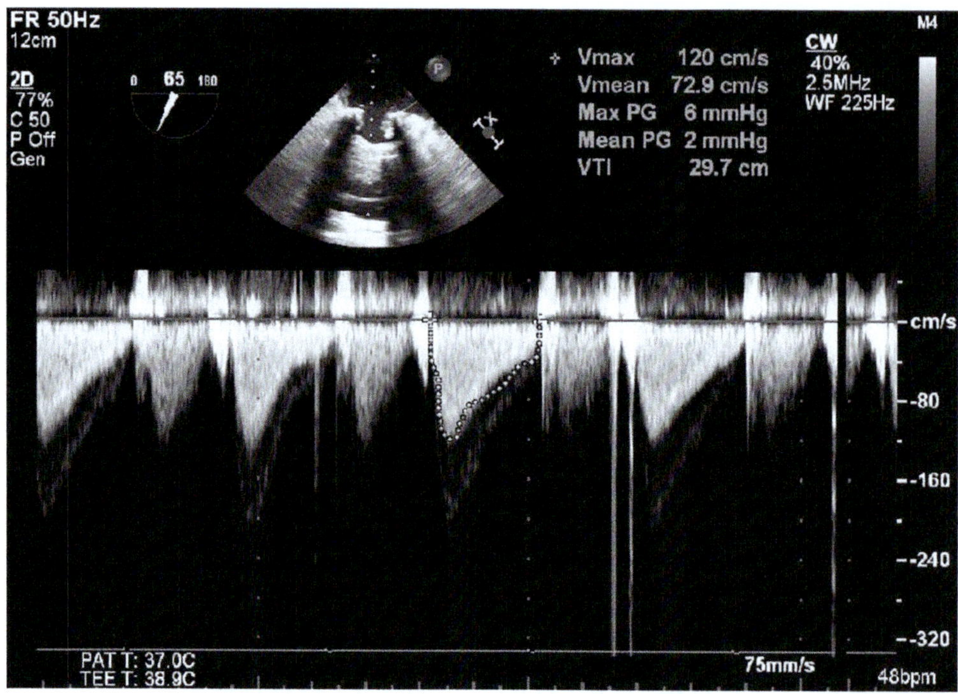

Fig. 11.62 Peak transvalvular gradient (6 mmHg) and mean transvalvular gradient (2 mmHg) immediately after implantation

Fig. 11.63 Two days after surgery, while the patient was on arteriovenous extracorporeal membrane oxygenation support, TEE (0° view) demonstrated severe biventricular dysfunction and severe mitral valve dysfunction. Both leaflets demonstrated very poor mobility and were severely restricted by overlying thrombus, which extended into the left atrium. Swirling sludge could be seen throughout the left atrium. The left atrial appendage had been ligated at the time of the original surgery

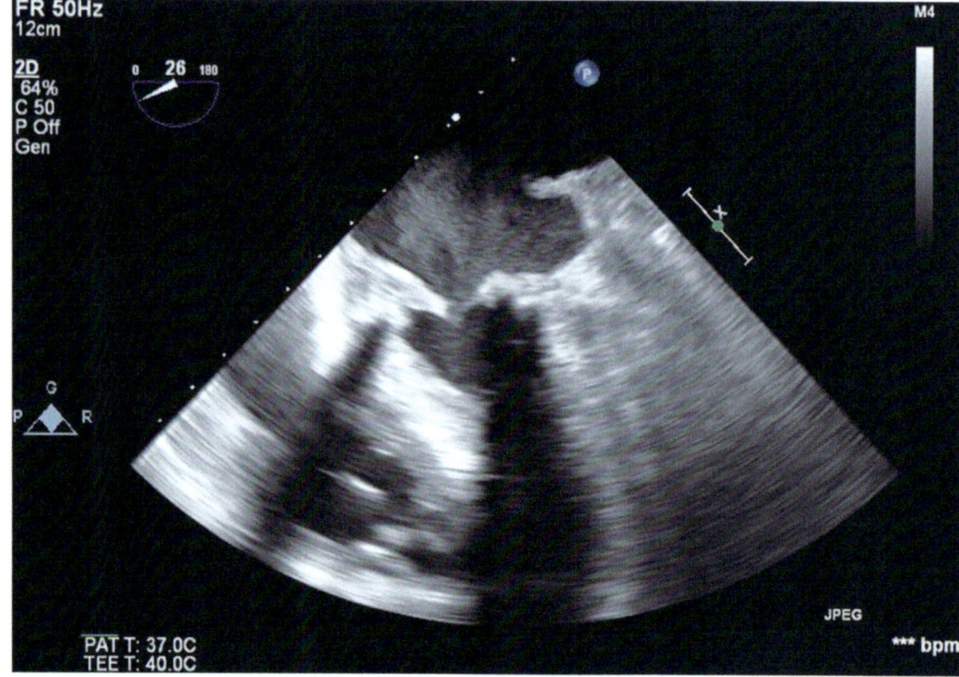

Fig. 11.64 TEE (138° view) performed at the same time as Fig. 11.63 also demonstrated severe biventricular dysfunction and severe mitral valve dysfunction. Both leaflets demonstrated very poor mobility and were severely restricted by overlying thrombus, which extended into the left atrium. Swirling sludge could be seen throughout the left atrium

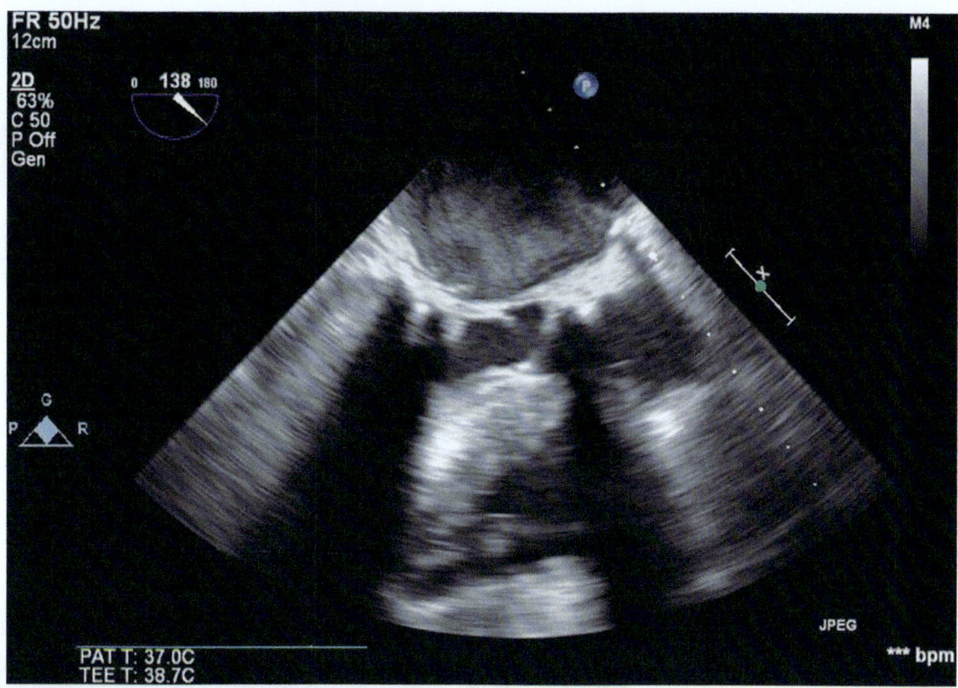

Fig. 11.65 Color Doppler imaging demonstrated only a small jet of turbulent forwards flow across the severely stenotic mitral valve

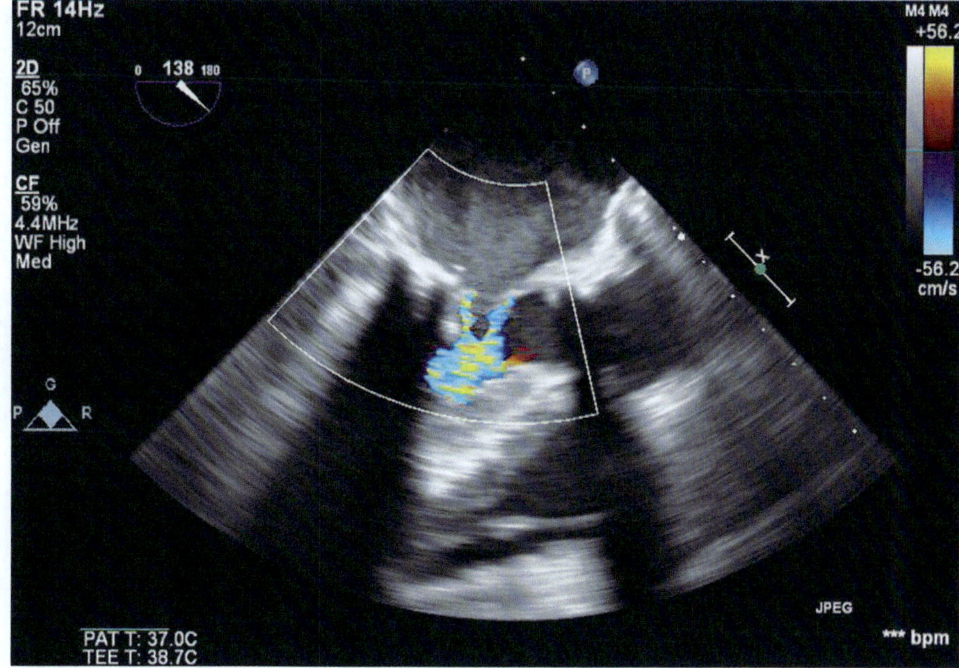

Fig. 11.66 3D reconstruction of the mitral valve showed a severely stenotic valve with only a slit-like valve orifice remaining

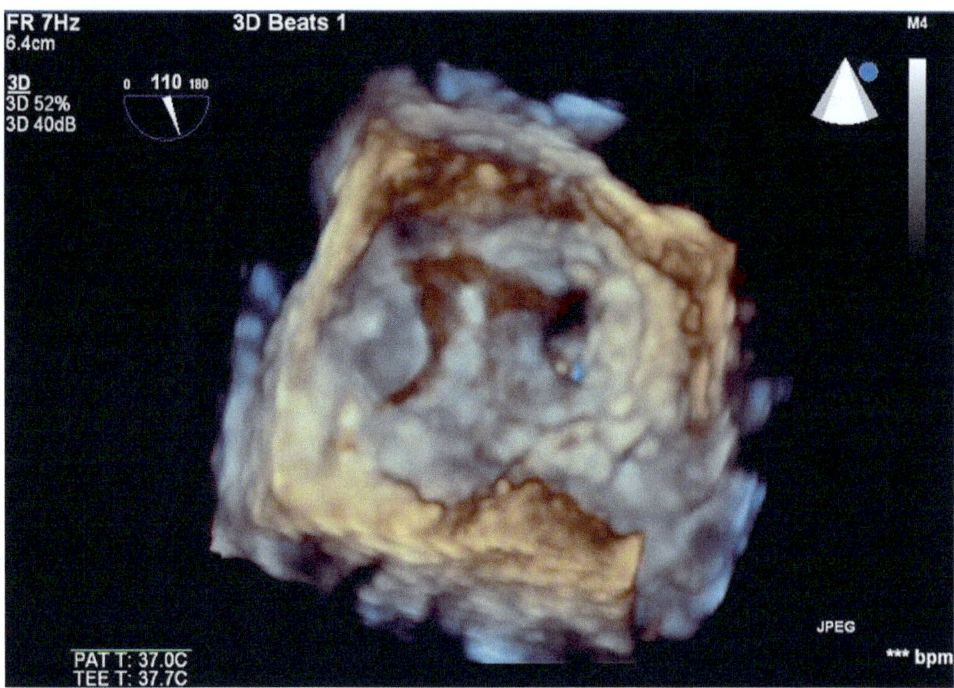

Fig. 11.67 Transvalvular gradients across the thrombosed valve had significantly increased to a peak and mean of 34 and 24 mmHg respectively

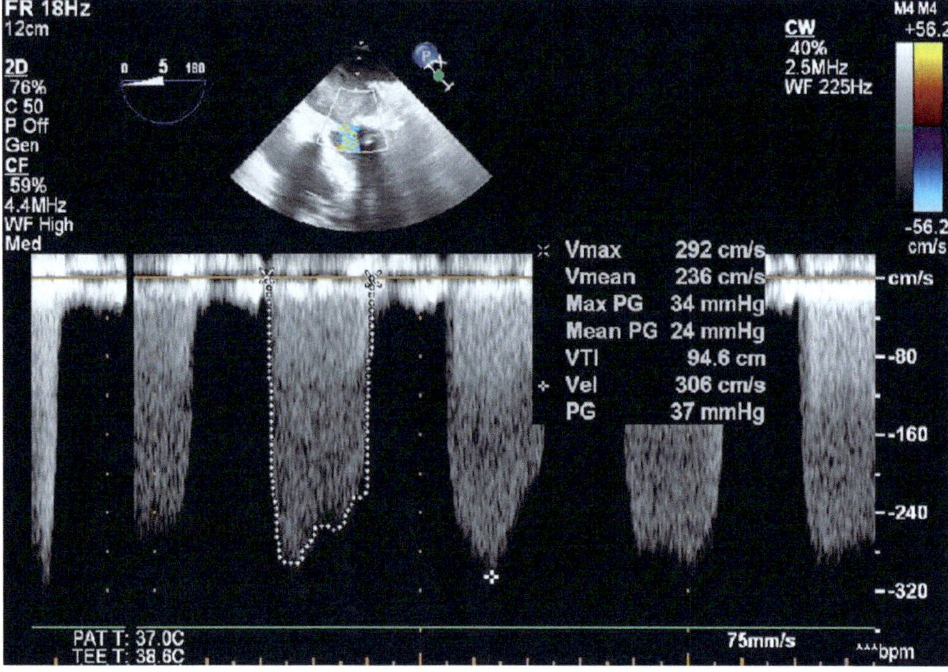

Fig. 11.68 After the thrombectomy, TEE (0° midesophageal view) demonstrated improved leaflet mobility, however a degree of restricted leaflet excursion persisted due to residual thrombus on the valve leaflets and annulus. Biventricular function remained severely impaired

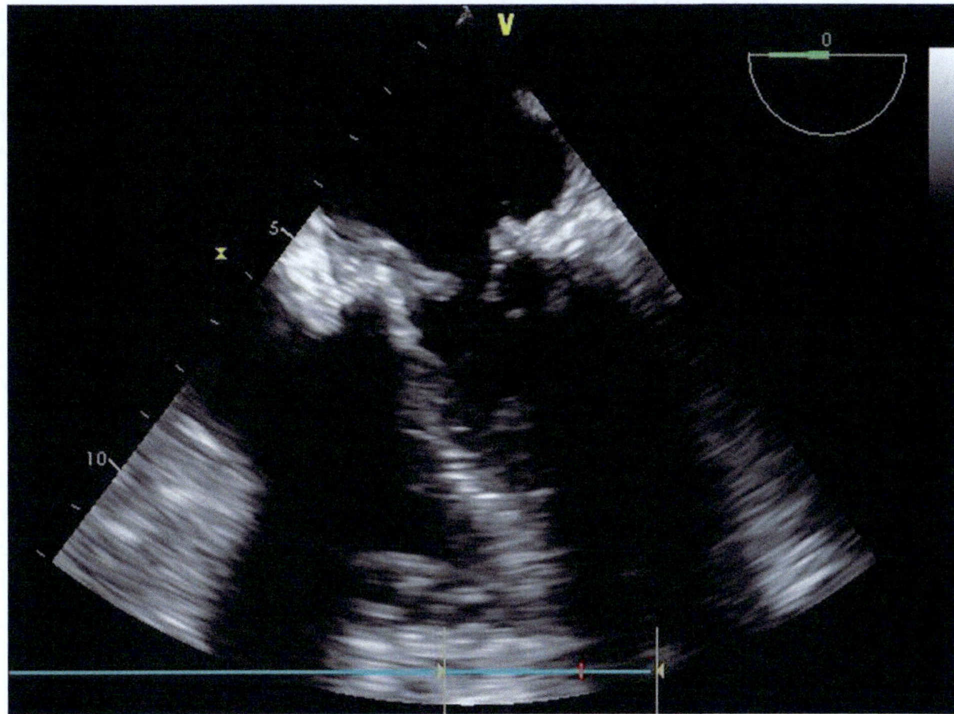

Fig. 11.69 Zoomed view of Fig. 11.68

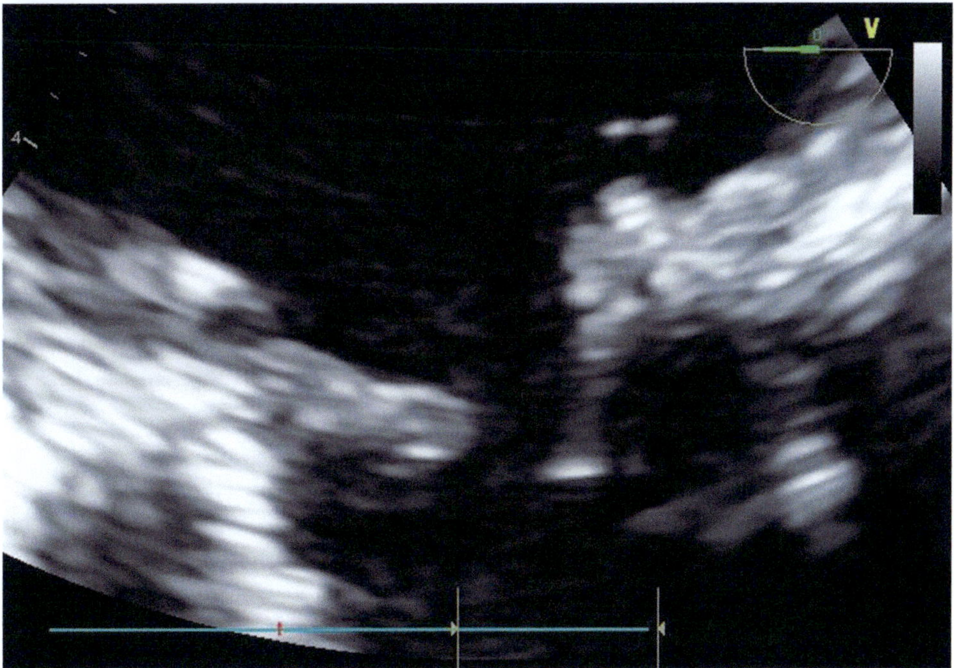

11.13 Case 13. Mitral Valve Thrombus

A 77-year-old man with a past history of recurrent deep vein thromboses and an inferior vena cava filter presented with severe mitral regurgitation due to a partial flail anterior mitral valve leaflet. He underwent a mitral valve replacement with 31-mm Magna pericardial prosthesis. Several days later, he developed shortness of breath, congestion on chest x-ray, and atrial fibrillation.

Transesophageal echocardiography revealed layered thrombus measuring up to 1 cm in diameter within the left atrium, along the interatrial septum and within the left atrial appendage. The lateral leaflet of the mitral bioprosthesis was fixed and thickened, probably related to superimposed thrombus (Figs. 11.70, 11.71, 11.72, and 11.73).

The patient was found to have a complex hypercoagulable state related to lupus anticoagulant and heterozygosity for Factor V Leiden deficiency. He was maintained on therapeutic anticoagulation, with gradual reduction of the left atrial thrombus burden and improvement in symptoms. The lateral leaflet remained restricted, but given his hypercoagulable state, he was managed conservatively.

Video 11.60 (a) TEE (0° view) showing that the lateral prosthetic valve leaflet is relatively fixed because of overlying thrombus, which also extends onto the annulus (AVI 6167 kb)

Video 11.60 (b) Zoomed view of Video 11.60a (AVI 8609 kb)

Video 11.61 Color Doppler imaging demonstrated significant turbulence in the flow across the valve, suggestive of valvular stenosis. Trivial regurgitation was noted (AVI 2146 kb)

Video 11.62 3D imaging of the trileaflet, bioprosthetic mitral valve prosthesis viewed from the left atrium. Significant restriction of lateral leaflet is noted, with relatively preserved excursion of the other two leaflets (AVI 1227 kb)

Fig. 11.70 (**a**) TEE (0° view) showing that the lateral prosthetic valve leaflet is relatively fixed because of overlying thrombus, which also extends onto the annulus. (**b**) Zoomed view

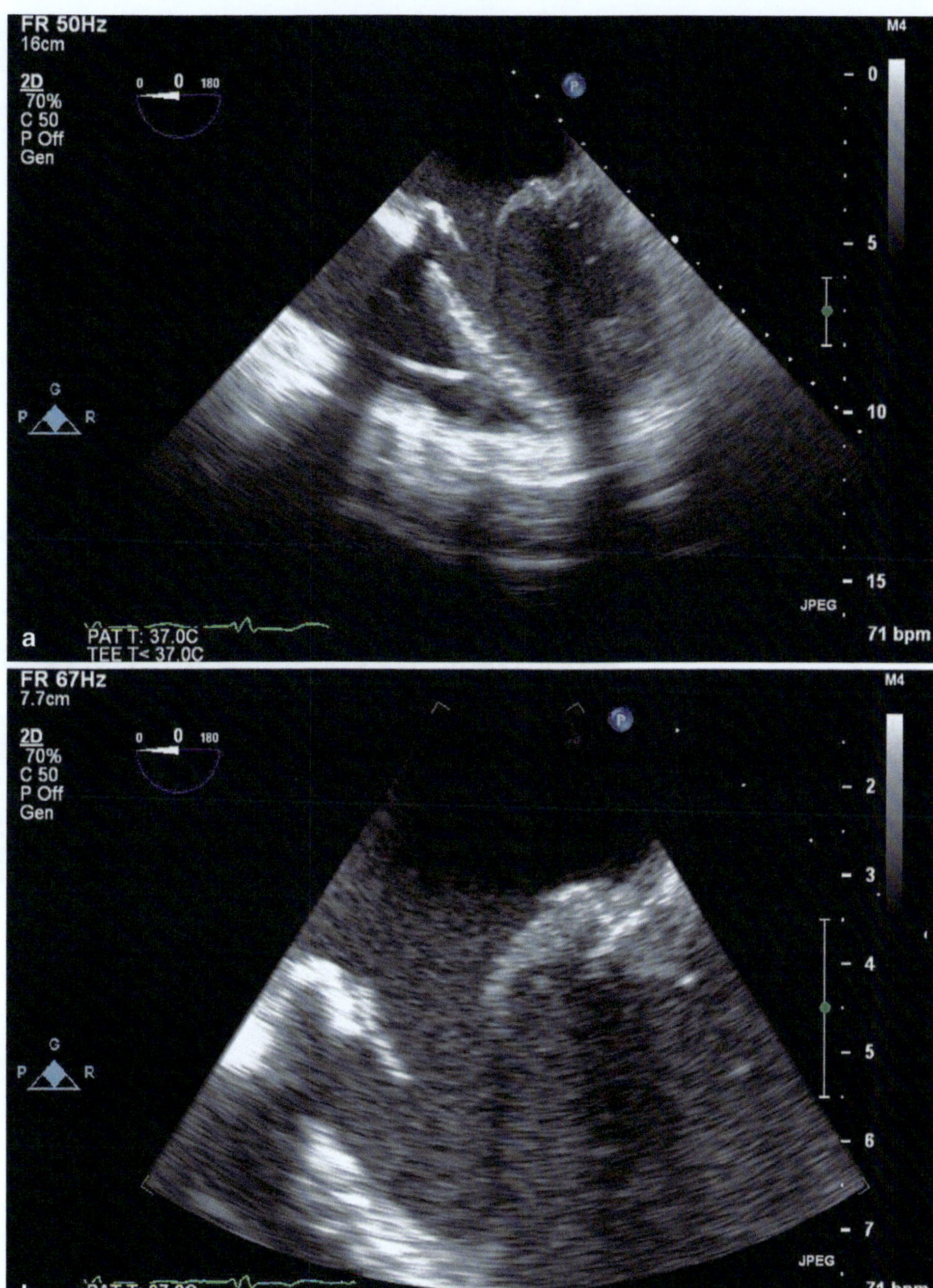

Fig. 11.71 Color Doppler imaging demonstrated significant turbulence in the flow across the valve, suggestive of valvular stenosis. Trivial regurgitation was noted

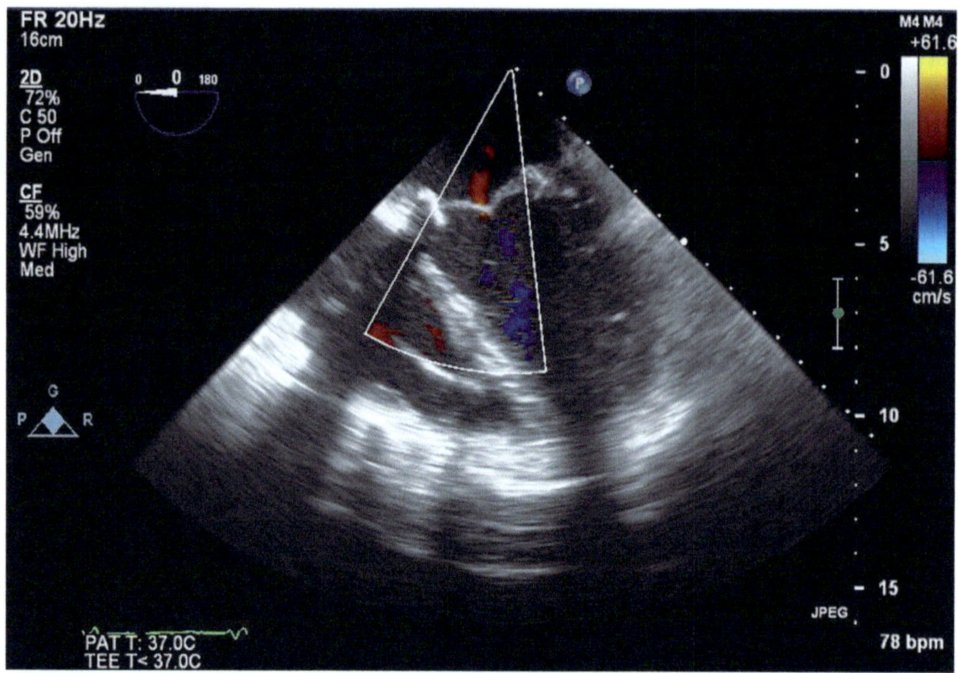

Fig. 11.72 3D imaging of the trileaflet, bioprosthetic mitral valve prosthesis viewed from the left atrium. Significant restriction of lateral leaflet is noted, with relatively preserved excursion of the other two leaflets

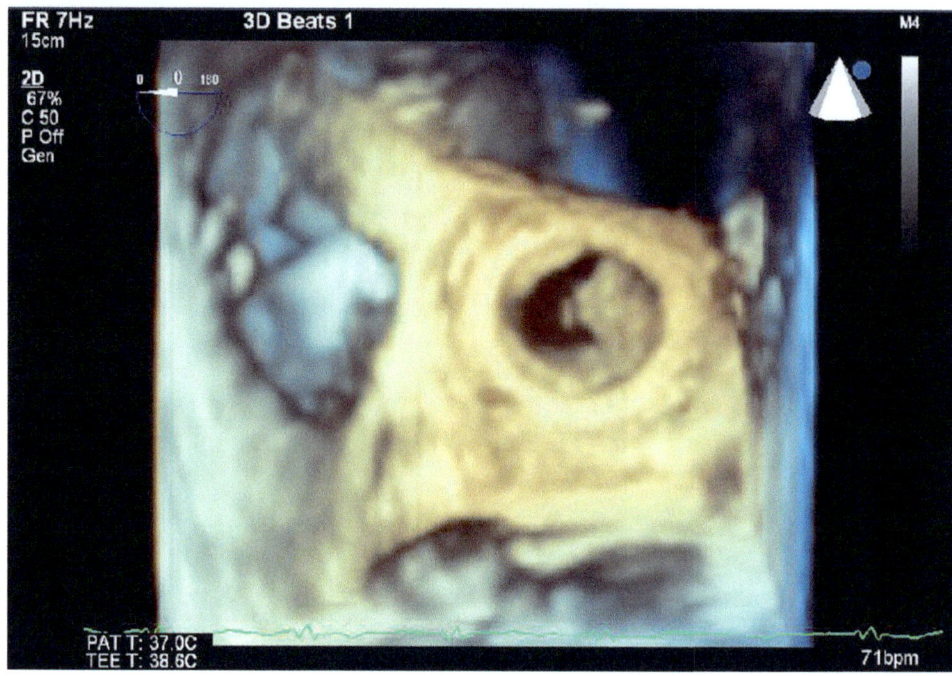

Fig. 11.73 Despite leaflet restriction, the transvalvular gradients were only mildly increased overall (peak, 11 mmHg; mean, 4 mmHg)

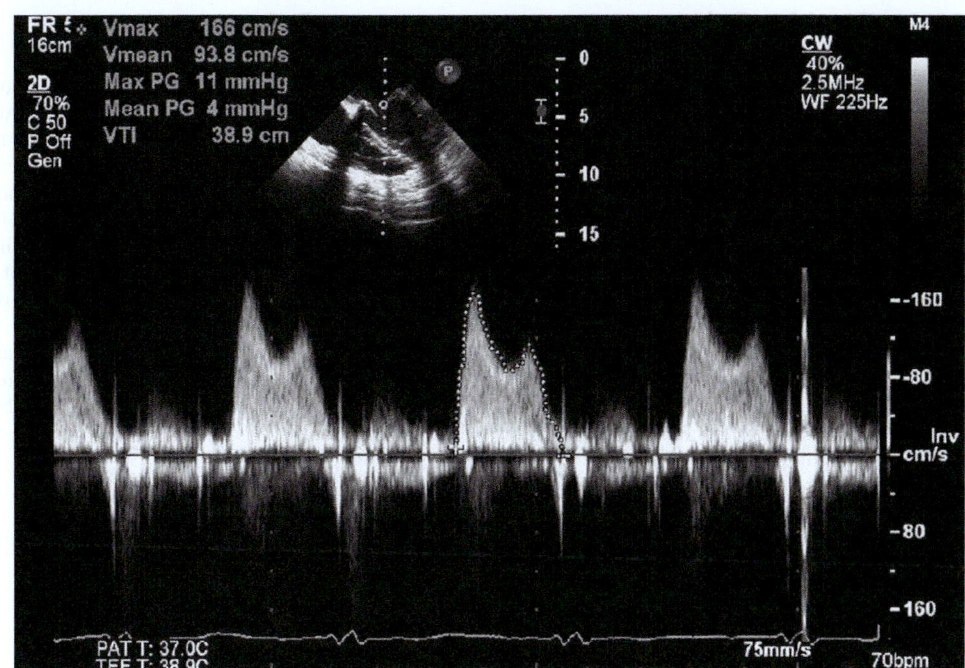

11.14 Teaching Points

- Hemolytic anemia in the setting of a paravalvular leak suggests that the defect is actually small. Turbulence of blood flow through the small communication results in hemolysis.
- Regardless of severity, the prognosis for ischemic mitral regurgitation is worse than for nonischemic mitral regurgitation. The recent changes in the AHA/ACC valve guidelines reflect this difference, reclassifying ischemic mitral regurgitation graded as 2+ and over as severe [1].
- Repair of the mitral valve is technically challenging. Overall, the highest rates of successful repair are achieved in valve centers of excellence by surgeons who perform high volumes of cases. A good replacement is always better than a poor repair, which may lead to premature redo surgery.
- A repair is usually preferred over a replacement because of both valve longevity and the avoidance of anticoagulation. Repair may not be feasible if the valve is stenotic, calcified, significantly thickened, or morphologically unsuitable. Valve surgery in the setting of ischemic mitral regurgitation remains controversial [2].
- Minimally invasive and percutaneous approaches for mitral valve surgery are gaining acceptance, although they lack long-term data regarding complication rates and durability. These approaches may be alternative treatment options for patients who are felt to be poor surgical candidates because of age or comorbidities.
- 3D/4D imaging has revolutionized our ability to diagnose and quantify prosthetic valve dysfunction [3].

References

1. Nishimura RA, Otto CM, Bonow RO, Carabello BA, Erwin 3rd JP, Guyton RA, et al. 2014 AHA/ACC guideline for the management of patients with Valvular Heart Disease: a report of the American College of Cardiology/American Heart Association Task Force on Practice Guidelines. Circulation. 2014;129:e521–643.
2. Kronzon I, Sugeng L, Perk G, Hirsh D, Weinert L, Garcia Fernandez MA, Lang RM. Real-time 3-dimensional transesophageal echocardiography in the evaluation of post-operative mitral annuloplasty ring and prosthetic valve dehiscence. J Am Coll Cardiol. 2009;53:1543–7.
3. Acker MA, Parides MK, Perrault LP, Moskowitz AJ, Gelijns AC, Voisine P, et al. Mitral-valve repair versus replacement for severe ischemic mitral regurgitation. N Engl J Med. 2014;370:23–32.

Applications of Stress Echocardiography in Mitral Valve Disease

12

Christine Jellis

Although stress echocardiography is primarily used to exclude inducible myocardial ischemia, it also has several useful applications related to mitral valve functional assessment. Its main role relates to assessment of contractile reserve, which can be used to optimally time mitral valve surgery in the setting of significant mitral regurgitation (MR). Clinically, stress echocardiography is most often used in the setting of myxomatous mitral valve prolapse with severe regurgitation but an absence of symptoms. Exercise stress echocardiography allows physicians to assess the patient's exercise capacity, investigate for exercise-induced pulmonary hypertension, and perhaps most importantly, assess the left ventricle's response to exercise. Unmasking of impaired functional capacity, inducible pulmonary hypertension, precipitation of atrial arrhythmias, worsening of MR severity, or failure of augmentation in left ventricular systolic function with exercise all may suggest that the patient will benefit from mitral valve surgery. Ideally, this surgery should involve mitral valve repair, so structural information regarding leaflet morphology or thickening, subvalvular apparatus, and the degree of calcification are important observations to include for preoperative planning.

At peak exercise, the left ventricular end-systolic cavity size should be visibly smaller than the cavity size at rest. Quantitatively, it has been shown that preserved contractile reserve is reflected by an increase in ejection fraction of at least 4 % owing to a reduction in end-systolic volume [1]. If this change in ejection fraction is not achieved, contractile reserve is said to be impaired. Clinically, this condition reflects an inability of the left ventricle to cope with the volume load of severe MR. It also may be related to underlying myocardial fibrosis, which prevents an increase in left ventricular stress function.

Exercise stress echocardiography also can be used to gain additional information regarding borderline-severe mitral stenosis. Impaired exercise capacity, a mean mitral transvalvular gradient of 10 mmHg or higher at peak stress, abnormally elevated peak-stress pulmonary pressures, or a combination of these findings supports a diagnosis of hemodynamically significant mitral stenosis that may warrant surgical intervention.

Electronic supplementary material The online version of this chapter (doi:10.1007/978-1-4471-6672-6_12) contains supplementary material, which is available to authorized users.

C. Jellis
Department of Cardiovascular Medicine, Cleveland Clinic,
9500 Euclid Avenue, Cleveland, OH 44195, USA
e-mail: jellisc@ccf.org

M. Desai et al. (eds.), *An Atlas of Mitral Valve Imaging*,
DOI 10.1007/978-1-4471-6672-6_12, © Springer-Verlag London 2015

12.1 Case 1. Preserved Contractile Reserve: Normal Left Ventricular Stress Response

A 44-year-old hospital administrator presents with posterior mitral valve leaflet prolapse and severe, anteriorly directed MR. Echocardiography was performed before and after 14 min of treadmill exercise stress. The ejection fraction increased from 65 to 73 % and the left ventricular end-systolic volume decreased from 45 to 22 mL, consistent with preserved contractile reserve. This case illustrates a normal ventricular response to exercise stress.

Video 12.1 Parasternal long-axis end-systolic image at rest, demonstrating posterior mitral valve leaflet prolapse (AVI 1240 kb)

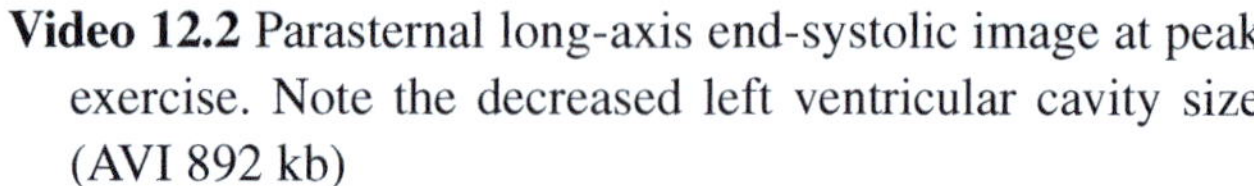

Video 12.2 Parasternal long-axis end-systolic image at peak exercise. Note the decreased left ventricular cavity size (AVI 892 kb)

Video 12.3 Parasternal short-axis end-systolic image at rest (AVI 1241 kb)

Video 12.4 Parasternal short-axis end-systolic image at peak exercise. Note the decreased left ventricular cavity size (AVI 932 kb)

Video 12.5 Apical two-chamber end-systolic image at rest (AVI 1273 kb)

Video 12.6 Apical two-chamber end-systolic image at peak exercise. Note the decreased left ventricular cavity size (AVI 849 kb)

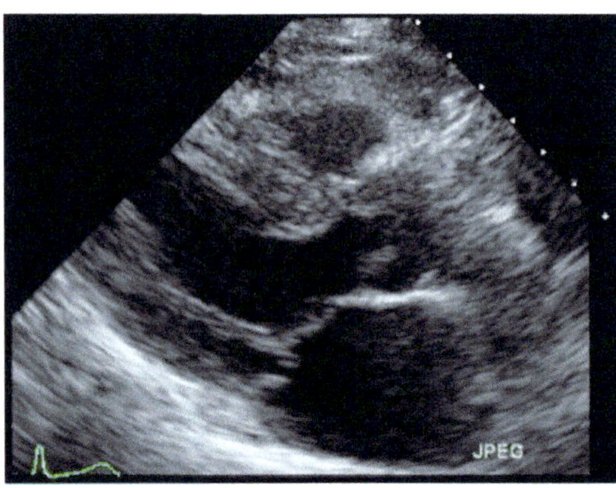

Fig. 12.1 Parasternal long-axis end-systolic image at rest, demonstrating posterior mitral valve leaflet prolapse

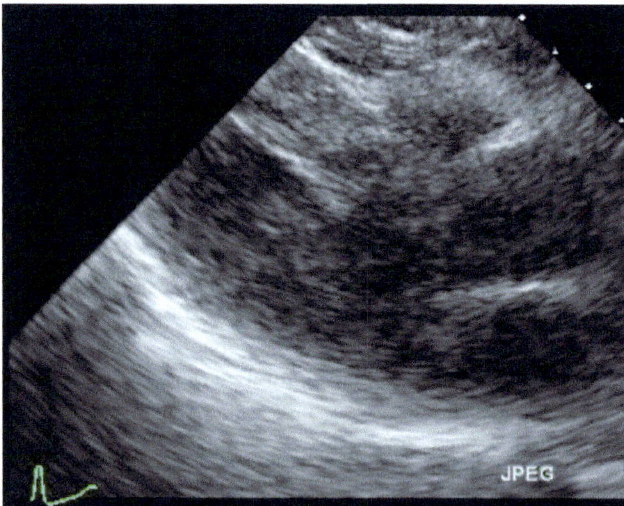

Fig. 12.2 Parasternal long-axis end-systolic image at peak exercise. Note the decreased left ventricular cavity size

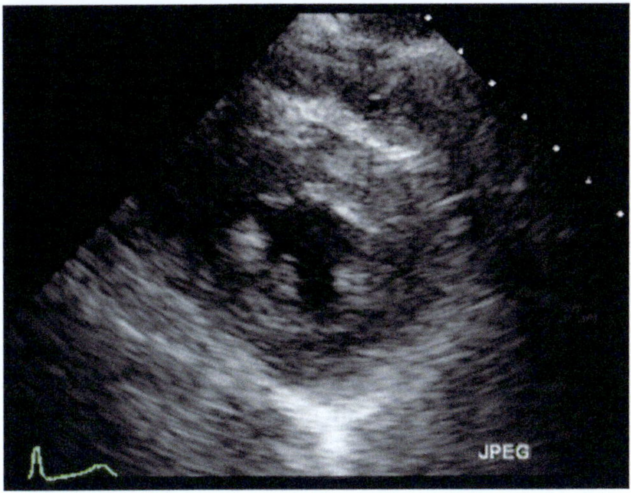

Fig. 12.3 Parasternal short-axis end-systolic image at rest

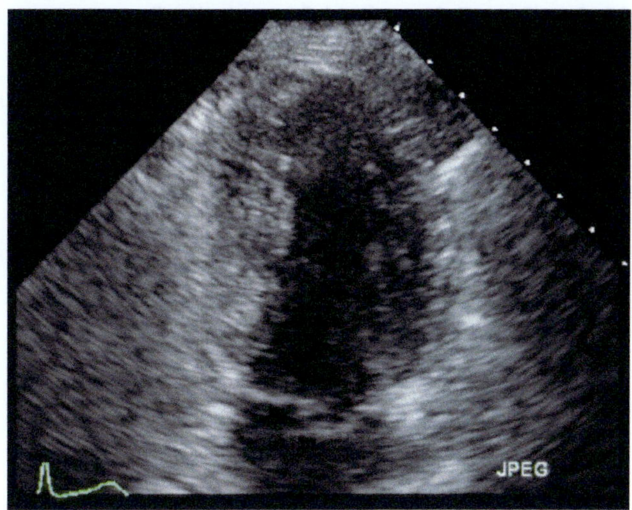

Fig. 12.5 Apical two-chamber end-systolic image at rest

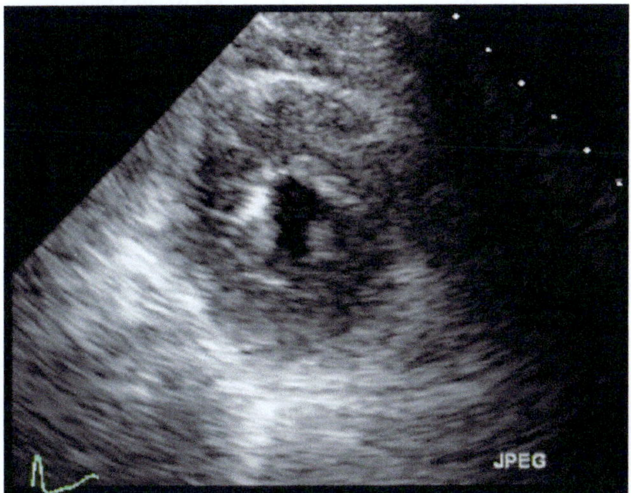

Fig. 12.4 Parasternal short-axis end-systolic image at peak exercise. Note the decreased left ventricular cavity size

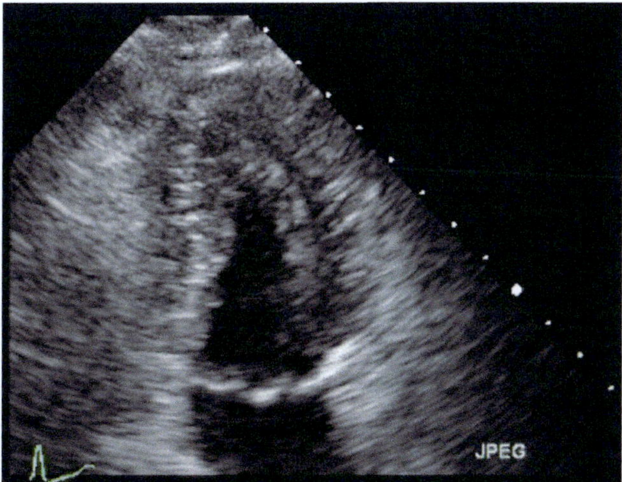

Fig. 12.6 Apical two-chamber end-systolic image at peak exercise. Note the decreased left ventricular cavity size

12.2 Case 2. Impaired Contractile Reserve: Increased Left Ventricular Size with Stress

A 52-year-old previously fit ballet instructor with known mitral valve prolapse and significant MR presented with increasing fatigue but no overt dyspnea or signs of heart failure. She was referred for exercise stress echocardiography to assess left ventricular contractile reserve and exercise capacity. She achieved 8 min of treadmill exercise according to the standard Bruce protocol. The test was ceased at 92 % of the maximum predicted heart rate because of dyspnea and fatigue.

Regional wall motion analysis did not demonstrate any focal abnormalities to suggest inducible ischemia, but the left ventricular size remained unchanged at peak exercise. This failure of augmentation in left ventricular function at peak stress reflected impaired contractile reserve. Color Doppler imaging also demonstrated a significant increase in the severity of her MR at peak stress. She was referred for consideration of mitral valve surgical repair.

Video 12.7 Apical four-chamber view with color Doppler demonstrating moderate (2+) mitral regurgitation at baseline (heart rate 62 bpm) (MOV 454 kb)

Video 12.8 Parasternal stress echocardiographic images before exercise (*left images*) and after exercise (*right images*). The images at the top show the long-axis view and the bottom images show the short-axis view at the level of the mid left ventricle. The left ventricular cavity increases with exercise stress, consistent with impaired contractile reserve (AVI 1799 kb)

Video 12.9 Apical four-chamber (*top*) and two-chamber (*bottom*) stress echocardiographic images before exercise (*left images*) and after exercise (*right images*). The left ventricular cavity size increases with exercise stress, consistent with impaired contractile reserve (AVI 1904 kb)

Video 12.10 Apical four-chamber view with color Doppler demonstrating severe (4+) mitral regurgitation in the early recovery phase even though the heart rate had nearly returned to the baseline of 68 bpm (MOV 432 kb)

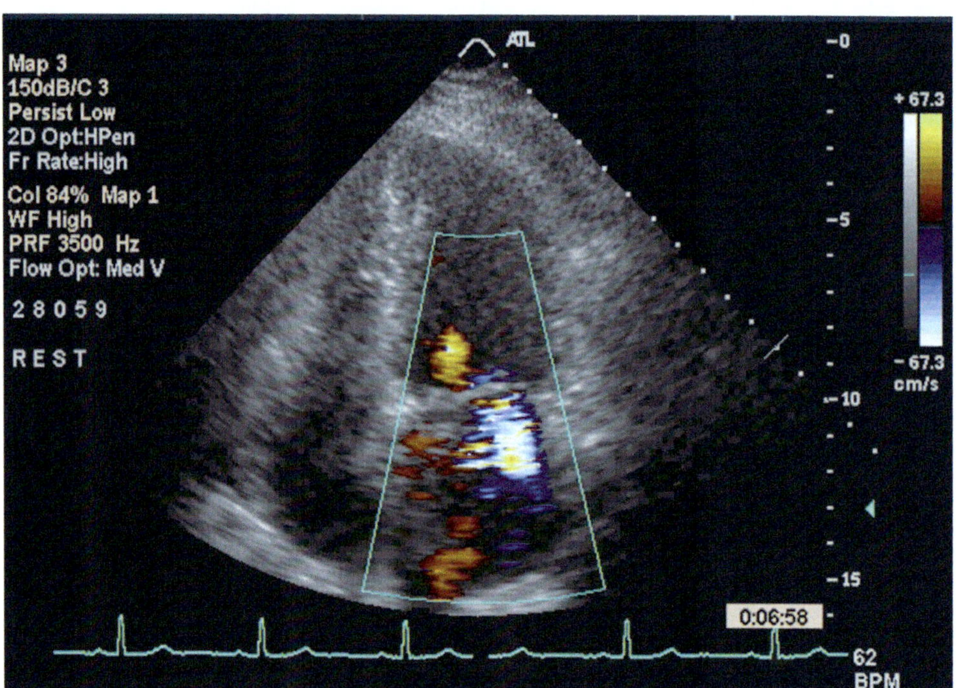

Fig. 12.7 Apical four-chamber view with color Doppler demonstrating moderate (2+) mitral regurgitation at baseline (heart rate 62 bpm)

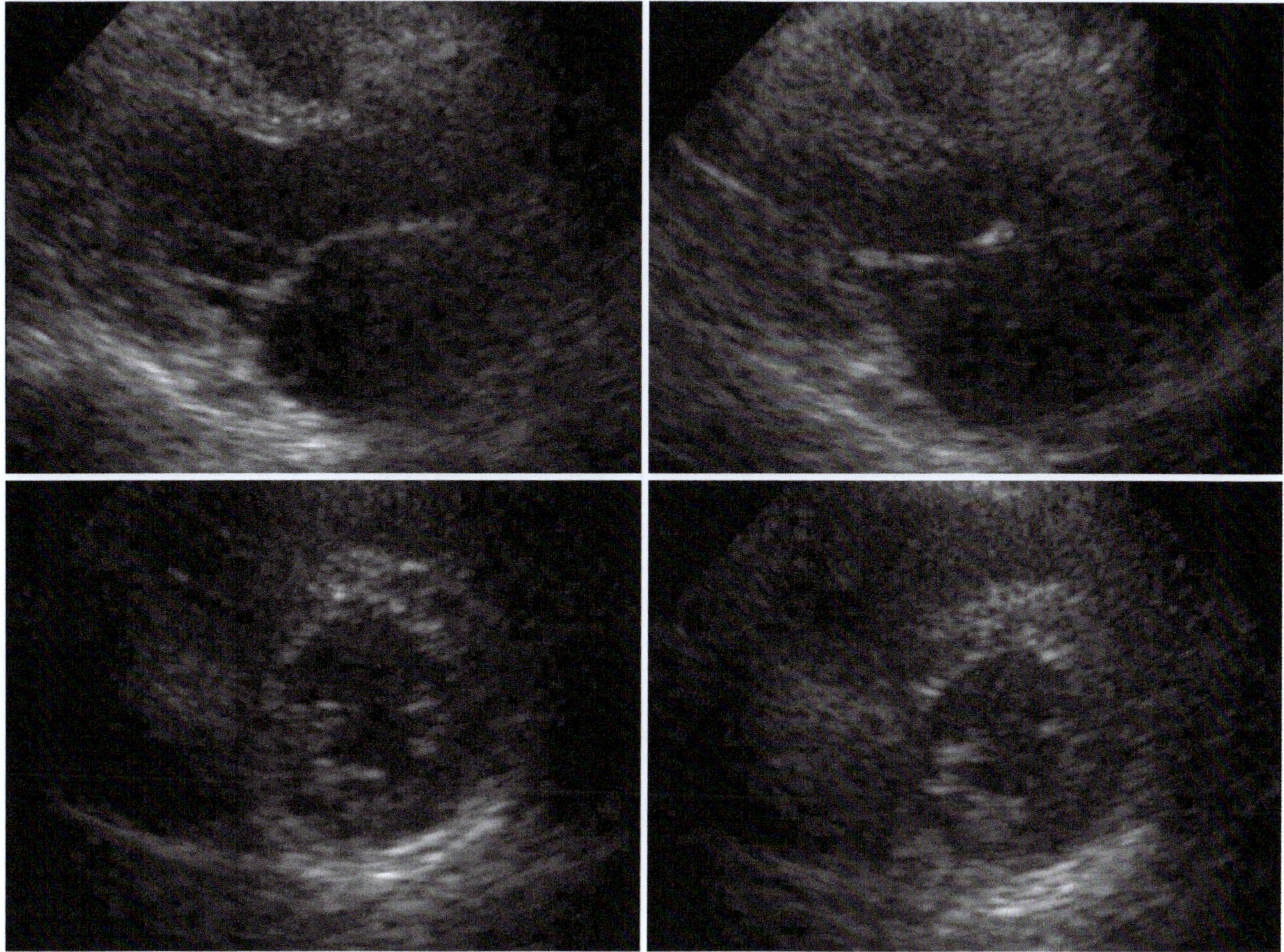

Fig. 12.8 Parasternal stress echocardiographic images before exercise (*left images*) and after exercise (*right images*). The images at the top show the long-axis view and the bottom images show the short-axis view at the level of the mid left ventricle. The left ventricular cavity increases with exercise stress, consistent with impaired contractile reserve

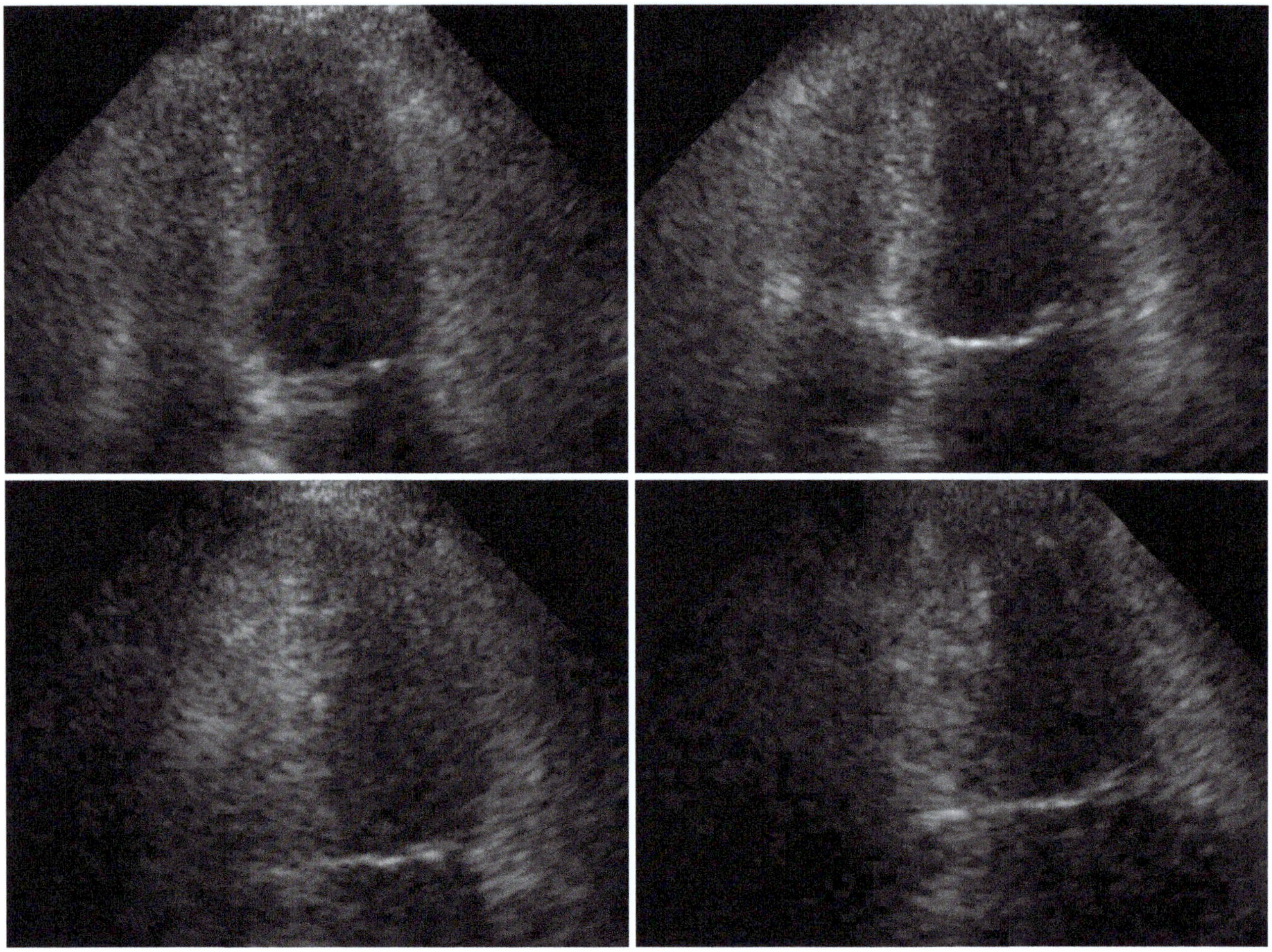

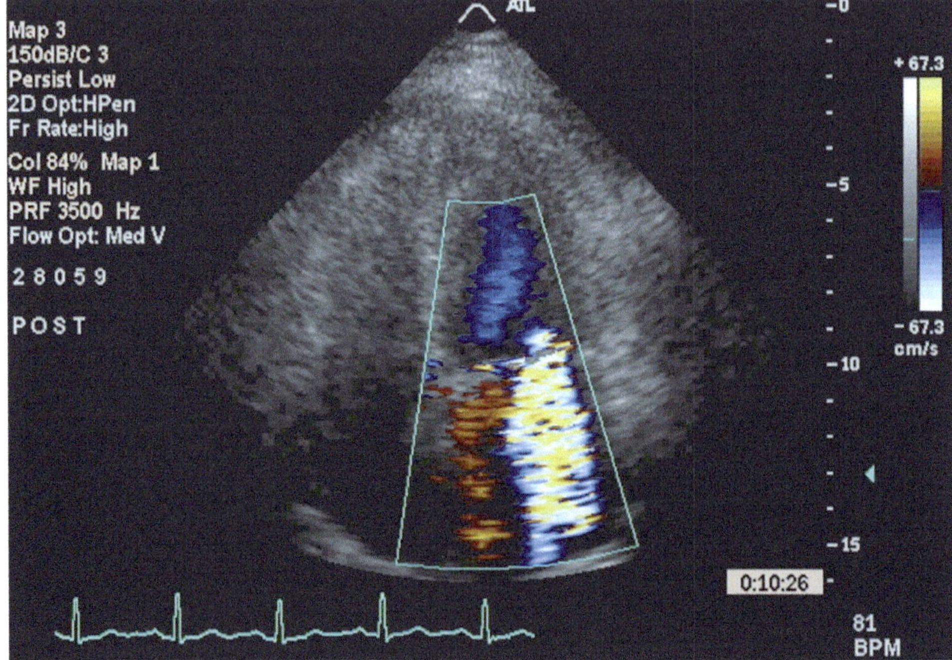

Fig. 12.9 Apical four-chamber (*top*) and two-chamber (*bottom*) stress echocardiographic images before exercise (*left images*) and after exercise (*right images*). The left ventricular cavity size increases with exercise stress, consistent with impaired contractile reserve

Fig. 12.10 Apical four-chamber view with color Doppler demonstrating severe (4+) mitral regurgitation in the early recovery phase even though the heart rate had nearly returned to the baseline of 68 bpm

12.3 Case 3. Increased Gradients After Stress

A 32-year-old female teacher presents for evaluation of palpitations and exercise-induced shortness of breath. She also complains of hand and arm numbness and increased fatigue. She reports dyspnea upon climbing one flight of stairs and states that the dyspnea is getting progressively worse. She describes occasional leg swelling, especially towards the end of the teaching day. The palpitations occur multiple times a day and are quite debilitating. She has a history of previous mitral valve repair with insertion of an annuloplasty ring for mitral valve prolapse.

The resting echocardiogram demonstrated normal left ventricular size and systolic function (EF=55 %). The right ventricle was mildly dilated, with mild systolic dysfunction. Peak and mean transvalvular gradients across the repaired mitral valve were 23 mmHg and 11 mmHg respectively. There was trivial valvular MR. Estimated right ventricular systolic pressure was 39 mmHg, consistent with mild pulmonary hypertension. The left atrium was severely dilated, with an indexed volume of 41 mL/m².

A stress echocardiogram was performed to assess functional capacity, peak pulmonary pressures, and mitral valve gradients at peak stress. She demonstrated a reduced exercise capacity of only 6.3 METs at a maximum heart rate of 76 %. With exercise, her peak right ventricular systolic pressure increased to 61 mmHg and her peak and mean mitral valve gradients rose to 53 and 35 mmHg respectively. At the submaximal predicted heart rate achieved, there was no evidence of inducible ischemia, and the left ventricular cavity size reduced appropriately with stress.

Her MR remained unchanged but her tricuspid regurgitation increased from mild (1+) at baseline to moderate (2+) with exercise.

Based upon the stress echocardiography findings, she was referred for redo surgery. Given her young age and concern regarding valve longevity and further repeat sternotomy, a mechanical mitral valve prosthesis was selected.

Video 12.11 Parasternal long-axis view at rest, with color Doppler imaging demonstrating a repaired mitral valve with an annuloplasty ring and trivial valvular mitral regurgitation (AVI 1849 kb)

Video 12.12 (a) Parasternal long-axis view before exercise (AVI 8020 kb)

Video 12.12 (b) The same view after exercise, demonstrating a decrease in left ventricular size with stress, indicative of preserved contractile reserve. No regional wall motion abnormalities are seen that would suggest underlying myocardial ischemia, although this exercise was at a submaximal predicted heart rate (AVI 1331 kb)

Video 12.13 (a) Apical four-chamber view before exercise (AVI 1344 kb)

Video 12.13 (b) The same view after exercise, demonstrating a decrease in left ventricular size with stress, indicative of preserved contractile reserve. No regional wall motion abnormalities are seen that suggest underlying myocardial ischemia, although this exercise was at a submaximal predicted heart rate (AVI 973 kb)

Video 12.14 (a) Color Doppler imaging of the tricuspid valve at rest demonstrates mild to moderate (1–2+) tricuspid regurgitation (AVI 2068 kb)

Video 12.14 (b) This regurgitation increases to moderately severe (3+) after exercise stress (AVI 2169 kb)

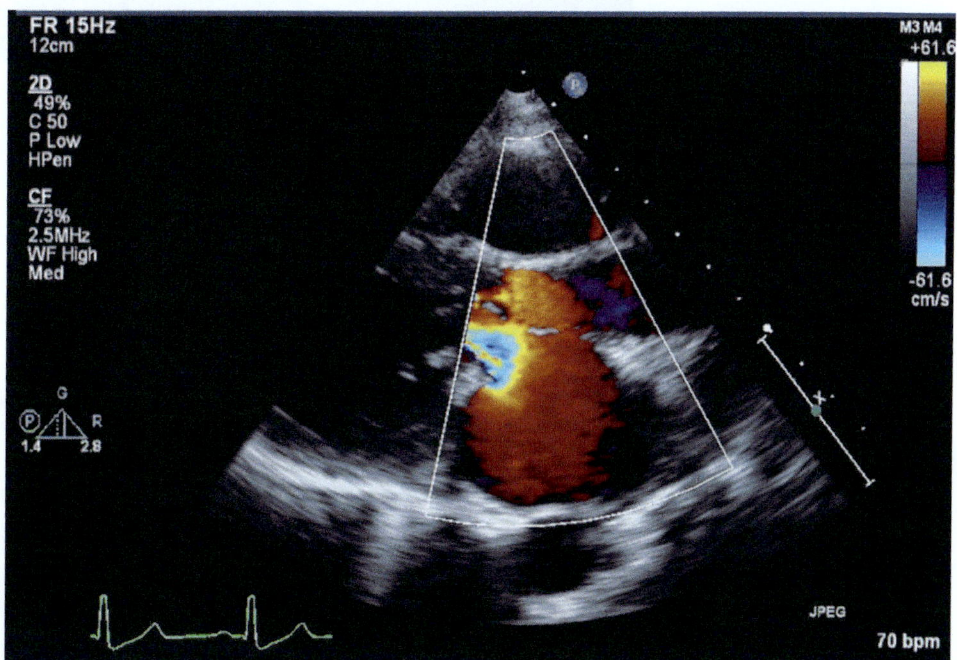

Fig. 12.11 Parasternal long-axis view at rest, with color Doppler imaging demonstrating a repaired mitral valve with an annuloplasty ring and trivial valvular mitral regurgitation

Fig. 12.12 (**a**) Parasternal long-axis view before exercise. (**b**) The same view after exercise, demonstrating a decrease in left ventricular size with stress, indicative of preserved contractile reserve. No regional wall motion abnormalities are seen that would suggest underlying myocardial ischemia, although this exercise was at a submaximal predicted heart rate

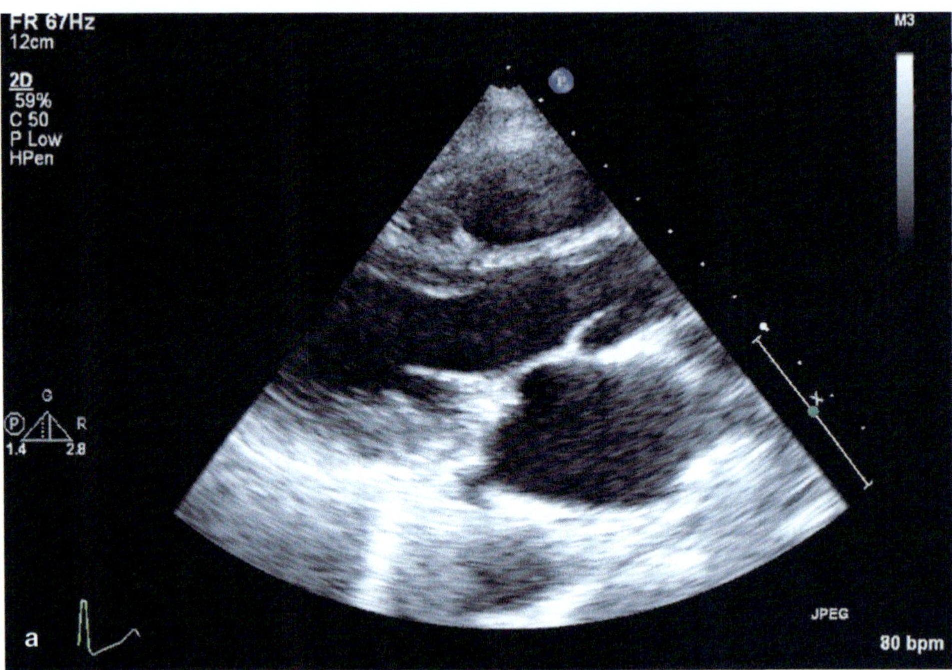

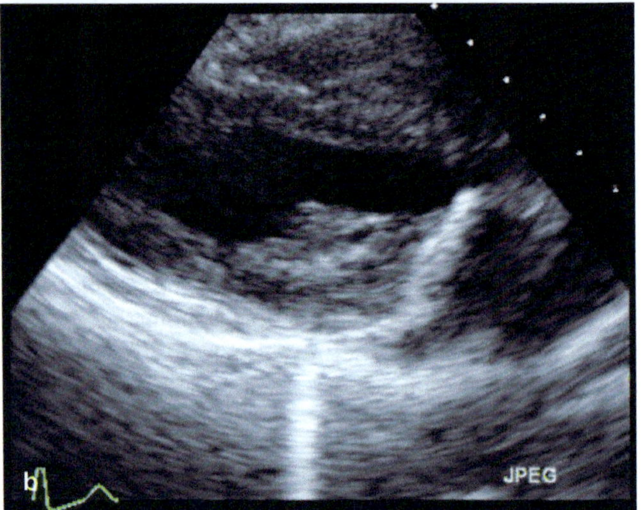

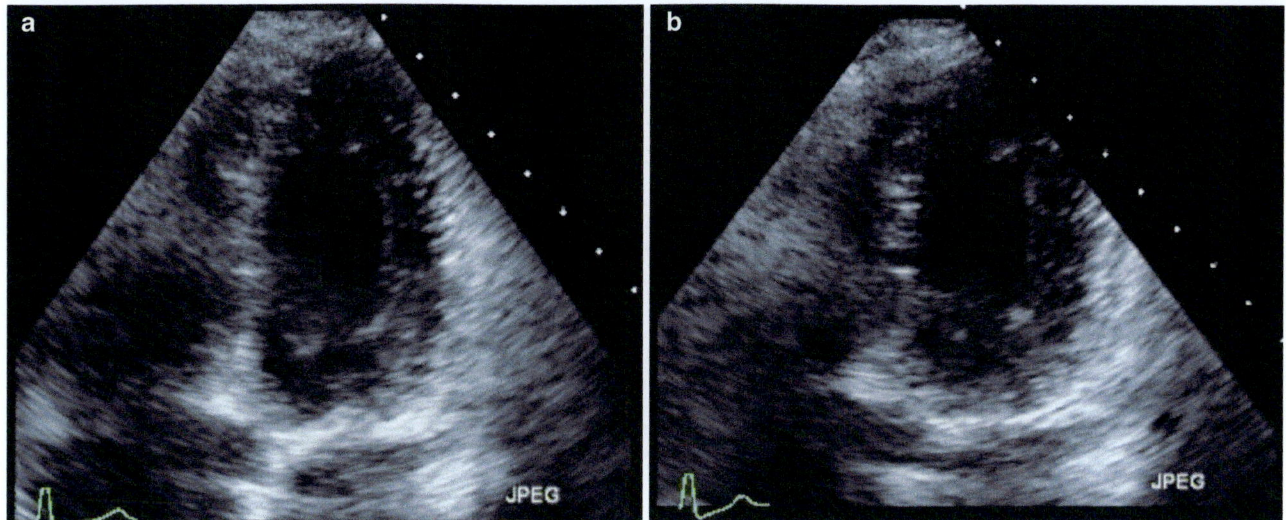

Fig. 12.13 (**a**) Apical four-chamber view before exercise. (**b**) The same view after exercise, demonstrating a decrease in left ventricular size with stress, indicative of preserved contractile reserve. No regional wall motion abnormalities are seen that suggest underlying myocardial ischemia, although this exercise was at a submaximal predicted heart rate

Fig. 12.14 (**a**) Continuous-wave Doppler through the mitral valve at rest demonstrates borderline-severe mitral stenosis with a peak gradient of 23 mmHg and a mean gradient of 11 mmHg. (**b**) With exercise stress, the transvalvular gradients significantly increase to peak 53 mmHg and mean 35 mmHg

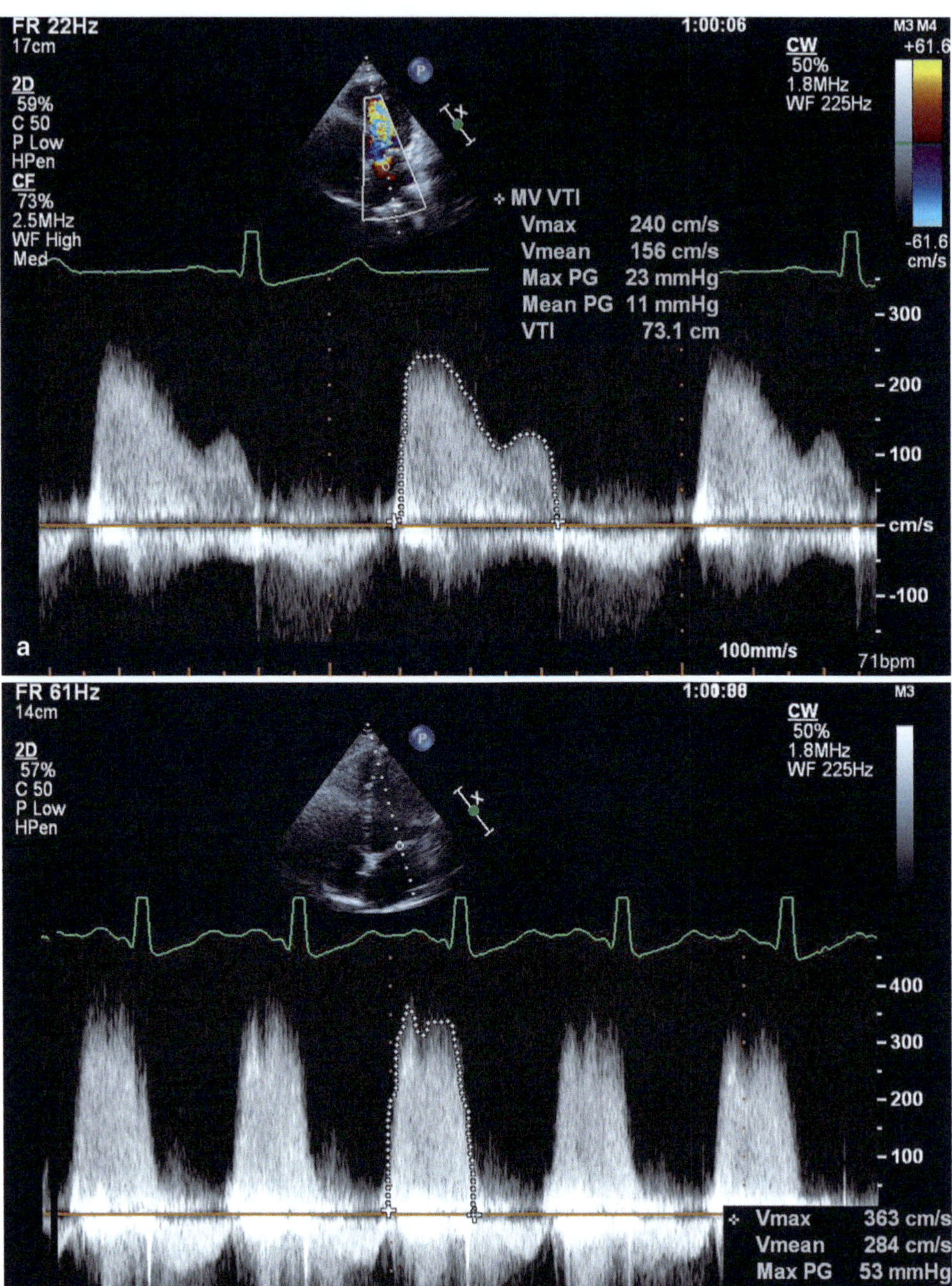

Fig. 12.15 (**a**) Color Doppler imaging of the tricuspid valve at rest demonstrates mild to moderate (1–2+) tricuspid regurgitation. (**b**) This regurgitation increases to moderately severe (3+) after exercise stress

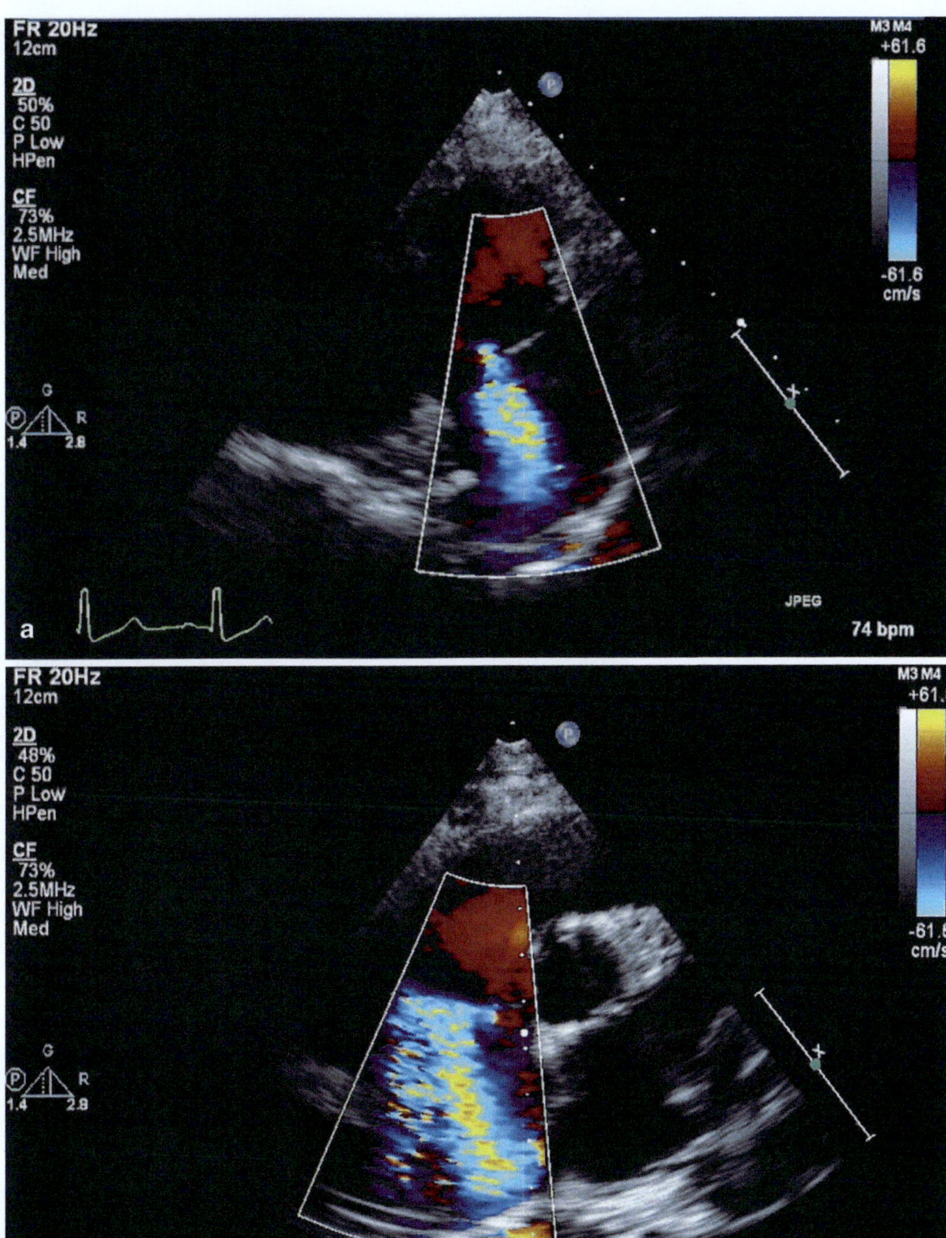

Fig. 12.16 (**a**) The estimated right ventricular peak systolic pressure at rest is 39 mmHg, assuming a right atrial pressure of 5 mmHg. (**b**) After exercise, the peak pressure increases significantly to 61 mmHg

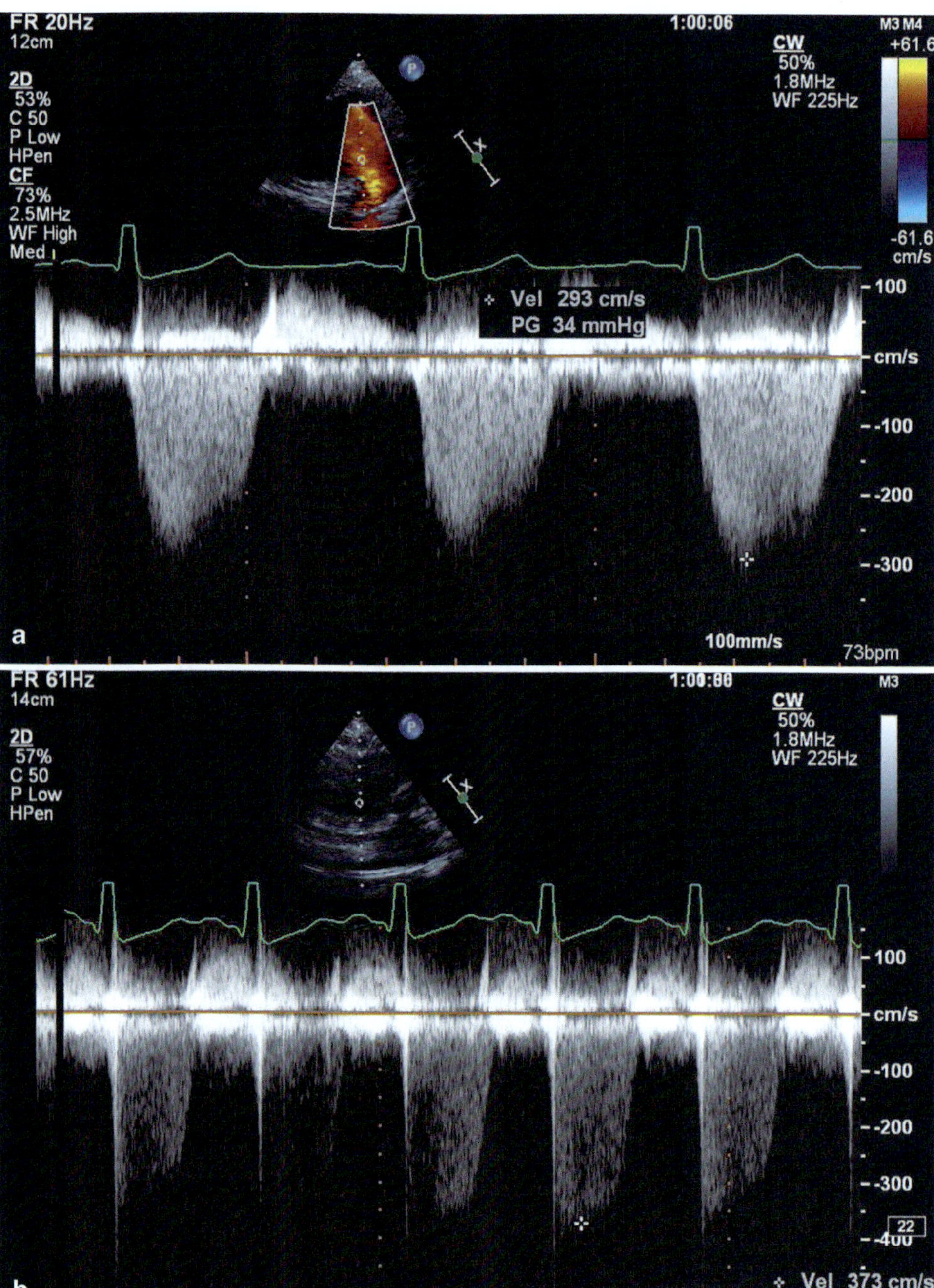

12.4   Teaching Points

- Stress echocardiography is a useful technique for the evaluation of mitral valve disease that might be borderline in severity or not clearly symptomatic.
- Assessment of contractile reserve, exercise capacity, pulmonary pressures, transvalvular gradients, exercise-induced arrhythmias, and MR severity with exercise are all important components to consider when optimizing the timing of surgery and may be relevant to both acute surgical outcomes and long-term prognosis.

References

1. Leung DY, Griffin BP, Stewart WJ, Cosgrove 3rd DM, Thomas JD, Marwick TH. Left ventricular function after valve repair for chronic mitral regurgitation: predictive value of preoperative assessment of contractile reserve by exercise echocardiography. J Am Coll Cardiol. 1996;28:1198–205.

Suggested Reading

Lancellotti P, Magne J. Stress echocardiography in regurgitant valve disease. Circ Cardiovasc Imaging. 2013;6:840–9.

Lancellotti P, Magne J. Stress testing for the evaluation of patients with mitral regurgitation. Curr Opin Cardiol. 2012;27:492–8.

Magne J, Lancellotti P, Piérard LA. Exercise pulmonary hypertension in asymptomatic degenerative mitral regurgitation. Circulation. 2010;122:33–41.

Naji P, Griffin BP, Asfahan F, Barr T, Rodriguez LL, Grimm R, et al. Predictors of long-term outcomes in patients with significant myxomatous mitral regurgitation undergoing exercise echocardiography. Circulation. 2014;129:1310–9.

Nishimura RA, Otto CM, Bonow RO, Carabello BA, Erwin 3rd JP, Guyton RA, et al. 2014 AHA/ACC guideline for the management of patients with valvular heart disease: a report of the American College of Cardiology/American Heart Association Task Force on Practice Guidelines. Circulation. 2014;129:e521–643.

Picano E, Pibarot P, Lancellotti P, Monin JL, Bonow RO. The emerging role of exercise testing and stress echocardiography in valvular heart disease. J Am Coll Cardiol. 2009;54:2251–60.

Supino PG, Borer JS, Schuleri K, Gupta A, Hochreiter C, Kligfield P, et al. Prognostic value of exercise tolerance testing in asymptomatic chronic non-ischemic mitral regurgitation. Am J Cardiol. 2007;100:1274–81.

Cardiac Masses and Miscellaneous

13

Teerapat Yingchoncharoen

13.1 Case 1. Mitral Valve Myxoma

A 59-year-old man presented with acute dysarthria and left hemiparesis, which lasted for 15 min and spontaneously resolved. He had no risk factors for cardiovascular diseases and had a negative family history for stroke or other premature cardiovascular diseases. Cardiac examination revealed a grade 3/6 systolic murmur at the left parasternal border.

13.1.1 Learning Points

Although cardiac myxoma is the most common benign cardiac tumor, those that originate from the heart valve are rare [1]. Mitral valve myxoma, conventionally defined as a myxoma arising from the mitral leaflet, annulus, commissures, junction area, or subvalvular apparatus (chordae or papillary muscle), is considered rare, with up to 64 myxomas described in 42 articles from 2006 to 2011 [2]. This case represented a mitral valve myxoma originated from the papillary muscle and chordae, which is considered exceedingly rare. This case also highlights the role of multimodality imaging in diagnosis and treatment planning. Cardiac MRI provided complementary data on tissue characteristics of the tumor and anatomic definition for surgical planning (Figs. 13.1, 13.2, 13.3, 13.4, 13.5, 13.6, and 13.7). Cardiac myxomas that are located in the left ventricular chamber are associated with higher embolization risk, partly owing to higher mobility and left ventricular pressure [3], so surgical resection should be performed promptly once the diagnosis is established. Follow-up echocardiography should be performed to detect recurrence [4].

Video 13.1 Transthoracic echocardiography (TTE) parasternal long-axis view showed a 3.7×3.6-cm, highly mobile echodensity with frond-like projections in the left ventricle, attached to the posterior mitral valve leaflet and subvalvular apparatus (AVI 5351 kb)

Video 13.2 TTE apical four-chamber view showed the mass (*arrows*) of the mitral valve (AVI 4775 kb)

Electronic supplementary material The online version of this chapter (doi:10.1007/978-1-4471-6672-6_13) contains supplementary material, which is available to authorized users.

T. Yingchoncharoen
Department of Cardiovascular Medicine, Cleveland Clinic,
9500 Euclid Avenue, Cleveland, OH 44195, USA
e-mail: teerapatmdcu@gmail.com

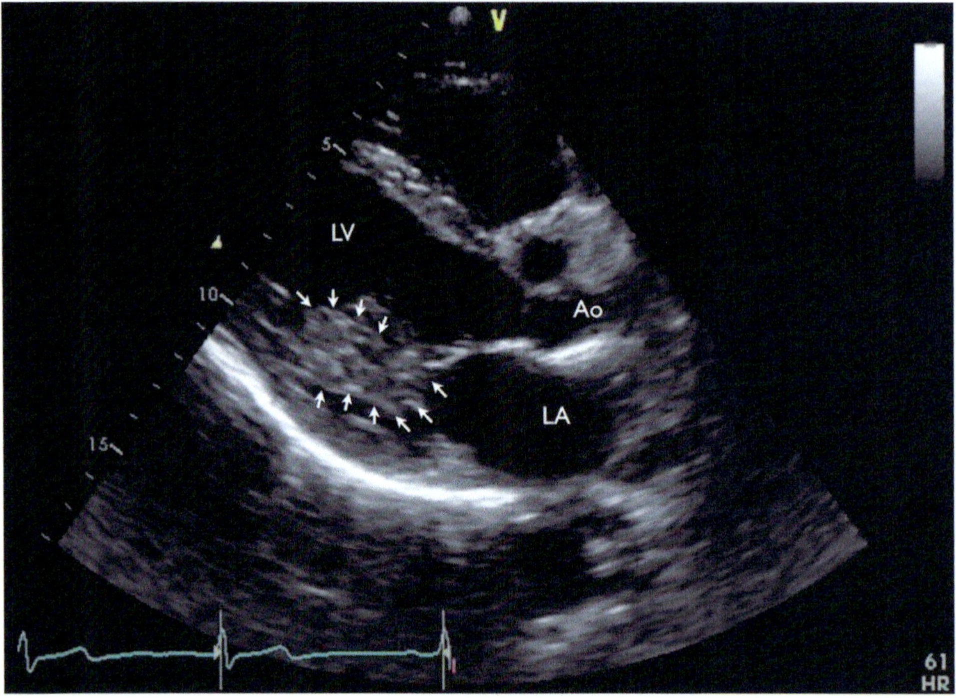

Fig. 13.1 Transthoracic echocardiography (TTE) parasternal long-axis view showed a 3.7×3.6-cm, highly mobile echodensity (*arrows*) with frond-like projections in the left ventricle (LV), attached to the posterior mitral valve leaflet and subvalvular apparatus. *Ao* aorta, *LA* left atrium

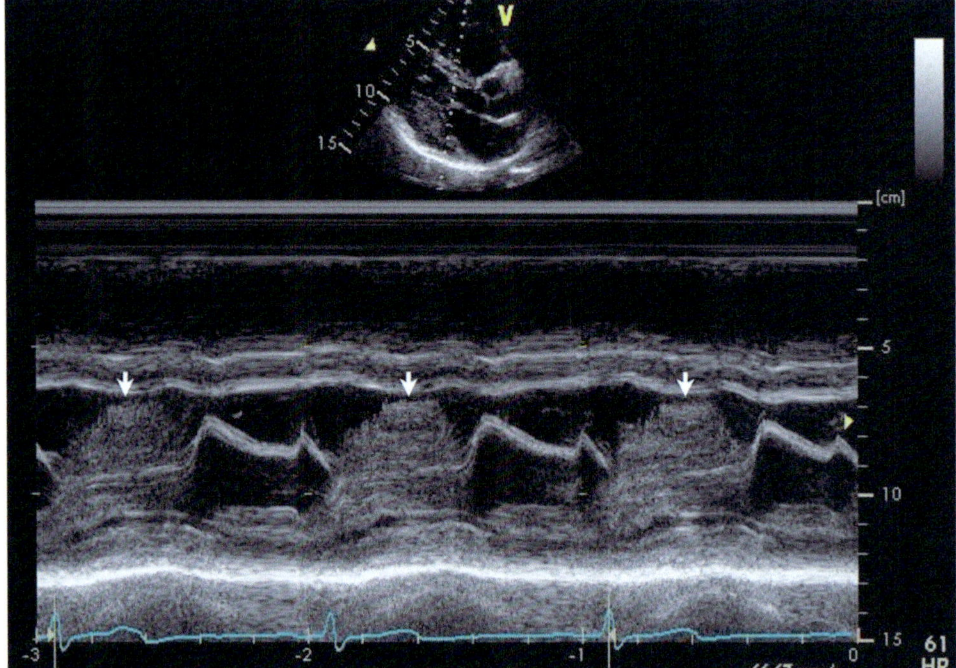

Fig. 13.2 M-mode echocardiography at the mitral valve showed the presence of an echodensity intermittently protruding into the left ventricular outflow tract during systole (*arrows*)

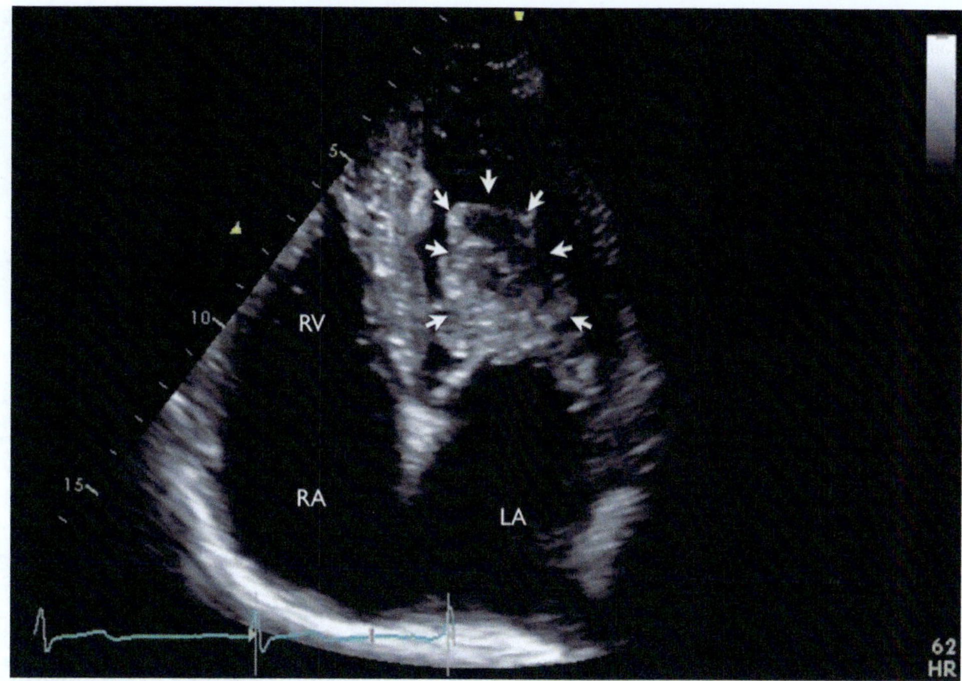

Fig. 13.3 TTE apical four-chamber view showed the mass (*arrows*) of the mitral valve. *RA* right atrium, *RV* right ventricle

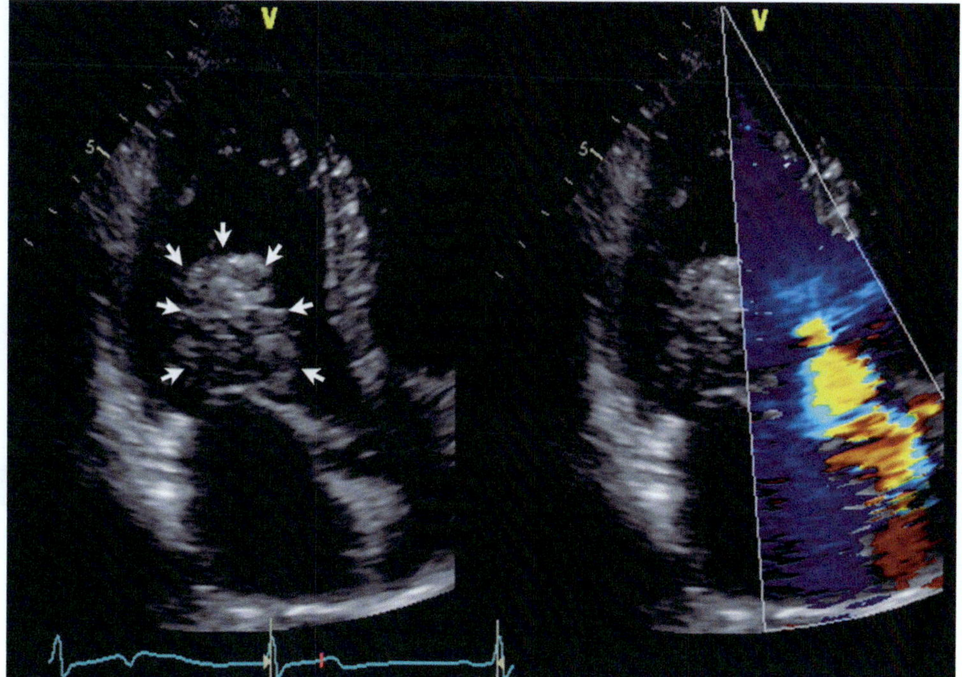

Fig. 13.4 TTE apical five-chamber view showed that the mass (*arrows*) protruded into the left ventricular outflow tract (LVOT) during systole. The mass also caused flow acceleration in the LVOT, corresponding to the patient's systolic murmur

Fig. 13.5 (**a–d**) Cardiac MRI confirmed the findings, with tissue characteristics consistent with cardiac myxoma. *SSFP* steady-state free precession

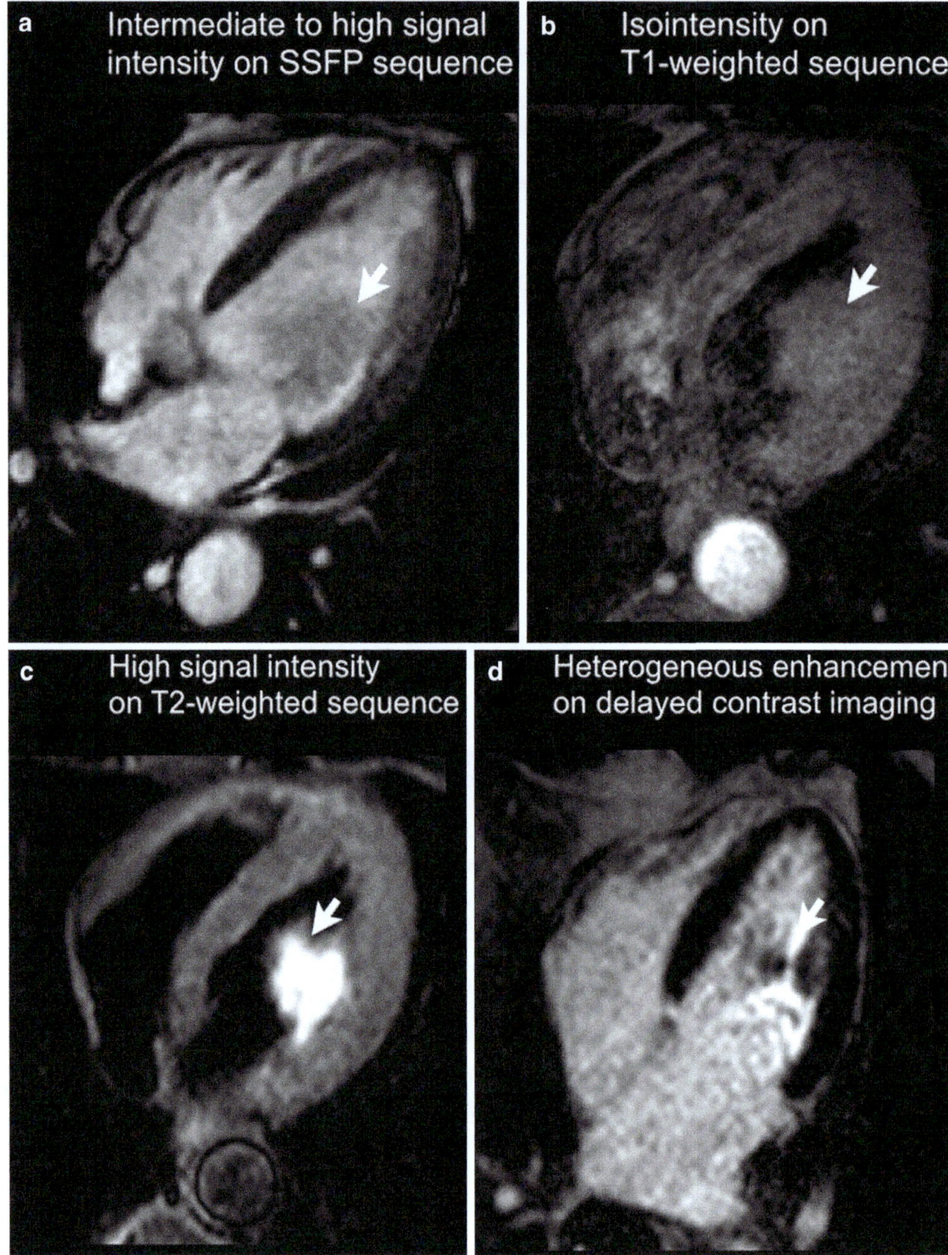

Fig. 13.6 Intraoperative findings showed that the mass (*arrow*) was attached to the head of the posteromedial papillary muscle and several chords going to the P2 segment of the posterior mitral valve leaflet (*Courtesy of* Dr. Joseph Sabik, Cleveland Clinic)

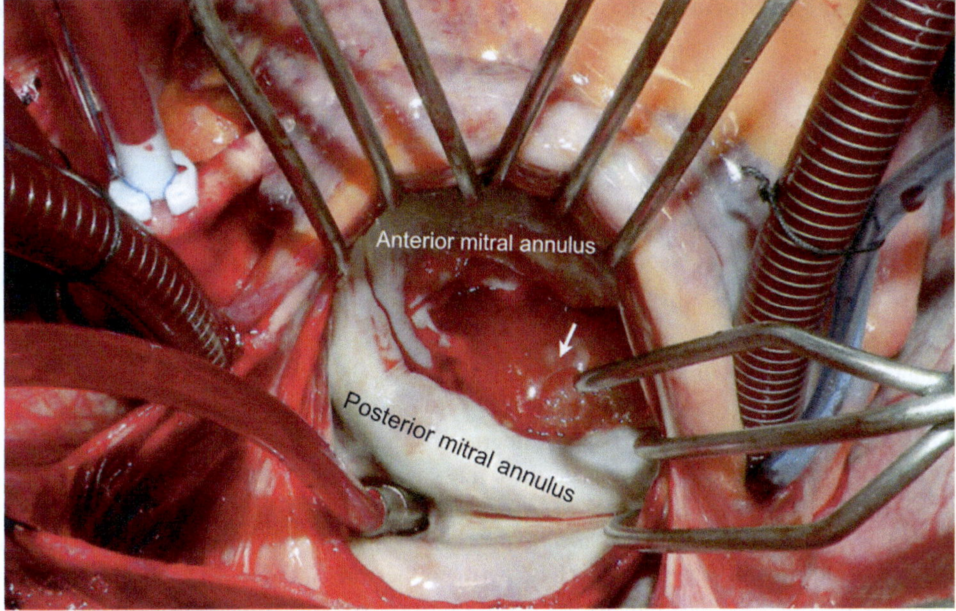

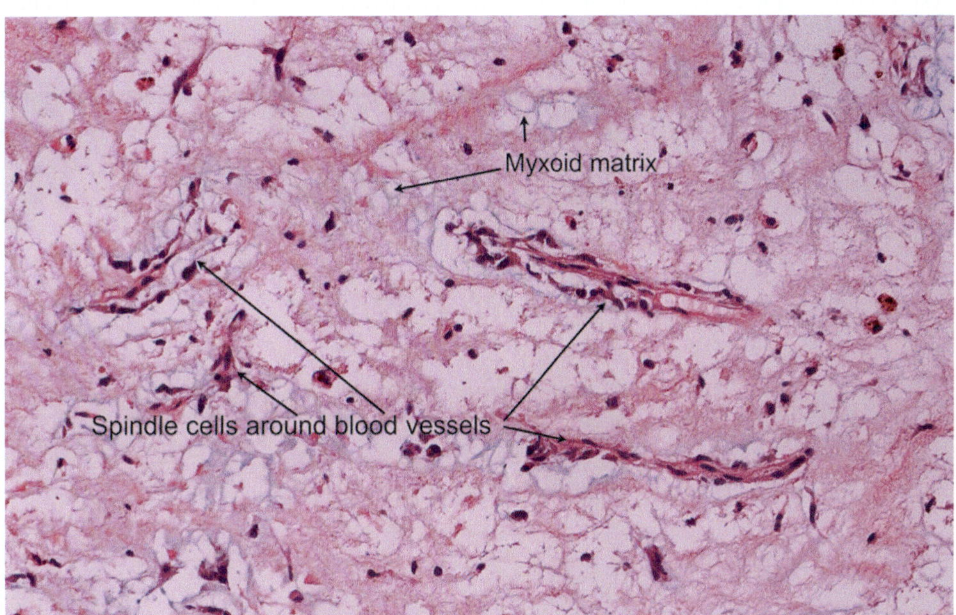

Fig. 13.7 Pathology confirmed the diagnosis of mitral valve myxoma. (*Arrow* indicates mass.) (*Courtesy of* Dr. Carmela Tan and Dr. Rene Rodriguez, Cleveland Clinic)

13.2   Case 2. Blood Cyst

An 84-year-old man with past medical history of hypertension and dyslipidemia was sent for echocardiographic evaluation because of near syncope.

13.2.1   Learning Points

Blood cysts are congenital in origin and most frequently have been found as a postmortem finding in fetuses and infants less than 6 months of age [5]. Histologically, they are diverticuli lined with flat, endothelium-like cells on both sides, containing bloody fluid. Echocardiographic findings include a thin-walled, well-circumscribed mass with an echolucent core (Figs. 13.8, 13.9, 13.10, and 13.11). The presence of microbubbles inside the cystic cavity during diastole (confirming the passage of blood between the ventricular cavity and the cyst lumen) has been described as a pathognomonic sign of the presence of a blood cyst [6]. The cyst is most commonly present at an atrioventricular valve; it occurs less often in semilunar valves and is also found at papillary muscle [7] or the atrialized right ventricular portion of Ebstein's anomaly.

There is no consensus regarding optimal management of asymptomatic blood cysts. The natural history is not known. (They regress spontaneously in most patients, but cyst growth also been reported.) Conservative management with echocardiographic follow-up is suggested for asymptomatic patients with a small cyst. Surgical resection should be performed for masses that interfere with cardiac function.

Video 13.3 TTE parasternal long-axis view showed a thin-walled, well-circumscribed mass with an echolucent core in the posteroinferior wall area (AVI 878 kb)

Video 13.4 TTE parasternal long-axis view zoomed at the mass (*arrow*) confirmed the same findings (AVI 841 kb)

Video 13.5 TTE short-axis view zoomed at the mass attached to the anterolateral papillary muscle (AVI 858 kb)

Video 13.6 TTE apical four-chamber view confirmed the thin-walled, well-circumscribed mass with an echolucent core attached to the anterolateral papillary muscle, findings consistent with a blood cyst (AVI 853 kb)

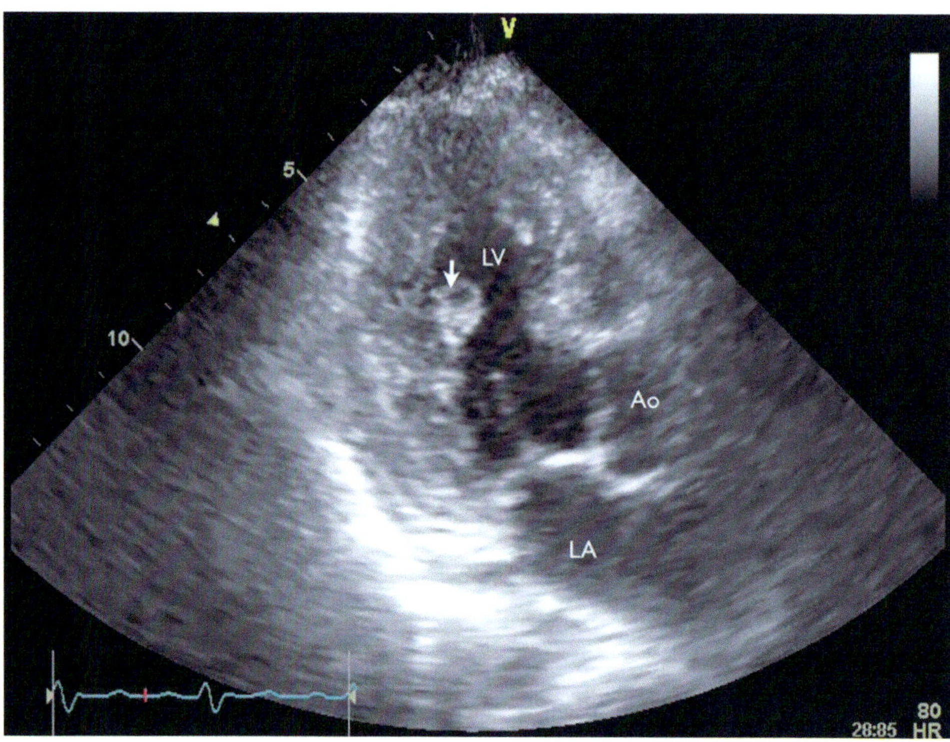

Fig. 13.8 TTE parasternal long-axis view showed a thin-walled, well-circumscribed mass with an echolucent core in the posterioinferior wall area (*arrow*)

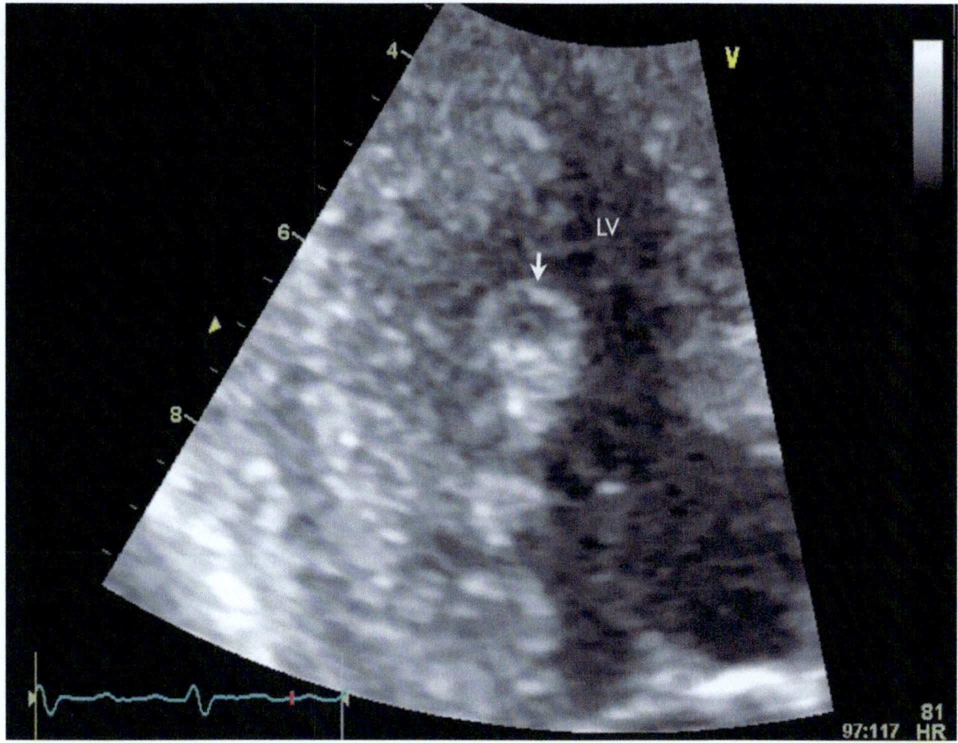

Fig. 13.9 TTE parasternal long-axis view zoomed at the mass (*arrow*) confirmed the same findings

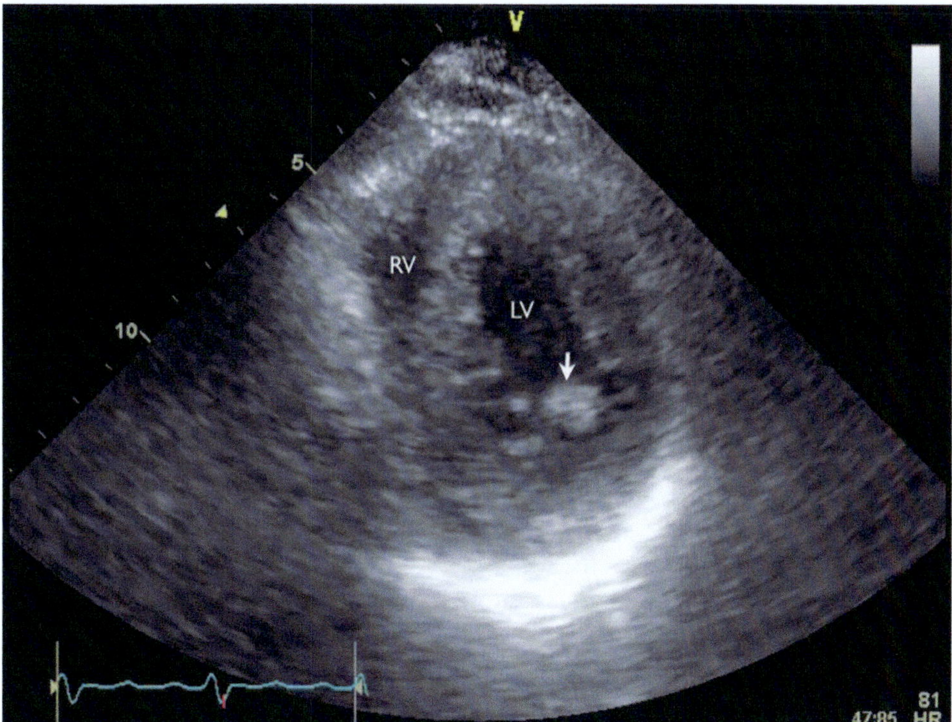

Fig. 13.10 TTE short-axis view zoomed at the mass attached to the anterolateral papillary muscle (*arrow*)

Fig. 13.11 TTE apical four-chamber view confirmed the thin-walled, well-circumscribed mass with an echolucent core attached to the anterolateral papillary muscle, findings consistent with a blood cyst (*arrow*)

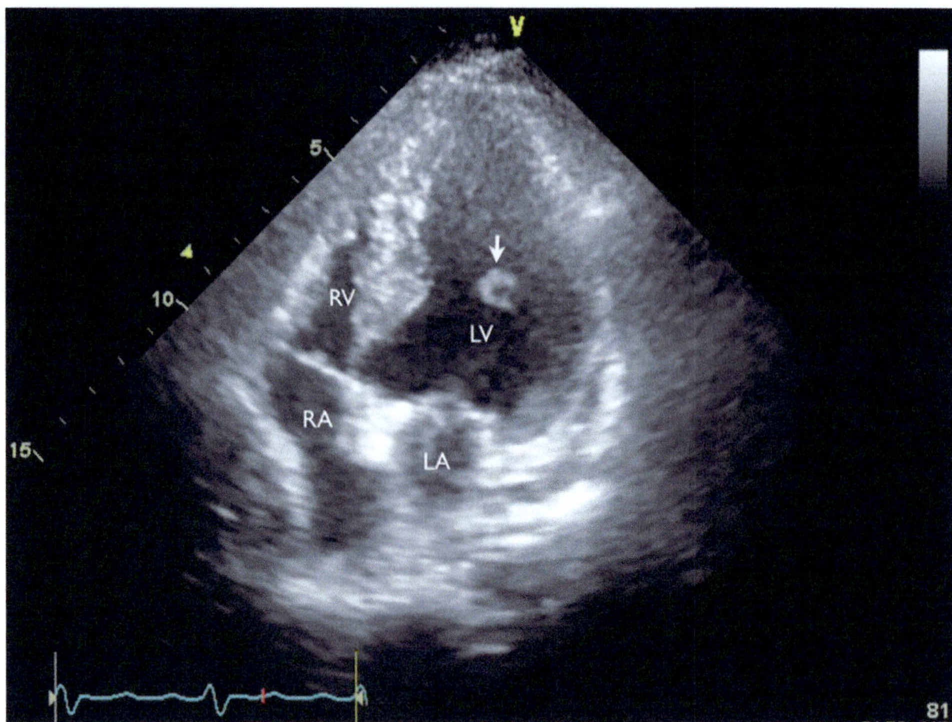

13.3 Diastolic Mitral and Tricuspid Regurgitation

A 75-year-old man with shortness of breath on exertion was found to have complete heart block and underwent implantation of a permanent pacemaker. On examination, a 3/6 systolic murmur with short diastolic murmurs was heard at the lower left parasternal border.

13.3.1 Learning Points

Diastolic mitral and tricuspid regurgitation is a common finding in patients with atrioventricular conduction abnormalities. It is caused by delayed ventricular contraction following atrial contraction. The high ventricular pressure during atrial relaxation with incomplete atrioventricular valve closure results in reverse regurgitation (Figs. 13.12, 13.13, 13.14, and 13.15).

Video 13.7 A TTE apical four-chamber view with color Doppler flow imaging showed typical systolic mitral regurgitation but also a short regurgitation jet from the left ventricle to the left atrium during diastole, consistent with diastolic mitral regurgitation (AVI 114027 kb)

Video 13.8 A TTE apical four-chamber view with color Doppler flow imaging showed typical systolic tricuspid regurgitation but also a short regurgitation jet from the right ventricle to the right atrium during diastole, consistent with diastolic tricuspid regurgitation (AVI 112410 kb)

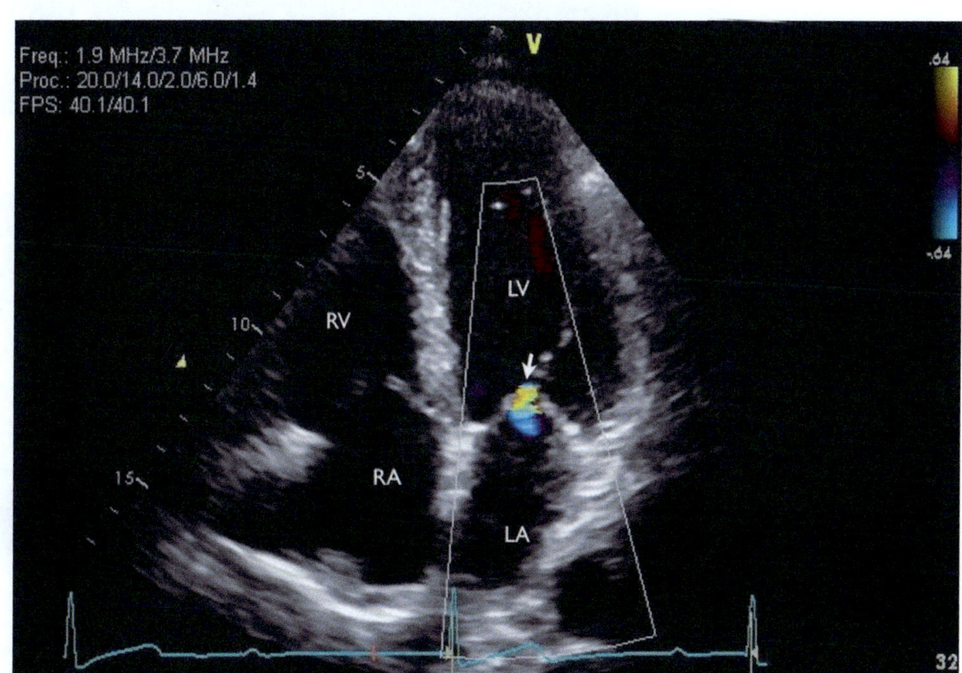

Fig. 13.12 A TTE apical four-chamber view with color Doppler flow imaging showed typical systolic mitral regurgitation but also a short regurgitation jet from the left ventricle to the left atrium during diastole, consistent with diastolic mitral regurgitation (*arrow*)

Fig. 13.13 Continuous-wave Doppler of mitral inflow showed systolic (*arrowheads*) and diastolic (*arrows*) mitral regurgitation

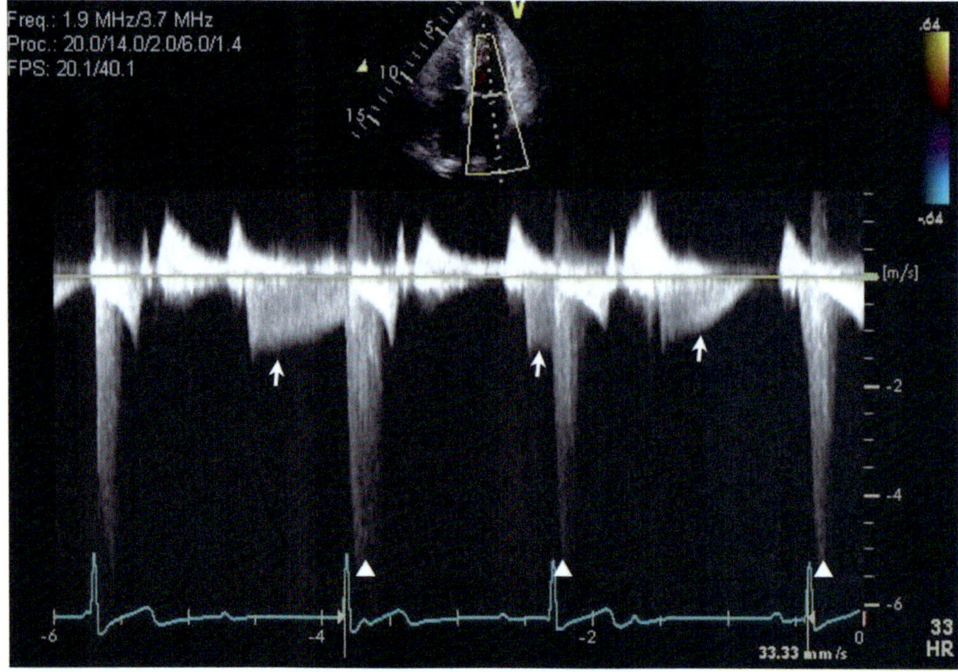

Fig. 13.14 A TTE apical four-chamber view with color Doppler flow imaging showed typical systolic tricuspid regurgitation but also a short regurgitation jet from the right ventricle to the right atrium during diastole, consistent with diastolic tricuspid regurgitation (*arrow*)

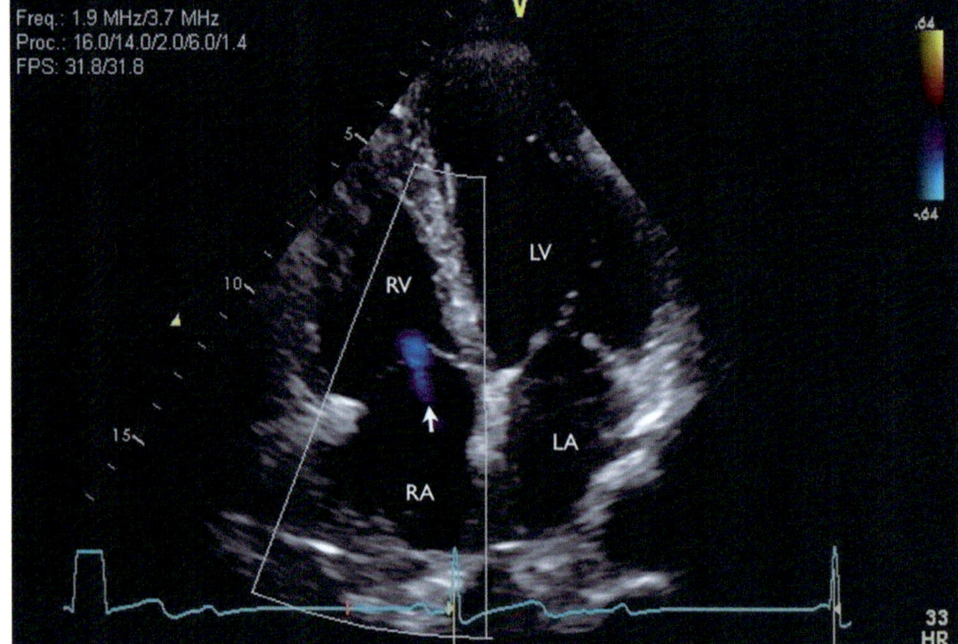

Fig. 13.15 Continuous-wave Doppler of mitral inflow showed systolic (*arrowheads*) and diastolic (*arrows*) tricuspid regurgitation

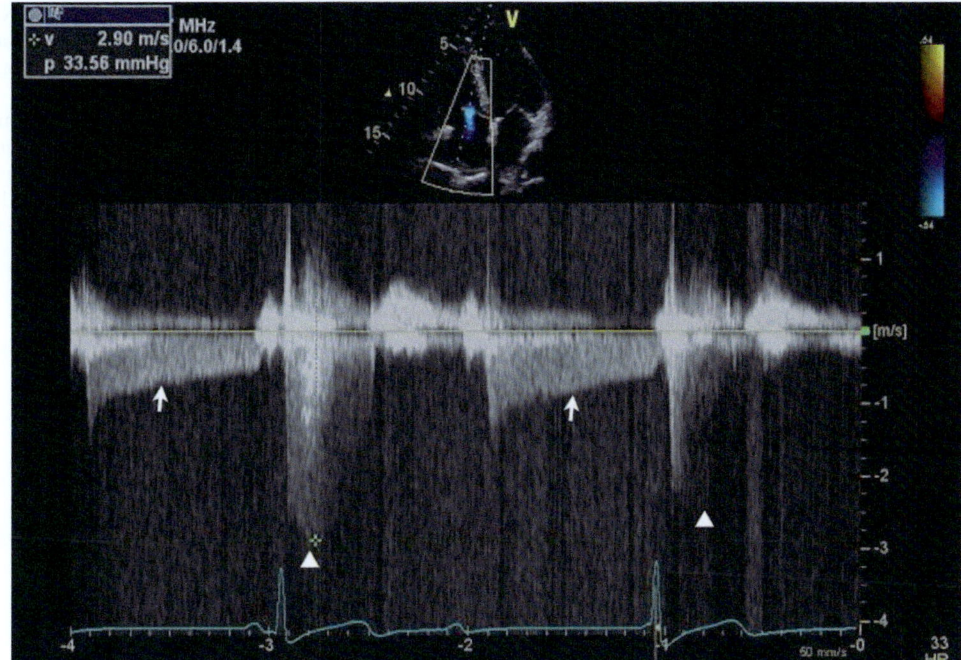

References

1. Jaleski TC. Myxoma of the heart valves: report of a case. Am J Pathol. 1934;10:399–406.
2. Yuan SM. Mitral valve myxoma: clinical features, current diagnostic approaches, and surgical management. Cardiol J. 2012;19:105–9.
3. Hata M, Gummert JF, Borgermann J, Hakim-Meibodi K. Mitral chordae myxoma–chordae replacement with a premeasured gore-tex loop using a minimally invasive video-assisted approach. J Cardiothorac Surg. 2013;8:227.
4. Kuroczynski W, Peivandi AA, Ewald P, Pruefer D, Heinemann M, Vahl CF. Cardiac myxomas: short- and long-term follow-up. Cardiol J. 2009;16:447–54.
5. Yamamoto H, Nakatani S, Niwaya K, Ohnishi T, Uematsu M, Kitakaze M. Images in cardiovascular medicine. Giant blood cyst of the mitral valve: echocardiographic and intraoperative images. Circulation. 2005;112:e341.
6. Migliore F, Scarabeo V, Corfini A, Piovesana P. Microbubbles contrast inside the cyst: a pathognomonic sign of mitral valve blood cyst. J Cardiovasc Med (Hagerstown). 2010;11:294–6.
7. Park MH, Jung SY, Youn HJ, Jin JY, Lee JH, Jung HO. Blood cyst of subvalvular apparatus of the mitral valve in an adult. J Cardiovasc Ultrasound. 2012;20:146–9.

Index

CPI Antony Rowe
Eastbourne, UK
September 02, 2024